DENTAL COLLECTION

Atlas of Laser Applications in Dentistry

ATLAS OF LASER APPLICATIONS IN DENTISTRY

Donald J. Coluzzi, DDS
Associate Clinical Professor
Division of Clinical General Dentistry
Department of Preventive and Restorative Dental Sciences
School of Dentistry
University of California, San Francisco
San Francisco, California

Robert A. Convissar, DDS
Director of Laser Dentistry
Department of Dental and Oral Medicine
New York Hospital Medical Center of Queens
Flushing, New York

Private Practice in Laser, Cosmetic, and Restorative Surgery
New York City, New York

quintessence books

Quintessence Publishing Co, Inc

Chicago, Berlin, Tokyo, London, Paris, Milan, Barcelona, Istanbul,
São Paulo, Mumbai, Moscow, Prague, and Warsaw

Library of Congress Cataloging-in-Publication Data

Coluzzi, Donald J.
Atlas of laser applications in dentistry / Donald J. Coluzzi and Robert A. Convissar.
p. ; cm.
Includes bibliographical references.
ISBN-13: 978-0-86715-476-4 (hardcover)
1. Lasers in dentistry--Atlases. I. Convissar, Robert A. II. Title.
[DNLM: 1. Lasers--therapeutic use. 2. Oral Surgical Procedures --methods. 3. Laser Surgery--methods. WU 26 C726a 2007]
RK685.L37C65 2007
617.6'05--dc22

2006030029

Quintessence Publishing Co, Inc
4350 Chandler Drive
Hanover Park, Illinois 60133
www.quintpub.com

Editor: Bryn Goates
Production: Sue Robinson
Cover and internal design: Dawn Hartman

Printed in Canada

TABLE OF CONTENTS

Preface *viii*

1 An Overview of Lasers in Dentistry *1*

Laser Fundamentals
Delivery and Emission Modes
Tissue Interaction and Safety
Advantages and Disadvantages

2 Biologic Justification for Laser Use *9*

Incision, Excision, and Ablation
Gingival Surgery
Nonsurgical Periodontal Therapy
Regenerative Periodontal Surgery
Endodontics
Operative Dentistry

3 Periodontal Laser Therapy *25*

Nonsurgical Periodontal Therapy
Frenectomy
Gingivectomy
Gingival Graft
Regenerative Periodontal Surgery

4 Adjunctive Laser Surgery in Implant Dentistry 47

Implant Uncovering Surgery
Implant Placement
Peri-implantitis Treatment
Implant Problem Solving

5 Laser Use in Operative Dentistry 73

Class I Restoration
Class II Restoration
Class III Restoration
Class IV Restoration
Class V Restoration

6 Laser Applications in Fixed Prosthodontics 91

Gingival Retraction
Recontouring of the Gingival Margin for Crown Lengthening
Edentulous Site Preparation
Osseous Recontouring for Crown Lengthening

7 Laser Applications in Removable Prosthodontics 117

Treatment of Inflamed Soft Tissues
Soft Tissue Denture Base Modification
Torus Reduction

8 Esthetic Laser Dentistry 133

Esthetic Crown Lengthening
Hyperpigmentation Removal
Laser-Activated Tooth Whitening

9 Endodontic Laser Therapy 153

Pulp Capping
Root Canal Disinfection
Endodontic Treatment
Apicoectomy
Desensitization

10 Laser Use in Oral Surgery, Oral Medicine, and Oral Pathology 169

Drug-Induced Gingival Hyperplasia
Aphthous Ulcer
Herpetic Lesion
Pericoronitis
Gingival Abscess
Kaposi Sarcoma Lesion
Lichen Planus
Premalignant Lesion
Biopsy

11 Laser Applications in Pediatric Dentistry 195

Exposure of Unerupted Teeth
Frenectomy
Gingivectomy
Drainage of a Gingival Abscess
Strip Crown Restoration
Restoration of Leaking Sealants
Pulpotomy

PREFACE

In the early 1960s, dental researchers studied the effects of using pulsed red light from a ruby laser for tooth preparation. Unfortunately, these early attempts resulted in surface cracking and thermal damage to the enamel and dentin. Shortly thereafter, physicians began employing laser energy for soft tissue surgeries. By 1977, the first successful case of laser use in the oral cavity was reported by Shafir and Slutzki. The first laser instrument developed specifically for general dentistry, a 3 W neodymium-doped yttrium aluminum garnet (Nd:YAG) laser, was not introduced, however, until 1989. Since that time laser dentistry has experienced tremendous innovation; today, dentists can choose from over half a dozen laser wavelengths manufactured by a dozen companies. Dental lasers have evolved into bona fide clinical instruments capable of providing treatment results comparable to or, for many procedures, superior to those provided by conventional techniques and instruments.

Currently, there are more than two dozen indications for laser use, ranging from simple excision of gingival tissue to caries removal and tooth preparation. When compared to treatment with conventional instrumentation, dentists and hygienists can use laser devices to significantly reduce pathogens, provide superior hemostasis, decrease healing periods and postoperative sequelae, and ensure better patient comfort.

The case presentations in this book demonstrate more than 100 examples of clinical applications for dental lasers:

- For periodontal procedures, lasers can remove diseased gingiva and bone, reduce bacteria, prepare a superior environment for reattachment of connective tissue to root surfaces, and shape and sculpt both hard and soft tissues for predictable healing.
- Utilizing lasers for placement and uncovering of implants offers the clinician advantages, such as improved visualization of the surgical field and reduced risk of infection. In addition, treatment of peri-implantitis with lasers has been proven to provide excellent results.

- For operative dentistry, the erbium family of lasers can selectively remove caries, often without anesthesia, for minimally invasive tooth preparations.
- In both fixed and removable prosthodontics, lasers can prepare and contour supporting tissues, as well as greatly aid impression techniques.
- Cosmetic periodontal procedures for esthetic treatment plans can be performed with lasers while maintaining the health and function of the patient's dentition.
- In endodontics, lasers can disinfect root canal systems, prepare canals for better obturation, and improve the outcome of apical surgery.
- In oral surgery, oral medicine, and oral pathology, lasers can be used to provide safe and effective patient care.
- Laser instruments can be used in pediatric patients as young as 1 day old with optimal results and reduce stress for both the young patients and the dentist.

Each case presented in this book is accompanied by suggested instrument settings and techniques so that the clinician can readily incorporate the information into treatment planning.

This book presents the most current applications for surgical lasers in dentistry, but the list of applications is by no means complete. Ongoing research in the field of laser dentistry will validate the use of current laser wavelengths for other clinical procedures as well as the use of new laser wavelengths that are being developed.

This atlas could not have been created without the support of many people. We would like to thank all of our colleagues in the field of laser dentistry who supplied cases for the book. Finally, we could not possibly have been able to manage such an undertaking without the love, support, patience, understanding, and compassion of our spouses, Catherine Coluzzi and Dr Ellen Goldstein, and our children, Craig, Alex, and Dana Convissar.

1

AN OVERVIEW OF LASERS IN DENTISTRY

Lasers have been in use in the medical community since the 1970s. In the 1980s, oral surgeons began using carbon dioxide (CO_2) lasers for soft tissue procedures,[1,2] and in 1989 the first laser specifically designed for use in dentistry was introduced.[3] Since that time, practitioners have found an increasing number of clinical applications for dental lasers.

Laser Fundamentals

The word *laser* is an acronym for *light amplification* by *stimulated emission* of *radiation*.

Light is a form of energy that exists as a particle, called a *photon*, and travels in a wave. A wave of photons has three basic properties:

- *Velocity*: The speed of light.
- *Amplitude*: The vertical measurement of the height of the wave, from the zero axis to the peak, which describes the energy of that wave. For convenience, energy is measured in *millijoules*, one thousandth of a joule.
- *Wavelength*: The horizontal distance between any two corresponding points on the wave. In dentistry, useful wavelengths range between 450 and 10,600 nm (billionths of a meter).

Laser light is distinguished from ordinary light by two properties. Laser light is *monochromatic* because it only generates a laser beam of a single color, which is sometimes invisible. In addition, each wave of laser light is *coherent*, or identical in physical size and shape. The monochromatic, coherent wave of light energy that emerges from a laser device is a unique source of efficient energy. The laser beams emitted from some instruments are collimated over a long distance, but beams produced from optical fibers usually diverge at the fiber tip.

In 1916, Albert Einstein theorized that photoelectric amplification could emit a single frequency, or *stimulated emission*, which explains how a laser operates.[4] The gas or solid lasing medium in the core of a dental laser is surrounded by a pumping mechanism that supplies the initial photon energy via an electrical current or a rapid strobe lamp. The photons are stimulated and amplified by reflection and resonation until a laser light beam can be focused and emitted (Fig 1-1).

Laser light is a form of electromagnetic radiation with a spectrum ranging from gamma rays to radio waves. Current dental laser wavelengths range between 488 and 10,600 nm and are emitted in the form of nonionizing radiation, which, unlike ionizing radiation, is not mutagenic to cellular DNA components.[5]

In dentistry, there are four lasers in the visible light spectrum:

- *Argon (Ar) laser*: Blue wavelength of 488 nm
- *Ar laser*: Blue-green wavelength of 514 nm
- *Neodymium-doped yttrium aluminum garnet laser with a potassium titanyl phosphate (KTP) crystal*: Green wavelength of 532 nm
- *Low-level lasers*: Red nonsurgical wavelengths of 635 nm (for therapy) and 655 nm (for caries detection)

Ar lasers are no longer manufactured as dental surgical instruments, although they are still used for medical procedures.

Other dental lasers emit invisible laser light in the near, middle, and far infrared portions of the electromagnetic spectrum. These include low-level, nonsurgical devices between approximately 800 and 900 nm, as well as surgical instruments, in ascending wavelength order[6]:

- *Diode laser:* Wavelengths between 800 and 830 nm and a semiconductor active medium of aluminum, gallium, and arsenide
- *Diode laser*: Wavelength of 904 nm, with an active medium of gallium and arsenide
- *Diode laser*: Wavelength of 980 nm and a similar active medium of indium, gallium, and arsenide
- *Neodymium-doped yttrium aluminum garnet (Nd:YAG) laser*: Wavelength of 1,064 nm

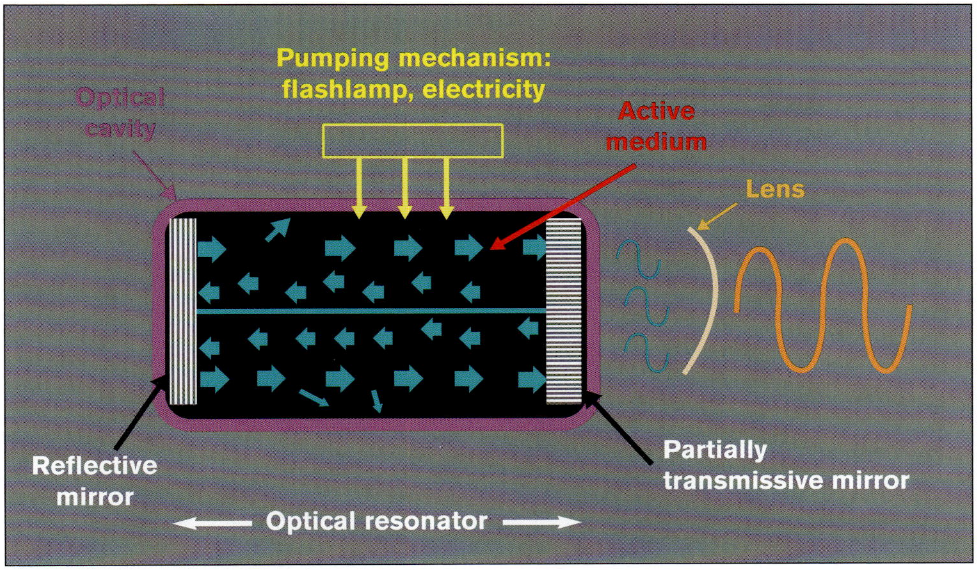

Fig 1-1 Basic laser components. The pumping mechanism provides the initial energy so that stimulated emission can occur within the active medium. The mirrors in the optical resonator collimate the photons to produce laser light.

- *Erbium-chromium–doped yttrium scandium gallium garnet (Er,Cr:YSGG) laser*: Wavelength of 2,780 nm
- *Erbium-doped yttrium aluminum garnet (Er:YAG) laser*: Wavelength of 2,940 nm
- *CO_2 laser*: Wavelength of 10,600 nm

Delivery and Emission Modes

Laser energy is delivered to the surgical site by various means. Shorter wavelength instruments, such as Ar, diode, and Nd:YAG lasers, have small, flexible fiber-optic systems with bare glass fibers that deliver the laser energy to the target tissue. Erbium (Er) and CO_2 devices are constructed with more rigid glass fibers, semiflexible hollow waveguides, or articulated arms to deliver the laser energy to the surgical site. Some of these systems employ small quartz or sapphire tips that attach to the laser device for contact with target tissue, while others do not directly contact the tissue. In addition, the Er family of dental lasers provides a cooling water spray for hard tissue procedures that can be switched off for soft tissue surgeries.

There are two basic modes of wavelength emission for dental lasers:

- *Continuous wave* emission means that laser energy is emitted continuously—as long as the laser is activated—and produces constant tissue interaction. CO_2, Ar, and diode lasers operate in this manner. Lasers that emit continuous wave energy are sometimes equipped with a mechanical shutter with a time circuit to produce *gated* or *super-pulsed* energy. This feature can minimize some of the undesirable residual thermal damage associated with continuous wave emission.
- *Free-running pulse* emission occurs with very short bursts of laser energy emitted every few ten-thousandths of a second. KTP, Nd:YAG, Er:YAG, and Er,Cr:YSGG devices operate as free-running pulsed lasers. Use of a laser with pulsed emission provides target tissue with thermal relaxation time in which to cool.

Regardless of the emission mode, all lasers produce a thermal effect on target tissues, and the operator must pay strict attention to the temperature of the surgical site and ensure that the laser energy is correctly controlled.[7]

Tissue Interaction and Safety

Because of the monochromaticity of laser energy, different laser wavelengths have different absorption coefficients when in contact with dental tissue (Fig 1-2); laser energy can be transmitted or absorbed based on the composition of target tissue.[8] Water, which is present in all biologic tissue, best absorbs the two Er wavelengths, followed by CO_2 wavelength. Conversely, water allows the transmission of the shorter wavelength lasers, including Ar, diode, and Nd:YAG. Apatite crystal, which forms the structure of teeth and bone, readily absorbs CO_2 wavelength and, to a lesser degree, those in the Er family. Apatite does not, however, absorb the shorter wave-

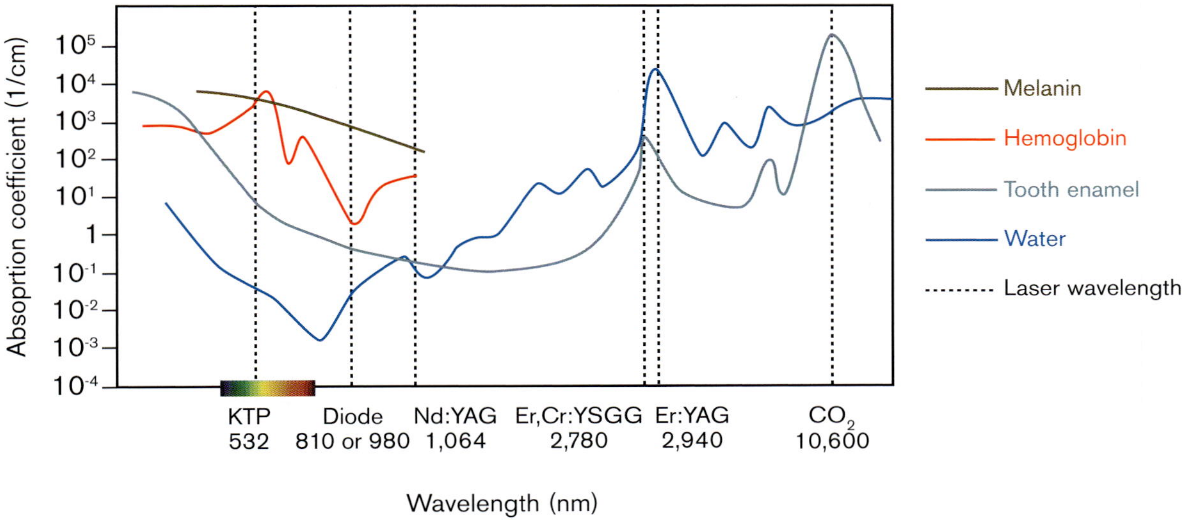

Fig 1-2 Approximate net absorption curves of various components of dental tissue (ie, water, hemoglobin, melanin, and tooth enamel) graphed against dental laser wavelengths.

lengths of Ar, diode, and Nd:YAG. Hemoglobin and other blood components, and the tissue pigment melanin, absorb the short wavelength lasers (Ar, diode, and Nd:YAG).

Because human dental tissues are composed of a combination of water, apatite crystal, blood, and tissue pigment, the clinician must choose the best laser for each treatment. For soft tissue treatments, the practitioner can use any dental laser regardless of wavelength, because all dental lasers are absorbed by one or more of the soft tissue components. For hard tissue surgery, however, the only lasers are from the Er family. Er lasers use extremely short pulse durations and can easily ablate layers of calcified tissue with minimal thermal effects.

In addition to unique absorptive optical properties, all wavelengths have different penetration depths through tissue. The Er family of lasers is absorbed on the surface of the target tissue, whereas diode lasers can reach several thousand microns deeper into the tissue.

The clinician can treat a variety of dental pathologies using different lasers, and, when there is a choice between different laser parameters, the underlying principle is to use the least amount of laser energy to perform the treatment objective.[9] Lasers primarily interact with dental structures photothermally. The temperature of the target tissue increases as laser light is absorbed,[10] and, when the tissue reaches 100°C, the inter- and intracellular water boils away, causing either soft tissue vaporization or explosive expansion and disruption of hard tissue. The possibility of significant tissue damage occurs only if the laser energy continues to be absorbed by the tissue, which leads to carbonization. Both target and nontarget tissues are subjected to the harmful effects of laser energy. The variable properties of laser usage, such as energy, beam diameter, and duration of exposure, must be carefully monitored to achieve a successful treatment.

Numerous safety regulations govern the operation of a dental laser, including wearing wavelength-specific protective eyewear, using a high-volume plume evacuation system, having a designated safety officer present, restricting access to the laser surgery area, minimizing reflective surfaces in the laser surgery area, and following normal protocol for infection control.[11,12]

Advantages and Disadvantages

Lasers offer both selection and precision when interacting with diseased tissues. The clinician can reduce the amount of bacteria and other pathogens in the surgical field when lasers are used.[13–15] In the case of soft tissue procedures, lasers achieve hemostasis and reduce need for sutures.[16,17] Laser devices offer advantages over conventional high-speed rotary handpieces when interacting with tooth structues[18–20]; the erbium lasers provide some selectivity in removing diseased tooth structure, since caries has a much higher water content than healthy tissue and, therefore, more readily absorbs laser energy.[21,22] Moreover, osseous tissue removal and recontouring proceed easily with the Er lasers.[23,24]

Current laser devices do present some disadvantages. They are relatively costly and require extensive training. Because a majority of dental instruments are both side- and end-cutting, the use of dental lasers requires a modification in clinical technique. Some procedures that require a side-cutting and shaping action cannot be performed with lasers, and surgical access can be compromised with some dental laser systems. One additional drawback to the Er family of lasers is the inability to remove defective ceramic or cast metal restorations. Finally, no single laser wavelength can be used to optimally treat all dental diseases.

Summary

This introduction to laser use in dentistry has presented the basic science behind laser devices and their interaction with dental tissues. Before using dental lasers, practitioners must be familiar with how lasers work, have clinical experience, and receive proper laser training.[25] Laser instrumentation requires some procedures to be performed much differently than with conventional instrumentation, but the indications for laser use continue to expand and further benefit patient care.[26]

References

1. Frame JW. Carbon dioxide laser surgery for benign oral lesions. Br Dent J 1985;158:125–128.
2. Pick RM, Pecaro BC, Silberman CJ. The laser gingivectomy. The use of the CO_2 laser for the removal of phenytoin hyperplasia. J Periodontol 1985;56:492–496.
3. Myers TD, Myers ED, Stone RM. First soft tissue study utilizing a pulsed Nd:YAG dental laser. Northwest Dent 1989;68(2):14–17.
4. Einstein A. Zur Quantum Theorie Der Stralung. Verk Deutsch Phys Ges 1916;18:318.
5. Myers TD. Lasers in dentistry. J Am Dent Assoc 1991;122:46–50.
6. Miserendino LJ, Pick RM (eds). Lasers in Dentistry. Chicago: Quintessence, 1995:27–38.
7. Manni JG. Dental Applications of Advanced Lasers. Burlington, MA: JGM Associates, 2004:1–18.
8. Frank K. Laser light and tissue: Biophysical aspects of medical laser application. In: Konov VI, Mueller GJ, Prokhorov AM (eds). First International Conference on Lasers and Medicine. San Jose, CA: International Society for Optical Engineering, 1990:37–45.
9. Dederich D. Laser tissue interaction. Alpha Omegan 1991;84:33–36.
10. White JM, Goodis HE, Yessik MJ, Myers TD. Histologic effects of a high repetition pulsed Nd:YAG laser on intraoral soft tissue. In: Wigdor HA, Featherstone JD, White JM (eds). Proceedings of Lasers in Dentistry. San Jose, CA: International Society for Optical Engineering, 1995:143–153.

11. American National Standard for Safe Use of Lasers in Health Care Facilities. Orlando: Laser Institute of America, 2002.
12. Piccione PJ. Dental laser safety. Dent Clin North Am 2004;48:795–807.
13. Moritz A, Gutknecht N, Doertbudak O. Bacterial reduction in periodontal pockets through irradiation with a diode laser: A pilot study. J Clin Laser Med Surg 1997;15:33–37.
14. Miyazaki A, Yamaguchi T, Nishikata J, et al. Effects of Nd:YAG and CO_2 laser treatment and ultrasonic scaling on periodontal pockets of chronic periodontitis patients. J Periodontol 2003;74:175–180.
15. Ando Y, Aoki A, Watanabe H, Ishikawa I. Bactericidal effect of erbium YAG laser on periodontopathic bacteria. Lasers Surg Med 1996;19:190–200.
16. Wilder-Smith P, Arrastia AM, Liaw LH, Berns M. Incision properties and thermal effects of three CO_2 lasers in soft tissue. Oral Surg Oral Med Oral Pathol Oral Radiol Endod 1995;79:685–691.
17. White JM, Goodis HE, Rose CL. Use of the pulsed Nd:YAG laser for intraoral soft tissue surgery. Lasers Surg Med 1991;11:455–461.
18. Fife CG, Zwahlen PG, Ludlow HE. Preparation time and pulpal temperature effects of Er:YAG laser treatment [abstract 1428]. J Dent Res 1998;77(special issue):284.
19. Aoki A, Ishikawa I, Yamada T, et al. Comparison between Er:YAG laser and conventional technique for root caries treatment in vitro. J Dent Res 1998;77:1404–1414.
20. DenBesten PK, White JM, Pelino J. The safety and effectiveness of an Er:YAG laser for caries removal and cavity preparation in children. Med Laser Appl 2001;16:215–222.
21. Hossain M, Nakamura Y, Yamada Y, Kimura Y, Matsumoto N, Matsumoto K. Effects of Er,Cr:YSGG laser irradiation in human enamel and dentin: Ablation and morphological studies. J Clin Laser Med Surg 1999;17:155–159.
22. Keller U, Hibst R, Geurtsen W, et al. Effects of Er:YAG laser in caries treatment: A clinical pilot study. Lasers Surg Med 1997;20:32–38.
23. Watanabe H, Yoshino T, Aoki A, Ishikawa I. Wound healing after irradiation of bone tissues by Er:YAG laser. In: Wigdor HA, Featherstone JD, Rechmann P (eds). Lasers in Dentistry III. San Jose, CA: International Society for Optical Engineering, 1997:39–42.
24. Ishikawa I, Aoki A, Takasaki AA. Potential applications of Erbium:YAG laser in periodontics. J Periodont Res 2004;39:275–285.
25. Myers TD, Sulewski JG. Evaluating dental lasers: What the clinician should know. Dent Clin North Am 2004;48:1127–1144.
26. Weiner GP. Laser dentistry practice management. Dent Clin North Am 2004;48:1105–1126.

Suggested Reading

Coluzzi DJ, Convissar RA (eds). Lasers in clinical dentistry. Dent Clin North Am 2004;48(4).

Convissar RA (ed). Lasers and light amplification in dentistry. Dent Clin North Am 2000;44(4).

Ishikawa I, Frame J, Aoki A (eds). Lasers in Dentistry, Revolution of Dental Treatment in the New Millennium. Amsterdam: Elsevier, 2003.

Manni JG. Dental Applications of Advanced Lasers. Burlington, MA: JGM Associates, 2004.

Miserendino LJ, Pick RM. Lasers in Dentistry. Chicago: Quintessence, 1995.

Tunér J, Hode L. Laser Therapy, Clinical Practice and Scientific Background. Sweden: Prima, 2002.

White JM. Curriculum guidelines and standards for dental laser education. In: Featherstone JD, Rechmann P, Fried D (eds). Lasers in Dentistry V. San Francisco: International Society for Optical Engineering, 1999:110–122.

2

BIOLOGIC JUSTIFICATION FOR LASER USE

Before using lasers, practitioners must understand the underlying biologic principles that justify their application in the oral cavity. Lasers have four types of tissue interaction: absorption, reflection, scatter, and transmission. Optimal therapeutic benefits result when the clinician uses the wavelength best absorbed by the target tissue; however, selecting the best laser for a given procedure depends on more than just matching the laser emission spectra to the tissue absorption spectra. The composition of the tissue surrounding the target tissue and the potential for damage or necrosis of the surrounding or underlying tissue also must be taken into account.

The remaining chapters of this text illustrate *how* to use lasers in each of the various dental disciplines—periodontics, implant dentistry, operative dentistry, prosthodontics, esthetics, endodontics, minor oral surgery, and pedodontics. This chapter discusses *why* lasers should be used, from a biologic viewpoint. As the field of laser dentistry expands, new uses are continually being discovered. The Table of Contents provides an overview of some of the current uses of lasers in dentistry.

Incision, Excision, and Ablation

Most soft tissue laser procedures can be categorized as one of three simple processes: incision, excision, or ablation. Whether the clinician is reducing a soft tissue tuberosity (excision) to enhance results of treatment involving a removable prosthesis, conducting a small biopsy of a large palatal lesion (incision), or removing an area of lichen planus from the buccal mucosa (ablation), the basic process is the same no matter which wavelength is used.

There are differences, however, in how the various lasers interact with oral tissues. The most significant distinctions among soft tissues are variations in pigmentation, vascularity, water content, and thickness. As an example of how these differences impact wavelength selection between carbon dioxide (CO_2), neodymium-doped yttrium aluminum garnet (Nd:YAG), and diode lasers, consider two patients in need of a gingivectomy: the first patient has light pink gingiva (Fig 2-1) while the second patient has dark melanotic gingiva (Fig 2-2). Because the CO_2 laser is absorbed by water, a difference in pigmentation would not affect its cutting efficiency, and both the pink and melanotic gingiva would respond equally well to the CO_2 wavelength.

For the same patients, the use of Nd:YAG and diode lasers reveals a significant difference in the cutting efficiency between the two clinical situations. Because both diode and Nd:YAG lasers are absorbed by tissue pigments such as hemoglobin and melanin, the darker melanotic gingiva would absorb the Nd:YAG and diode wavelengths much more readily than would the pink gingiva. Moreover, the melanotic tissue might absorb the Nd:YAG or diode wavelengths more rapidly than the clinician would like, possibly damaging the tissue or creating a more extensive zone of thermal necrosis around the target tissue.

To avoid serious complications, laser parameters such as pulse duration, hertz, and joules need to be modified to suit the individual clinical situation. Laser parameters suggested by the manufacturers are for the "average" patient and must be adapted to accommodate many critical patient variables, such as tissue pigmentation.

Another clinical situation illustrates the effect of tissue vascularity and water content on laser efficiency. Two orthodontic patients (Figs 2-3 and 2-4) wearing full bands and archwires require gingivectomies to increase the gingivoincisal length of the teeth. The first orthodontic patient (see Fig 2-3) has immaculate home care, evident in healthy gingiva that is firm, pink, and stippled. For the second patient (see Fig 2-4), the combination of poor home care and an orthodontic appliance that traps plaque has led to gingival hyperplasia, characterized by hyperemic, red, and inflamed gingiva.

The patient variables in these clinical situations will influence the effectiveness of different laser wavelengths. The chromophore of hemoglobin absorbs diode and Nd:YAG wavelengths. Therefore, the greater vascularity of the hyperemic, swollen tissue of the second patient will be ablated more quickly than the healthy tissue of the first patient. In addition, because water absorbs the CO_2 wavelength, the greater water content of the swollen, hyperemic tissue of the second patient also would more readily absorb the CO_2 laser energy.

Tissue thickness also changes laser effectiveness, as is illustrated in two frenectomy cases. The first patient (Fig 2-5) has a very thin mandibular anterior frenum. The second patient (Fig 2-6) has a very thick, fibrous maxillary anterior frenum. Assuming that both frena have the same vascularity, water content, and pigmentation, the only difference is the amount of fibrous tissue to be cut. If CO_2 or erbium (Er) lasers are used to perform the frenectomies, both clinical situations will result in negligible thermal necrosis beneath the surgical sites, since both wavelengths have very shallow depths of penetration. If both frenectomies are performed with Nd:YAG or diode lasers, the results could be vastly different. The depth of penetration for both wavelengths ranges from 1 to 4 mm. Tissue underlying the thick, fibrous frenum would be unaffected, since there is a sufficient bulk of frenal tissue to absorb the deep-penetrating laser energy. The surgical area underlying the thin, fragile frenum, however, might result in a large area of thermal necrosis due to the deep-penetrating laser energy.

These cases illustrate how the quality of the target tissue affects laser selection. With proper training, a clinician will be able to evaluate the types of cases described above and treat them with any laser wavelength by expertly adjusting the laser parameters to suit the tissues. Selection of the correct laser wavelength is not as critical to the success of these cases as selection of the proper laser parameters.

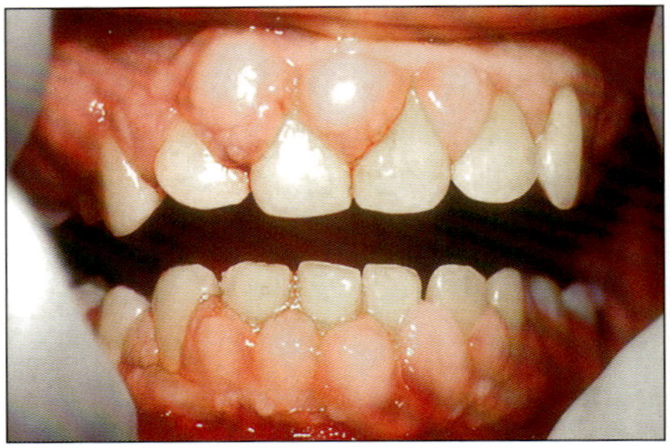

Fig 2-1 Cyclosporine-induced gingival hyperplasia in a kidney transplant patient with immaculate home care. Note the lack of calculus. The hyperplastic gingival tissue is healthy, firm, and fibrotic.

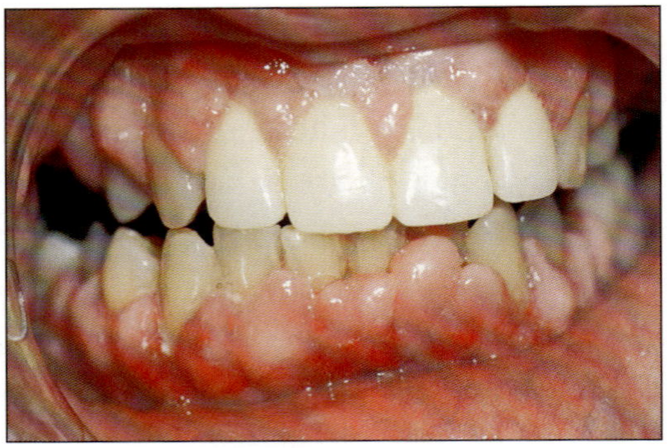

Fig 2-2 Cyclosporine-induced gingival hyperplasia in a kidney transplant patient with poor home care. Note the calculus and materia alba. The hyperplastic gingival tissue is edematous and hyperemic.

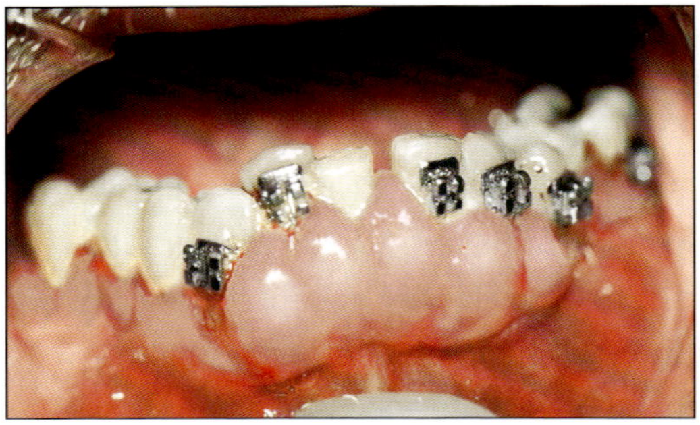

Fig 2-3 Orthodontic patient with excellent home care. The tissue, though hyperplastic, is firm, healthy, and fibrotic.

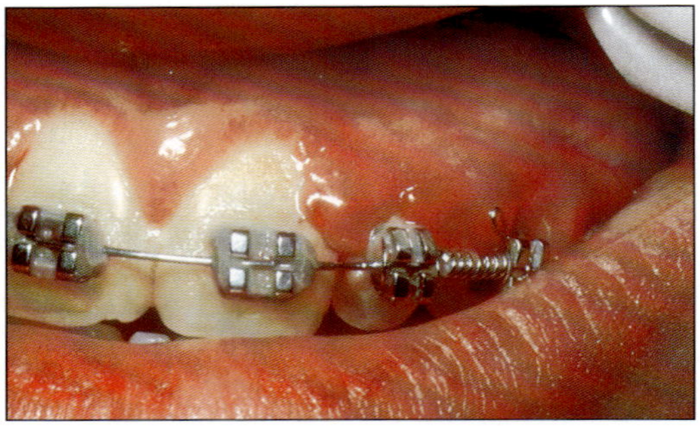

Fig 2-4 Orthodontic patient with poor home care. The soft tissue is edematous and friable.

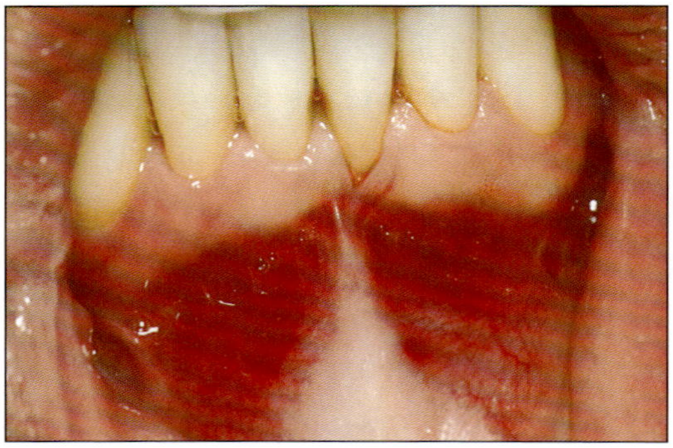

Fig 2-5 Thin, fragile mandibular anterior frenum. The thinness of the frenum will require very minimal ablation. Using too much energy or incorrect parameters could result in a large area of thermal necrosis in the surrounding and underlying soft tissue.

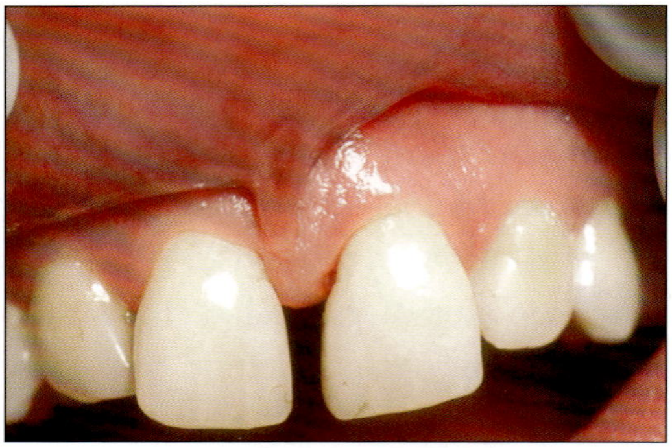

Fig 2-6 Thick, fibrous maxillary anterior frenum. Any wavelength will cut this frenum successfully. Because of its thick, fibrous quality, there is less danger of inadvertent thermal necrosis to the surrounding and underlying soft tissue during ablation.

Comprehensive training and education are crucial to any clinician that uses a laser because of the constant evolution of the technology, and therefore must be addressed both before the purchase of a laser and during its operational lifetime.

The cases illustrated in this book provide suggested laser wavelengths and parameters (watts, hertz, and spot sizes) for various procedures. Suggested laser parameters provided in this atlas or in laser manufacturer training manuals as well as laser default settings are for the "average" patient. Therefore, the practioner must evaluate the tissue variables of every patient individually with respect to water content, vascularity, and pigmentation before using the laser on a patient.

Gingival Surgery

According to the American Dental Association, dentists deliver more prosthodontic care than any other treatment modality except operative dentistry.[1] A review of the procedures listed in the Table of Contents indicates that most of the laser procedures in fixed, removable, and implant prosthetics are variations of a simple gingivectomy. The same may be said of most soft tissue procedures in pediatric dentistry and of many minor oral surgeries performed by general practitioners. Lasers offer many advantages over steel surgical instruments, including a dry and bloodless surgery, reduced bacteremia at the surgical site, reduced mechanical trauma, minimal postoperative swelling and scarring, and minimal postoperative pain.[2]

For the majority of procedures performed using laser instruments, the selection of wavelength is a matter of personal preference. However, for certain procedures the use of the correct laser wavelength can make the difference between success and failure. Some laser users prefer the CO_2 wavelength due to its high absorption in water and its lack of thermal penetration; others prefer Nd:YAG due to its absorption by tissue pigments and its deeper tissue penetration. Still other clinicians prefer diode lasers because of their compact size and portability. Many dentists use lasers from the Er family, which were originally developed for their efficacy in hard tissue ablation, for soft tissue procedures. A convincing argument can be made for or against the use of any of these laser wavelengths for specific procedures. Nevertheless, any well-trained dentist who understands both the physics and emission characteristics of each laser wavelength and the absorption spectra of the target tissue will be successful with most laser wavelengths.

Nonsurgical Periodontal Therapy

Because periodontal disease is a bacterial infection, nonsurgical periodontal therapy in the past decade has focused on bactericidal treatment. The use of systemic and locally delivered antibiotics to fight periodontal disease is well documented. Treatment protocols include systemic doxycycline[3–5] and metronidazole[6–8]; topical tetracycline-impregnated cords[9,10] and minocycline sphericals[11–14]; and small maintenance doses of tetracycline twice daily for 90 days or more.[15,16] Each therapy has the goal of eliminating bacteria from the periodontium and improving the patient's periodontal health. One essential criterion for wavelength selection for nonsurgical periodontal therapy, therefore, is proof of a bactericidal effect on periodontal tissues.

In a study by Moritz et al[17] using diode lasers in vivo, the Bleeding Index improved in 96.9% of the laser-treated population, compared with a 66.7% improvement in the nonlased population. They concluded that the diode laser provided a bactericidal effect, reduced inflammation, and supported healing of periodontal pockets through the elimination of bacteria. In a double-blind split-mouth study, Neill and Mellonig[18] assigned patients to one of three treatment regimens: scaling and root planing, Nd:YAG laser treatment with root planing, or a control group with no laser treatment or scaling. Their results showed that the patients who underwent laser treatment demonstrated significantly greater improvement in their Gingival Index and Bleeding Index than either of the other two groups. At 6 months postsurgery, the laser-treated group showed significant improvement in periodontal attachment gain.

Bader[19] describes laser curettage as reducing bacteria, enhancing hemostasis, and being less invasive than open-flap surgery. In this technique-sensitive procedure (see chapter 3), the laser is directed solely onto the soft tissue lining of the periodontal pocket. Because laser instruments are only end cutting, the energy is emitted from the fiber tip and not along the length of the fiber. When the cutting end is directed parallel to the root surface, the laser will remove the soft tissue bacteria and their exotoxins (eg, hyaluronidase, collagenase) that are responsible for breakdown of the periodontium.

Many studies describe this initial laser therapy as an *adjunct* to rather than a *replacement* for standard treatments.[17–20] Laser curettage of periodontal pockets will not be successful unless it is combined with standard scaling and root planing to remove bacteria and accretions from the root surface. The in vivo protocols of these studies showed the most significant improvement in the group of patients that had standard scaling performed with conventional instruments combined with laser treatment used solely on the soft tissue lining the pocket.

Bader[19] describes a technique in which the laser tip is moved circumferentially around the tooth rather than onto the root surface and is followed by hand instrumentation. Neill and Mellonig[18] emphasize that the fiber-optic tip should make light contact against the pocket epithelium rather than the root surface and be kept in a sweeping motion from the base of the pocket moving coronally. Laser energy must not be directed toward the root surface. Lasers are safe and effective instruments for adjunct nonsurgical periodontal therapy when used according to established protocols.

Regenerative Periodontal Surgery

The most difficult step that ultimately determines the success or failure of a surgical procedure is the removal of diseased tissue from the surgical site. The design, reflection, and resuturing of a full-thickness mucoperiosteal flap for any surgical procedure is relatively straightforward: the flap base must be wider than the flap crest to ensure adequate blood flow. However, if the diseased soft tissue and calcified accretions on the root surface are not removed, the surgical procedure will not be successful.

There are many techniques and instruments for removing diseased tissue. Historically, the instruments of choice have been curettes and other steel surgical instruments, though lasers are now being used for this procedure. Whatever laser wavelength is selected for regenerative periodontal surgery, it must not harm the root surfaces. Schwarz et al[21] compared the effects of a diode laser, an erbium-doped yttrium aluminum garnet (Er:YAG) laser, and conventional instrumentation in an in vivo study of teeth scheduled for extraction. The teeth were assigned to one of three groups: traditional scaling, Er:YAG treatment, or diode treatment. The results showed that the diode laser left the highest mean number of craters (14.6) on the root surface, scaling and root planing left a mean of 3 craters per sample, and the Er:YAG laser left no craters. The conclusion was that the Er:YAG wavelength provided selective subgingival calculus removal with minimal risk to the root surface, equivalent to that provided by traditional scaling and root planing. In vivo Er:YAG instrumentation produced nearly smooth root surfaces, with no cracks or thermal deffects.[21,22]

One of the most significant studies detailing the potential use of Er:YAG for periodontal regeneration was performed by Schwarz et al.[23] They studied the in vivo effects of the Er:YAG laser on the biocompatibility of periodontally diseased root surfaces and periodontal ligament fibroblasts. Their results demonstrated that the Er:YAG laser promotes the attachment of periodontal ligament fibroblasts on previously diseased root surfaces and that the surface structure of Er:YAG–instrumented roots offers better conditions for the adherence of periodontal fibroblasts than does the surface of roots treated only with scaling and root planing. The Er:YAG laser can promote periodontal regeneration by removing calculus from the root surface and leaving it smooth, which is ideal for successful attachment of new connective tissue fibers.

In a recent position paper on the use of lasers in periodontology, the American Academy of Periodontology concluded that "the Er:YAG laser demonstrated the best application of laser use directly on hard tissue, leaving the least thermal damage and creating a surface that suggests biocompatibility for soft tissue attachment. Studies have demonstrated the ability of the Er:YAG laser to remove lipopolysaccharides from root surfaces, facilitate removal of the smear layer after root planing, and remove calculus and cementum."[24] The Er:YAG laser is an excellent choice for regenerative periodontal surgery to prepare the root surface for new attachment of connective tissue.

After a soft tissue flap is reflected and the diseased tissue is removed from the surgical site, an epithelial exclusion technique must be performed.

This procedure prevents the epithelium from growing faster than the connective tissue and creating a long junctional epithelium. The principle of epithelial exclusion, in which connective tissue establishes a new attachment to the root surface, has been in the periodontal literature for over 50 years.[25]

A series of papers have addressed the question of whether lasers can be used in periodontics to retard epithelial downgrowth. The first paper, by Rossmann et al,[26] used monkeys to determine the capability of the CO_2 laser to prevent epithelial migration after surgery involving a soft tissue flap. In this split-mouth study, periodontal defects were produced bilaterally, and both sides were treated with open-flap debridement. On one side, the epithelium was removed with a CO_2 laser, while the other side served as the control. The results showed that epithelialization of the CO_2-irradiated side was delayed by at least 7 days, allowing for new connective tissue to grow. Moreover, the healing of the connective tissue was not retarded at all. It was concluded that the CO_2 laser can be used to delay the apical downgrowth of epithelium and that the technique was less technically demanding and more time efficient than other methods of epithelial retardation.

Israel et al[27] used the CO_2 laser in a human study in which they performed open debridement and notched teeth at the alveolar crest before resuturing. At the surgical uncovering 90 days later, every nonlased tooth had developed junctional epithelium from the root to the base of the notch. On the lased side, however, the tooth notch was filled with connective tissue and some repair cementum. Rossmann et al[28] refined this technique in a study on beagle dogs that found similar results. When their technique was performed clinically, in vivo human results demonstrated that CO_2 laser de-epithelialization produces new connective tissue attachment and some bone fill in previously diseased sites.[29] They concluded that this technique has shown significantly better results than those obtained through conventional osseous grafting alone.

The results of the CO_2 de-epithelialization studies and the Er:YAG root surface studies lead to the conclusion that the most effective technique for regenerative periodontal surgery would involve using both wavelengths. The Er:YAG laser would be used to debride the open surgical site, clean and disinfect the root surface, and prepare the root surface for the adhesion of fibroblasts. The CO_2 laser would then remove the epithelium to allow the fibroblasts to adhere and proliferate, creating new attachment.

This dual-wavelength technique shows tremendous promise in the field of regenerative periodontal surgery. Additional university- or hospital-based split-mouth studies involving a larger number of patients are necessary before this technique can be considered fully documented; however, there seems to be sufficient evidence to confirm a biologic justification for the use of this technique.

Endodontics

In the absence of bacterial contamination, teeth will retain their vitality and periapical lesions will not develop. In a landmark study, Kakehashi et al[30] took normal rats and germ-free rats and exposed their pulps. By day 8, the normal rats had nonvital, necrotic pulps and periapical abscesses, while the germ-free rats never lost pulp vitality, and no granulomas or abscesses formed. Other studies have compared the success rates of endodontic treatment using positive cultures to endodontic treatment using negative cultures. The success rate for teeth treated with negative cultures immediately before obturation was significantly higher than for teeth treated with positive cultures.[31,32] Most cases of endodontic failure are thought to involve a continuing infection of the root canal system.[33–36] Noncarious teeth that became devitalized as a result of trauma (rather than caries) often harbor pathogenic bacteria.[37,38] These studies demonstrate that bacteria must be present for endodontic infections and bony rarefactions at the apex of teeth to occur.

Both the in vivo and in vitro use of lasers have been shown to be bactericidal in root canals. Moritz et al[39] and Gutknecht et al[40] showed that the use of diode and Nd:YAG lasers eradicated bacteria in infected root canals. Schoop et al[41] subjected 220 extracted human teeth to bacteriologic evaluation. Their results showed a decisive bactericidal effect when an Er:YAG laser was introduced into an infected root canal. Mehl et al[42] inoculated 90 extracted anterior teeth with *Escherichia coli* or *Staphylococcus aureus* and effectively disinfected the canals using a Er:YAG laser.

Any laser wavelength can disinfect and deodorize a root canal system. However, if the goal of using a laser in endodontic therapy is more than just removing pathogens in the canal, the other treatment steps must be taken into account during laser selection. Once endodontic access and initial debridement of the canal are completed, the next critical steps are removing the smear layer and obturating the root canal system. Once the bacteria are removed from the root canal system and it is sealed off with gutta-percha, the periapical pathology will heal.

Removal of the smear layer is an important step in canal disinfection because the smear layer harbors bacteria and bacterial products and occludes the dentinal tubules in which bacteria multiply.[43] Smear layer removal ensures superior cleaning and disinfection of the root canal, and, if bacteria are not removed from the tubules, the success of the endodontic treatment is severely compromised. Takeda et al[44] compared the use of a 17% ethylenediaminetetraacetic acid (EDTA) solution, a 6% phosphoric acid solution, and Er:YAG lasers. Their results showed that the Er:YAG laser therapy was the most effective in removing the smear layer from root canal walls. In a separate study using extracted teeth, Takeda et al[45] showed that Er:YAG lasers efficiently cleaned the root canal walls by removing debris and opening dentinal tubules. A further study concluded that Er:YAG lasers effectively removed debris and smear layer from root canal walls.[46] When Er:YAG lasers were compared with other lasers, notably argon (Ar) and Nd:YAG wavelengths, they were shown to be the most effective wavelength and more effective than 17% EDTA solutions in removing the smear layer from root canal walls.[47]

For the final step in endodontic therapy—obturation of the canal—application of an Er:YAG laser to the root canal walls has been shown to increase the adhesion of epoxy-based root canal sealers. Pecora et al[48] tested 99 extracted maxillary molars with an Instron Universal machine to show that there was a statistically significant difference between laser-treated dentin and EDTA-treated dentin with respect to sealer adhesion to the dentin walls. Sousa-Neto et al[49] tested 40 extracted human molars with an Instron Universal machine to confirm that laser application significantly increased the adhesion of root canal sealers. Research has also responded to concerns about the effect of lasers on the periodontal ligament just beyond the apex of the tooth. The research has concluded that the effects of Er:YAG lasers are minimal because no discernable effects have been noted on the periodontal ligament.[50]

To summarize the value of lasers in endodontics, all wavelengths have been shown to be bactericidal. If removal of bacteria from the root canal system is the primary purpose for using a laser in endodontic therapy, any wavelength will suffice. If instrumentation, removal of the smear layer, and superior sealing of the canals are the goals of laser use in endodontic therapy, wavelengths from the Er family are the only ones that can perform those tasks.

Operative Dentistry

Dentists have long sought a painless and atraumatic method of removing caries without affecting surrounding healthy tissue. Laser use in operative dentistry was introduced in 1997 when the Food and Drug Administration (FDA) cleared the first Er:YAG laser for caries removal and cavity preparation. Since then, manufacturers of Er lasers have routinely touted the ability of this wavelength to remove diseased hard tissue without the need for anesthesia. Lasers in the Er family are versatile and include the Er:YAG laser with a wavelength of 2,940 nm and the erbium-chromium–doped yttrium scandium gallium garnet (Er,Cr:YSGG) laser with a wavelength of 2,780 nm. Anecdotal reports by laser users over the past decade conclude that operative procedures in primary teeth may be performed practically all of the time without anesthesia.[51,52] In permanent teeth, however, the ability to prepare teeth without anesthesia depends on their position in the arch. Anterior teeth generally may be prepared without anesthesia, but molars require anesthesia approximately 40% to 50% of the time.

Er family lasers are indicated for all classifications of caries in enamel, dentin, and cementum for both primary and permanent teeth. Er family lasers are capable of removing not only carious tooth structure but also many nonmetallic restorations, including resin composite, glass-ionomer, and compomer restorations. The one limitation of Er laser use is the removal of metallic and porcelain restorations. There is currently no laser wavelength that can remove amalgam, gold, or porcelain; these restorations must be removed in a conventional manner before caries removal is performed with a laser. The laser can, however, be used to make circumferential cuts in the tooth structure around metallic restorations before they are removed with hand instruments (see chapter 5).

Conclusion

When selecting a laser for a specific procedure, the dentist must consider the interaction among the wavelength, target tissue, and surrounding tissue. For certain procedures, the choice of wavelength is critical to the success of the procedure. However, for many dental procedures, any soft tissue laser will produce excellent results. In these cases, selection of a laser wavelength is a matter of personal preference, but setting the correct operating parameters (eg, joules, hertz, pulse duration) becomes critical to the success of the procedure.

References

1. 2000 Survey of Dental Practice. Chicago: American Dental Association, 2001.
2. Wigdor HA, Walsh JT Jr, Featherstone JD, Visuri SR, Fried D, Waldvogel J. Lasers in dentistry. Lasers Surg Med 1995;16:103–133.
3. Ng VW, Bissada NF. Clinical evaluation of systemic doxycycline and ibuprofen administration as an adjunctive treatment for adult periodontitis. J Periodontol 1998;69:772–776.
4. Asikainen S, Jousimies-Somer H, Kanervo A, Saxen L. The immediate efficacy of adjunctive doxycycline in treatment of localized juvenile periodontitis. Arch Oral Biol 1990;35(suppl):231S–234S.
5. Lee W, Aitken S, Kulkarni G, et al. Collagenase activity in recurrent periodontitis: Relationship to disease progression and doxycycline therapy. J Periodont Res 1991;26:479–485.
6. Jansson H, Bratthall G, Soderholm G. Clinical outcome observed in subjects with recurrent periodontal disease following local treatment with 25% metronidazole gel. J Periodontol 2003;74:372–377.
7. Rudhart A, Purucker P, Kage A, Hopfenmuller W, Bernimoulin JP. Local metronidazole application in maintenance patients. Clinical and microbiological evaluation. J Periodontol 1998;69:1148–1154.
8. Riep B, Purucker P, Bernimoulin JP. Repeated local metronidazole-therapy as an adjunct to scaling and root planing in maintenance patients. J Clin Periodontol 1999;26:710–715.
9. Latner L. Patient selection and clinical applications of periodontal tetracycline fibers. Gen Dent 1998;46:58–61.
10. Greenstein G. Treating periodontal diseases with tetracycline-impregnated fibers: Data and controversy. Compend Contin Educ Dent 1995;16:448–455.
11. Killoy WJ. Local delivery of antimicrobials: A new era in the treatment of adult periodontitis. Compend Contin Educ Dent 1999;20(4 suppl):13–18.
12. Williams RC, Paquette DW, Offenbacher S, et al. Treatment of periodontitis by local administration of minocycline microspheres: A controlled trial. J Periodontol 2001;72:1535–1544.

13. Dean JW, Branch-Mays GL, Hart TC, et al. Topically applied minocycline microspheres: Why it works. Compend Contin Educ Dent 2003;24:247–250.
14. van Steenberghe D, Rosling B, Soder PO, et al. A 15-month evaluation of the effects of repeated subgingival minocycline in chronic adult periodontitis. J Periodontol 1999;70: 657–667.
15. Caton J. Evaluation of Periostat for patient management. Compend Contin Educ Dent 1999;20:451–460.
16. Caton JG, Ciancio SG, Blieden TM, et al. Treatment with subantimicrobial dose doxycycline improves the efficacy of scaling and root planing in patients with adult periodontitis. J Periodontol 2000;71:521–532.
17. Moritz A, Schoop U, Goharkhay K, et al. Treatment of periodontal pockets with a diode. Lasers Surg Med 1998;22:302–311.
18. Neill ME, Mellonig JT. Clinical efficacy of the Nd:YAG laser for combination periodontitis therapy. Pract Periodontics Aesthet Dent 1997;9(6 suppl):1–5.
19. Bader H. Use of lasers in periodontics. Dent Clin North Am 2000;44:779–791.
20. Gutknecht N, Fischer J, Conrads G, et al. Bactericidal effect of the Nd:YAG lasers in laser supported curettage. In: Wigdor HA, Featherstone JD, Rechmann P (eds). Lasers in Dentistry III. San Jose, CA: International Society for Optical Engineering, 1997: 221–226.
21. Schwarz F, Sculean A, Berakdar M, Szathmari L, Georg T, Becker J. In vivo and in vitro effects of an Er:YAG laser, a GaAlAs diode laser, and scaling and root planing on periodontally diseased root surfaces: A comparative histologic study. Lasers Surg Med 2003; 32:359–366.
22. Schwarz F, Putz N, Georg T, Reich E. Effect of an Er:YAG laser on periodontally involved root surfaces: An in vivo and in vitro SEM comparison. Lasers Surg Med 2001;29: 328–335.
23. Schwarz F, Aoki A, Sculean A, Georg T, Scherbaum W, Becker J. In vivo effects of an Er:YAG laser, an ultrasonic system and scaling and root planing on the biocompatibility of periodontally diseased root surfaces in cultures of human PDL fibroblasts. Lasers Surg Med 2003;33:140–147.
24. Research, Science and Therapy Committee of the American Academy of Periodontology. Lasers in periodontics. J Periodontol 2002;73:1231–1239.
25. Goldman H. A rationale for the treatment of the intrabony pocket, one method of treatment—Subgingival curettage [abstract]. J Periodontol 1949;20:89.
26. Rossmann JA, McQuade MJ, Turunen DE. Retardation of epithelial migration in monkeys using a carbon dioxide laser: An animal study. J Periodontol 1992;63:902–907.
27. Israel M, Rossmann J, Froum S. Use of the carbon dioxide laser in retarding epithelial migration: A pilot histological human study utilizing case reports. J Periodontol 1995; 66:197–204.
28. Rossmann J, Parlar A, Ghaffar K, et al. Use of the carbon dioxide laser in guided tissue regeneration wound healing in the beagle dog [abstract]. J Dent Res 1996;75:31.
29. Israel M, Rossmann J. An epithelial exclusion technique using the CO_2 laser for the treatment of periodontal defects. Comp Contin Educ Dent 1998;19:86–88.
30. Kakehashi S, Stanley HR, Fitzgerald RJ. The effects of surgical exposures of dental pulps in germ-free and conventional laboratory rats. Oral Surg Oral Med Oral Pathol 1965;20:340–349.
31. Heling B, Shapira J. Roentgenologic and clinical evaluation of endodontically treated teeth, with or without negative culture. Quintessence Int 1978;9(11):79–84.
32. Zeldow B, Ingle J. Correlation of the positive culture to the prognosis of endodontically treated teeth: A clinical study. J Am Dent Assoc 1963;66:9–13.

33. Sundqvist G, Figdor D, Persson S, Sjögren U. Microbiologic analysis of teeth with failed endodontic treatment and the outcome of conservative re-treatment. Oral Surg Oral Med Oral Pathol Oral Radiol Endod 1998;85:86–93.
34. Nair P, Sjögren U, Krey G, Kahnberg KE, Sundqvist G. Intraradicular bacteria and fungi in root-filled, asymptomatic human teeth with therapy-resistant periapical lesions: A long-term light and electron microscopic follow-up study. J Endod 1990;61:580–588.
35. Sjögren U, Hagglund B, Sundqvist G, Wing K. Factors affecting the long-term results of endodontic treatment. J Endod 1990;16:498–504.
36. Sjögren U, Figdor D, Persson S, Sundqvist G. Influence of infection at the time of root filling on the outcome of endodontic treatment of teeth with apical periodontitis. Int Endod J 1997;30:297–306.
37. MacDonald J, Hare G, Wood A. The bacteriologic status of the pulp chambers in intact teeth found to be nonvital following trauma. Oral Surg Oral Med Oral Pathol 1957;10:318–322.
38. Wittgow W, Sabiston CB Jr. Microorganisms from pulpal chambers of intact teeth with necrotic pulps. J Endod 1975;1:168–171.
39. Moritz A, Gutknecht N, Schoop U, Goharkhay K, Doertbudak O, Sperr W. Irradiation of infected root canals with a diode laser in vivo: Results of microbiological examinations. Lasers Surg Med 1997;21:221–222.
40. Gutknecht N, Moritz A, Conrads G, Sievert T, Lampert F. Bactericidal effects of the Nd:YAG laser in in vitro root canals. J Clin Laser Med Surg 1996;14:77–80.
41. Schoop U, Moritz A, Kluger W, et al. The Er:YAG laser in endodontics: Results of an in vitro study. Lasers Surg Med 2002;30:360–364.
42. Mehl A, Folwaczny M, Haffner C, Hickel R. Bactericidal effects of 2.94 microns Er:YAG-laser radiation in dental root canals. J Endod 1999;25:490–493.
43. Fogel HM, Pashley DH. Dentin permeability: Effects of endodontic procedure on root slabs. J Endod 1990;16:442–445.
44. Takeda FH, Harashima T, Kimura Y, Matsumoto K. A comparative study of the removal of smear layer by three endodontic irrigants and two types of laser. Int Endod J 1999;32:32–39.
45. Takeda FH, Harashima T, Kimura Y, Matsumoto K. Efficacy of Er:YAG laser irradiation in removing debris and smear layer on root canal walls. J Endod 1998;24:548–551.
46. Takeda FH, Harashima T, Eto J, Kimura Y, Matsumoto K. Effect of Er:YAG laser treatment on the root canal walls of human teeth: An SEM study. Endod Dent Traumatol 1998;14:270–273.
47. Takeda FH, Harashima T, Kimura Y, Matsumoto K. Comparative study about the removal of smear layer by three types of laser devices. J Clin Laser Med Surg 1998;16:117–122.
48. Pecora JD, Cussioli AL, Guerisoli DM, Marchesan MA, Sousa-Neto MD, Brugnera-Junior A. Evaluation of Er:YAG laser and EDTAC on dentin adhesion of six endodontic sealers. Braz Dent J 2001;12:27–30.
49. Sousa-Neto MD, Marchesan MA, Pecora JD, et al. Effect of Er:YAG laser on adhesion of root canal sealers. J Endod 2002;28:185–187.
50. Kimura Y, Yonaga K, Yokoyama K, Kinoshita J, Ogata Y, Matsumoto K. Root surface temperature increase during Er:YAG laser irradiation of root canals. J Endod 2002;28:76–78.
51. Gimbel C. Hard tissue laser procedures. Dent Clin North Am 2000;44:931–954.
52. Cozean C, Arcoria C, Pelagalli J, Powell GL. Dentistry for the 21st Century? Erbium:YAG laser for teeth. J Am Dent Assoc 1997;128:1080–1087.

3

PERIODONTAL LASER THERAPY

The first periodontal laser surgeries were performed with medical carbon dioxide (CO_2) lasers in 1985.[1] The initial laser instruments were cumbersome and could not be used to access all areas of the oral cavity. In addition, those early units were only useful for soft tissue ablation and could cause thermal damage to teeth and bone.[2,3] Today, laser instruments have more sophisticated delivery systems, which allow for easier placement of the laser beam anywhere in the oral cavity and therefore increase the visibility of surgical sites. Moreover, the erbium (Er) family of wavelengths can readily contour osseous structures without damaging tooth structure. These qualities make dental lasers extremely useful for treatment of periodontal disease.

A fundamental change in the understanding of the pathogenesis of periodontal disease has shifted emphasis from patient risk factors to include the microbial component as well.[4,5] Lasers drastically decrease the bacteria at surgical sites, which benefits both the patient and practitioner in managing periodontal problems. In numerous studies, the argon (Ar), diode, neodymium-doped yttrium aluminum garnet (Nd:YAG), Er family, and CO_2 wavelengths have all demonstrated significant bacterial reduction at surgical sites.[6–10] The diode, Nd:YAG, and CO_2 lasers provide excellent hemostasis and, in some cases, can even "weld" together the edges of soft tissue flaps, thus lessening the need for sutures.[11–13] Er family wavelengths have limited coagulation abilities, but acceptable bleeding control can be accomplished by increasing the pulse rate and shutting off the water spray.[14]

Protocols combining conventional scaling and root planing with laser periodontal pocket therapy have been documented as reducing periodontal pockets and increasing periodontal attachment[15–17]; one abstract involving a

Nd:YAG laser reported the formation of a new periodontal ligament attachment following laser treament.[18] When used carefully at low power and parallel to the root surface, lasers cause no harm to the teeth or the periodontium.[19,20] Though some research has documented adverse effects when using Nd:YAG and diode lasers on root surfaces, those in vitro studies used lasers perpendicular rather than parallel to the root surface. As with any procedure, proper clinical technique is critical to ensure success.

Er family lasers have indications for use in removing calculus and other root-surface accretions, although care must be taken that these wavelengths do not ablate cementum.[21] Er family wavelengths effectively ablate bone with minimal thermal damage to adjacent tissues. One study reported that the healing rate for osseous surgery may be more rapid following use of an erbium-doped yttrium aluminum garnet (Er:YAG) laser than following the use of a bur with water spray in a high-speed turbine handpiece.[22]

Soft tissue contouring to improve gingival and mucosal architecture, including frenum repositioning, can be readily achieved with any dental laser.[23]

Preventing apical epithelia from proliferating from adjacent surfaces to the surgical site promotes new attachment of the periodontal ligament to the root. In protocols where lasers are used instead of barrier membrane techniques, definitive histologic results reported in three animal models (ie, beagles, monkeys, and humans) have shown that CO_2 lasers successfully prevent epithelial downgrowth and encourage new soft tissue attachment rather than long junctional epithelial attachments.[24–27] When compared to treatment involving only conventional scaling and root planing, the Er:YAG wavelength has been shown in multiple studies to be superior in preparing root surfaces for attachment of periodontal fibroblasts.[28–31]

Because periodontal therapy has evolved from scaling, root planing, and excisional surgery to include antimicrobial and regenerative treatments, the dental laser has emerged as a proven modality with superior results.[32,33]

Nonsurgical Periodontal Therapy: Case 1

Periodontal therapy in the posterior maxilla in an adult male patient.

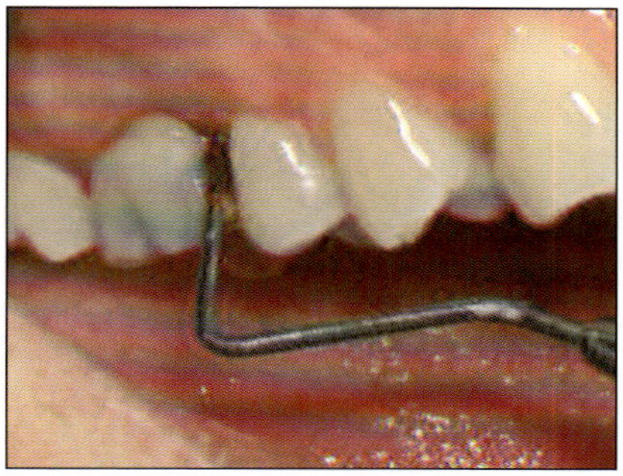

Fig 3-1a Periodontal probing of an area of advanced disease with deep pocketing.

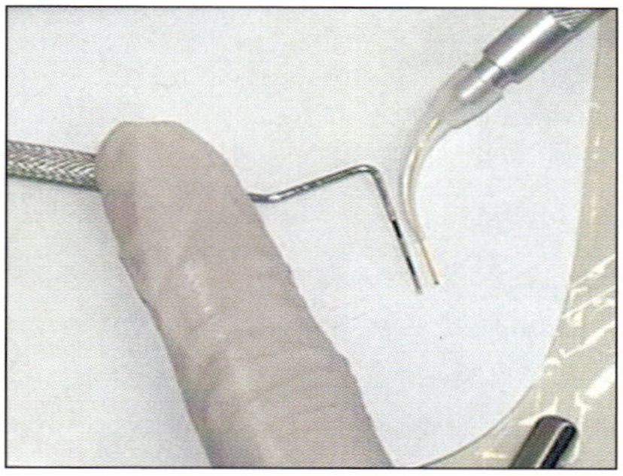

Fig 3-1b Calibration of the laser fiber against a periodontal probe. When short wavelength lasers such as diode or Nd:YAG are used, the length of the bare optic fiber must be set 1 mm shorter than the depth of the periodontal pocket.

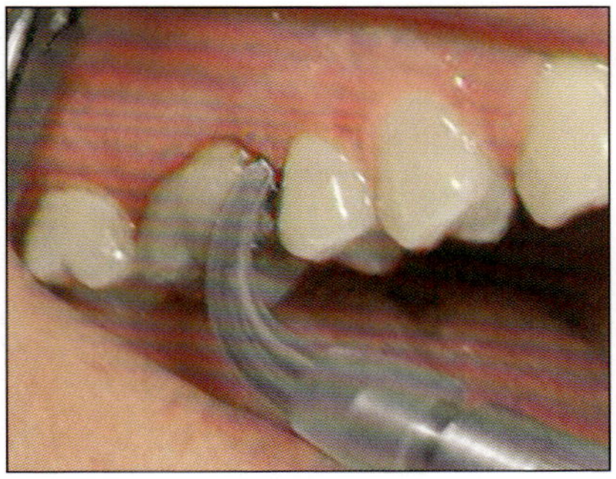

Fig 3-1c The laser fiber is placed into the periodontal pocket 1 mm short of the probed depth.

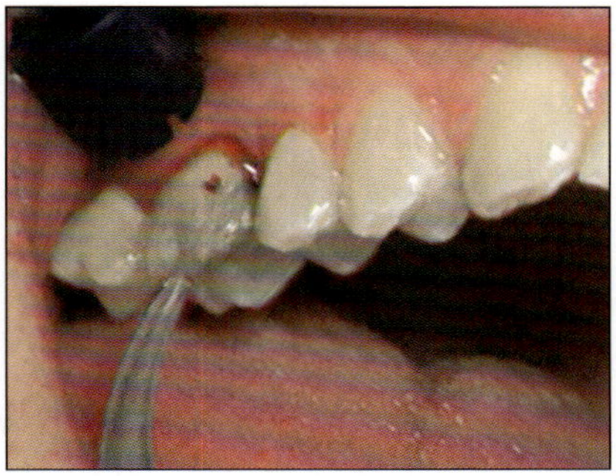

Fig 3-1d Immediate postoperative view following removal of the fiber from the periodontal pocket. The granulomatous tissue at the tip of the laser fiber must be removed with dry gauze before the laser fiber is placed back into the periodontal pocket.

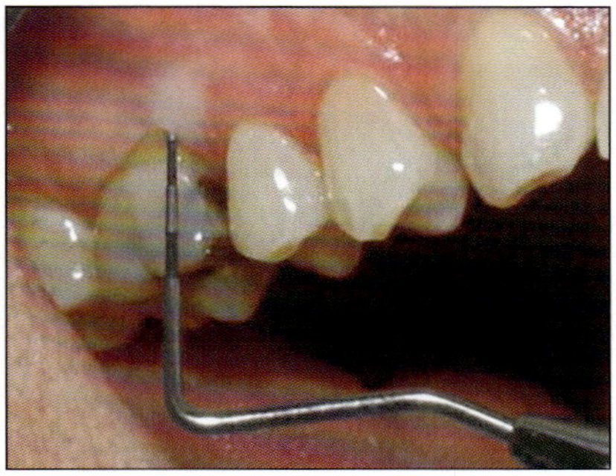

Fig 3-1e Periodontal probing 1 year following treatment. The absence of pathology and the lack of significant pocket depth is evident.

Purpose of the procedure	Treatment of a periodontal pocket

Use of a bactericidal dental laser in the periodontal pocket decreases the pathogenic microbial population, removes the diseased epithelial lining of the pocket, and restores the tissues to health.

Wavelength and settings

Diode laser, 810 nm, set to 0.4 W, continuous wave, with a 300 µm fiber.

Alternate wavelengths that may be used

A Nd:YAG or an ultrapulsed CO_2 laser can also be used to perform the procedure.

Clinical tip

When performing nonsurgical periodontal therapy, the clinician must ensure that the fiber tip is free of debris and has a sharp cleave. Fig 3-1d shows granulomatous tissue on the fiber tip, which must be removed with dry gauze. The tip must also be evaluated to see if it needs recleaving. To do this, shine the laser tip onto a white piece of a paper (eg, a bracket table cover) and evaluate the spot shape. If the spot is not perfectly round and it has either a "comet-tail" or oval appearance, the fiber tip should be recleaved.

Nonsurgical Periodontal Therapy: Case 2

Periodontal therapy in the anterior mandible in an adult patient.

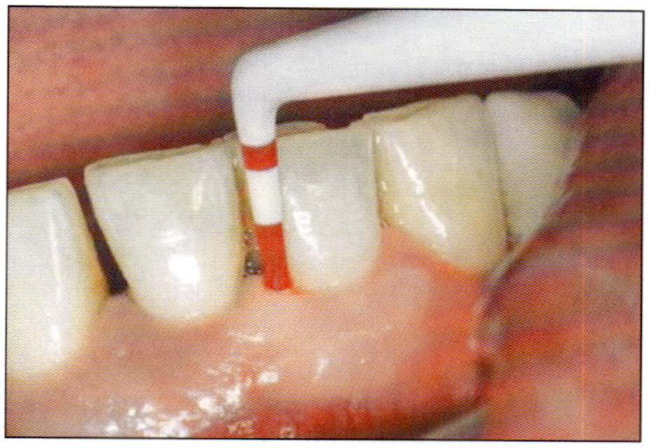

Fig 3-2a Periodontal probing in the anterior mandible reveals a deep periodontal pocket.

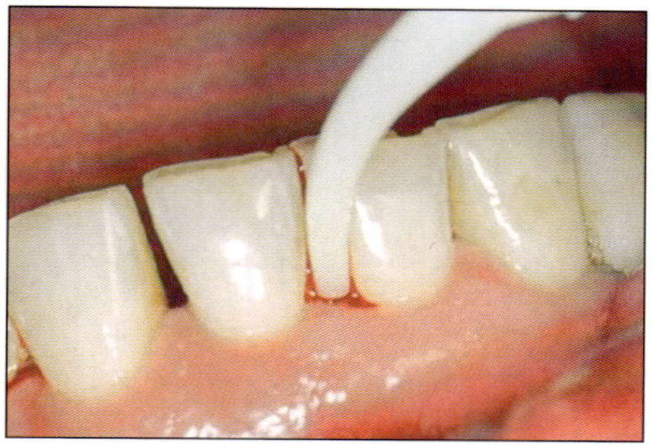

Fig 3-2b A properly calibrated Nd:YAG laser fiber is placed into the pocket 1 mm short of the probing depth.

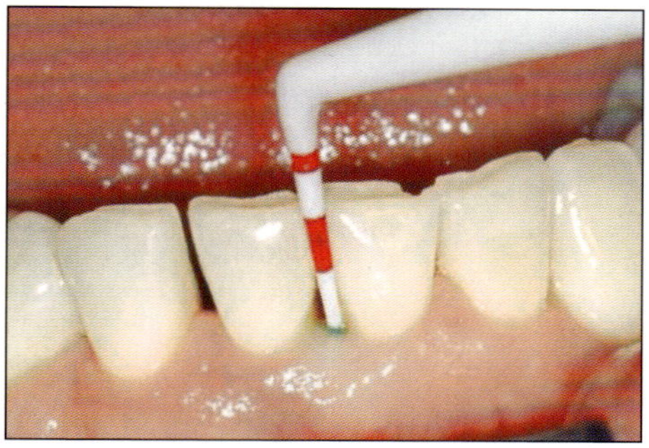

Figs 3-2c Postoperative view at 6 months showing healthy pink and stippled tissue. The probing depth has been reduced.

Purpose of the procedure

Treatment of a periodontal pocket

Use of a bactericidal dental laser in the periodontal pocket reduces the pathogenic microbial population, removes the diseased epithelial lining of the pocket, and restores the tissues to health.

Wavelength and settings

Nd:YAG laser, 1064 nm, set to 1.8 W, 30 mJ, 60 Hz, with a 300 μm fiber.

Alternate wavelengths that may be used

A diode or an ultrapulsed CO_2 laser can also be used to perform this procedure.

Nonsurgical Periodontal Therapy: Case 3

Periodontal therapy in the posterior mandible in an adult patient.

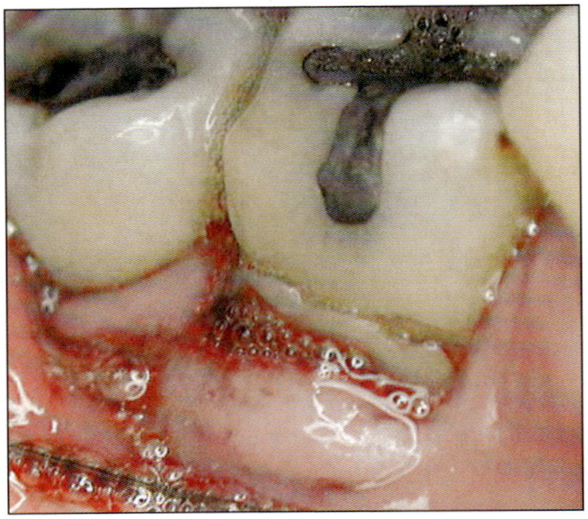

Fig 3-3a A mandibular molar with a periodontal abscess involving the furcation on the buccal surface. Note the exudate at the gingival margin. The defect has a probing depth of over 8 mm.

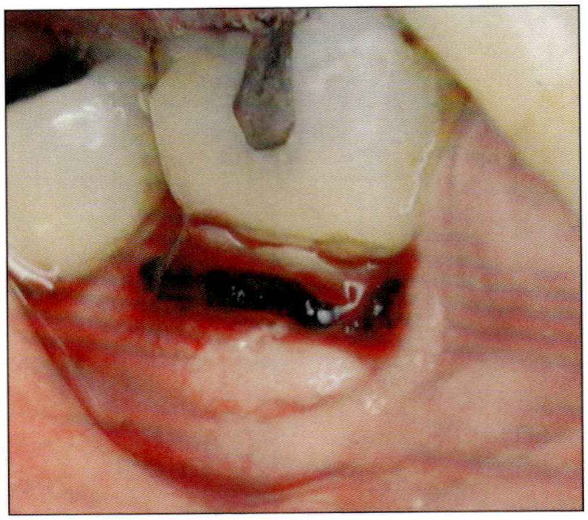

Fig 3-3b Immediate postoperative view following laser debridement of the affected area.

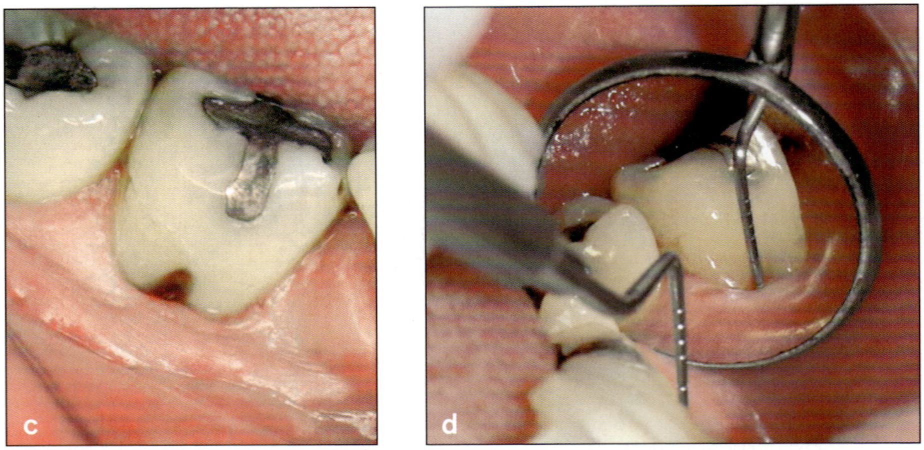

Figs 3-3c and 3-3d Postoperative views of the molar show significant improvement of the tissue at 2 weeks *(c)* and complete healing at 7 months *(d)* after treatment. (Case courtesy of Dr Kenneth Luk, Hong Kong, China.)

Purpose of the procedure	Treatment of a periodontal pocket

Use of a bactericidal dental laser in the periodontal pocket decreases the pathogenic microbial population, removes the diseased epithelial lining of the pocket, and restores the tissues to health.

Wavelength and settings

Diode laser, 810 nm, digitally pulsed for an average power of 2.7 W, with a 400 μm fiber.

Alternate wavelengths that may be used

An Nd:YAG or an ultrapulsed CO_2 laser can also be used to perform this procedure.

Clinical tip

For nonsurgical periodontal therapy, it is important to use very low power settings. The purpose of these procedures is not to cut but to disinfect or decontaminate the tissue. When using a laser with fiber-optic delivery, such as Nd:YAG and diode, the laser fiber is placed into the pocket 1 mm short of the probing depth. For lasers without fiber-optic delivery, such as CO_2 lasers, the laser tip is placed at the entrance to the pocket. With either delivery system, the laser is walked around the pocket, in a manner similar to that used when measuring probing depths.

Frenectomy: Case 1

Repositioning of a mandibular frenum in an adult patient.

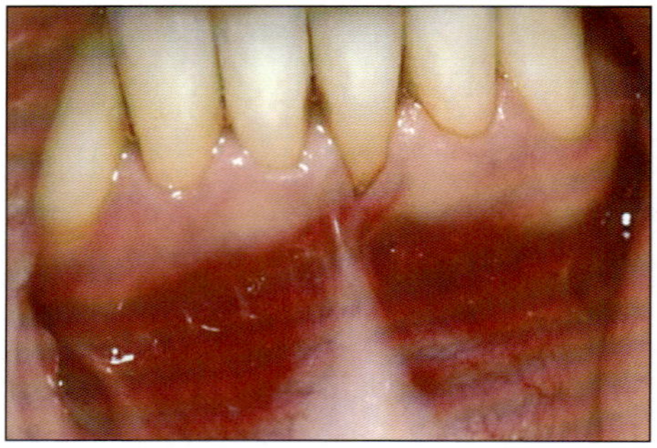

Fig 3-4a A mandibular labial frenum creates significant pull on the anterior gingiva. Note the gingival recession around the mandibular left central incisor.

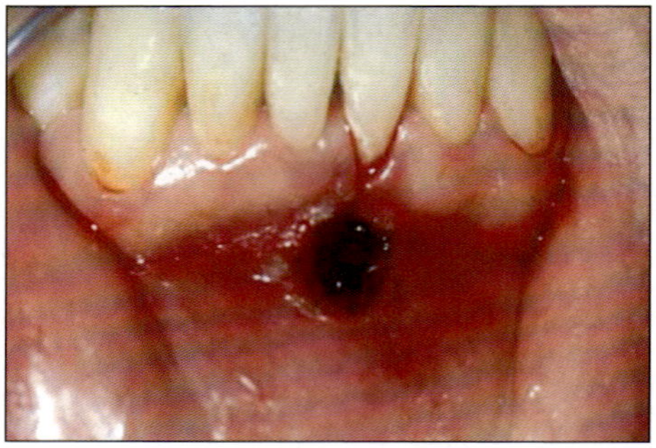

Fig 3-4b A CO_2 laser was used to ablate the frenum.

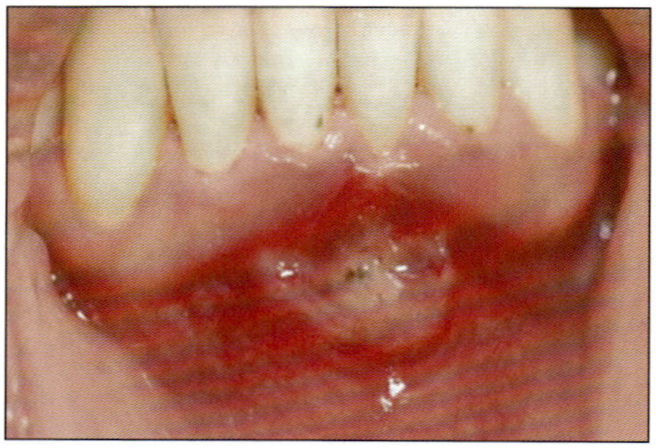

Fig 3-4c One-week postoperative view showing significant healing of the surgical site and a healthier gingival margin at the mandibular left central incisor.

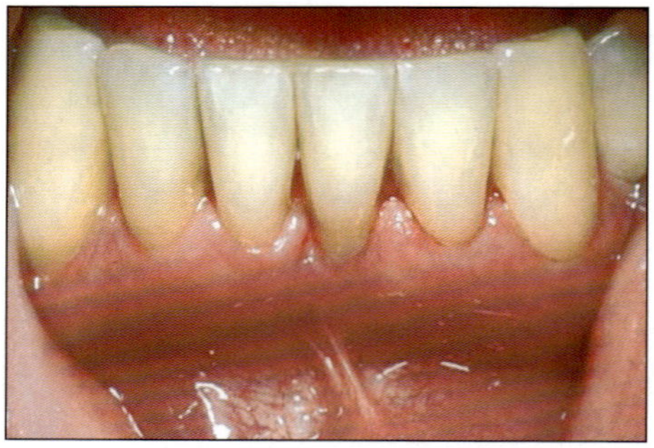

Fig 3-4d Two weeks following treatment, the surgical site is completely healed, the marginal tissue is free from frenal strain.

Purpose of the procedure

Repositioning of a labial frenum

The frenectomy reduces frenal strain and encourages the health of the gingiva.

Wavelength and settings

CO_2 laser set to 3 W, continuous wave, with an 800 μm ceramic tip in a contra-angle handpiece.

Alternate wavelengths that may be used

Any laser can be used to perform this procedure.

Frenectomy: Case 2

Repositioning of a mandibular labial frenum in an adult patient.

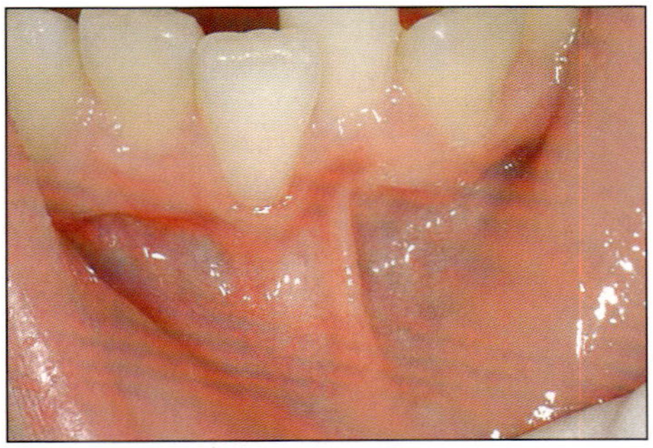

Fig 3-5a An aberrant frenum pulls the gingiva around the mandibular left central incisor.

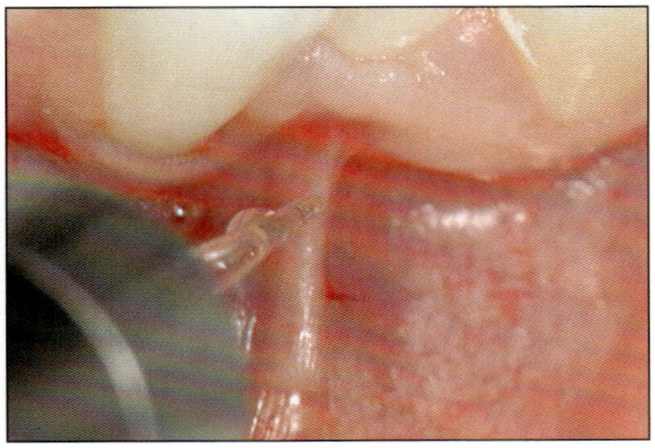

Fig 3-5b An Er:YAG laser ablates the frenal attachment.

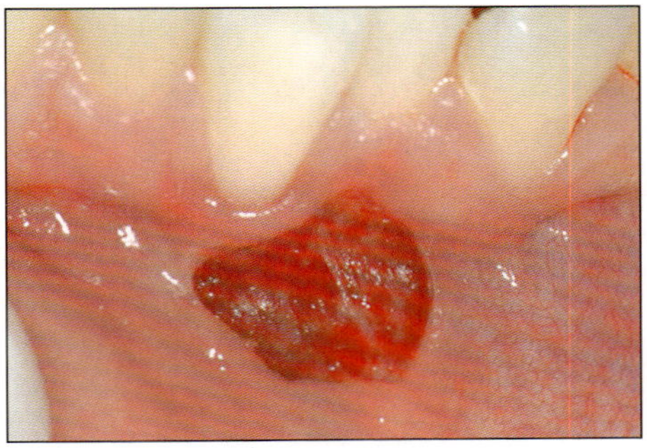

Fig 3-5c Immediate postoperative view following frenal ablation.

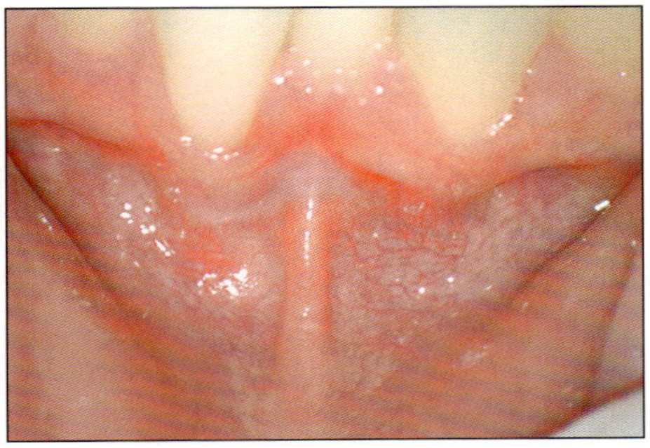

Fig 3-5d Two-week postoperative view of the healed and repositioned frenum.

Purpose of the procedure

Repositioning of a labial frenum

The frenectomy reduces frenal strain on the anterior labial gingiva.

Wavelength and settings

Er:YAG laser set to 30 mJ, 50 Hz, with a tapered tip and no water spray.

Alternate wavelengths that may be used

Any laser can be used to perform this procedure.

Clinical tip

When a frenectomy is performed via laser ablation, neither sutures nor surgical packing is necessary because the surgical site heals by secondary intention. The laser makes an incision down to the periosteum, and often the clinician uses a curette on the periosteum and bone to ensure that all of the muscle fibers have been severed.

Frenectomy: Case 3

Removal of a maxillary labial frenum in an adult patient.

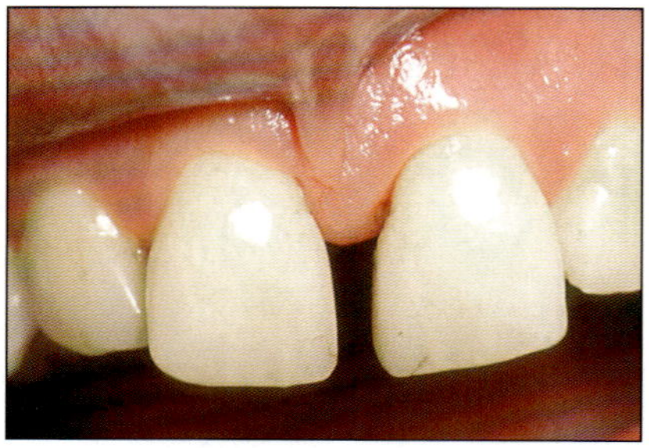

Fig 3-6a Preoperative view of thick, fibrous maxillary labial frenum.

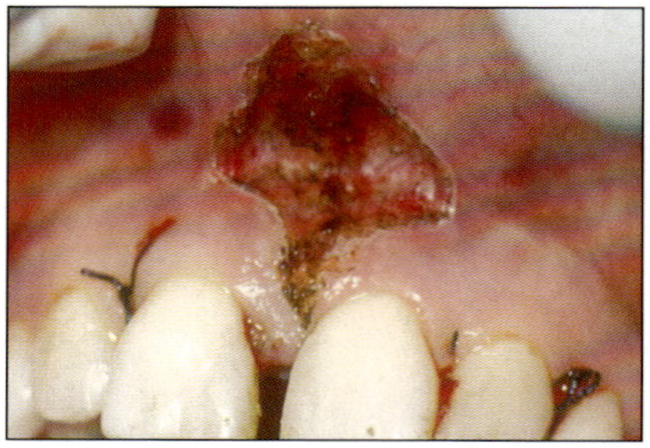

Fig 3-6b Immediate postoperative view of frenectomy site.

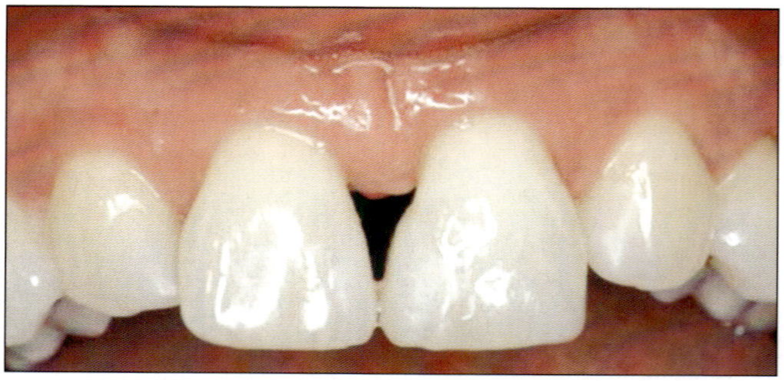

Fig 3-6c View of frenectomy 1 year following treatment. Without the use of orthodontic devices, the diastema between the maxillary central incisors spontaneously closed once the thick frenum was removed.

Purpose of the procedure	Removal of an aberrant frenum
The diastema between the maxillary central incisors closes once the frenectomy is removed.	

Wavelength and settings

CO_2 laser set to 3 W, continuous wave, with an 800 μm ceramic tip in a contra-angle handpiece.

Alternate wavelengths that may be used

Any laser can be used to perform this procedure.

Gingivectomy: Case 1

Removal of inflamed tissue over a maxillary left canine in a young patient.

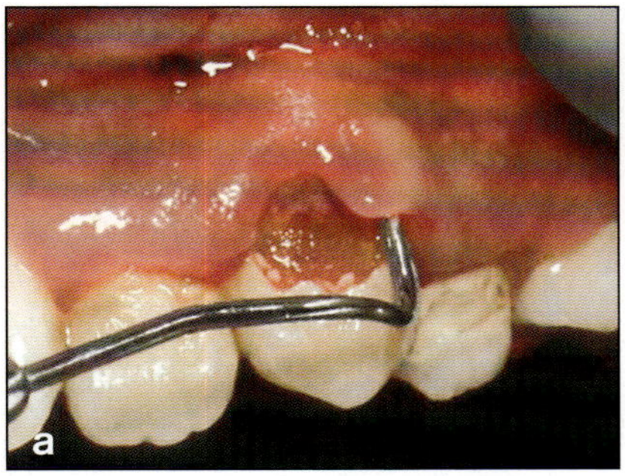

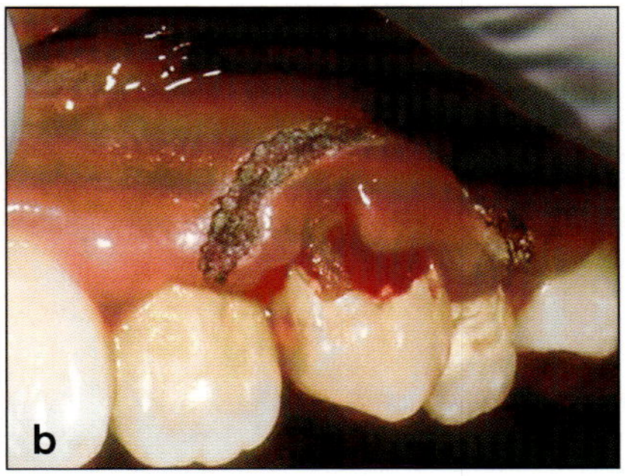

Fig 3-7a Periodontal probing of inflamed marginal gingiva that has become unattached. The tissue is interfering with access to the facial caries on the canine.

Fig 3-7b The laser outlined the planned gingivectomy over the maxillary left canine.

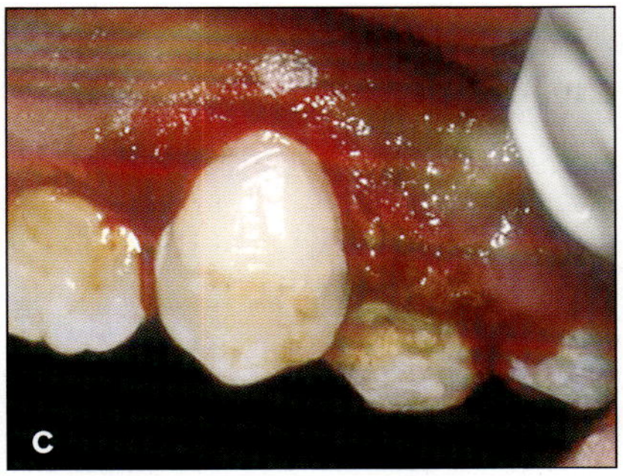

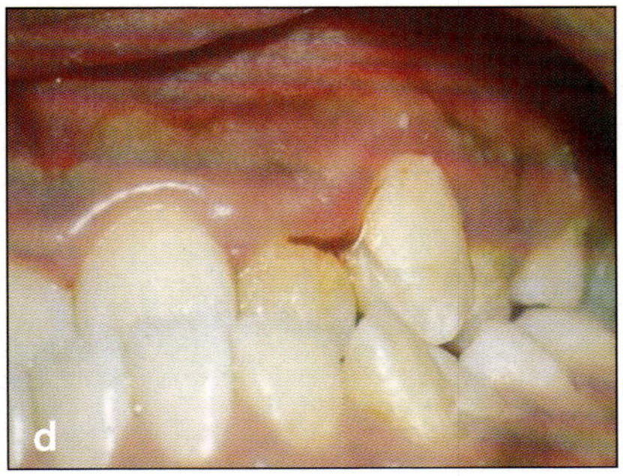

Fig 3-7c Immediate postoperative view following the gingivectomy and operative dental procedures.

Fig 3-7d One-week postoperative view of the surgical site. The gingiva was restored to an excellent anatomic form.

Purpose of the procedure

Gingivectomy

Removing unhealthy gingiva restores the anatomic contour of the soft tissue margins.

Wavelength and settings

CO_2 laser; settings for lesion outlining: 3 W, pulsed at a 50% duty cycle; setting for soft tissue ablation: 3 W, continuous wave, with an 800 μm ceramic tip in a contra-angle handpiece.

Alternate wavelengths that may be used

Any laser can be used to perform this procedure.

Clinical tip

When a gingivectomy is performed, the clinician must first outline the intended margins of the surgical site with a laser set to low power. Fig 3-7b shows the ablation outline of a CO_2 laser used in a pulsed mode. At this stage, the clinician examines the outline and can change it if necessary. Once the shape is verified, the dots of the pulsed CO_2 outline are connected as the gingiva is ablated.

Gingivectomy: Case 2

Full maxillary gingivectomy to reduce periodontal pockets in a male patient.

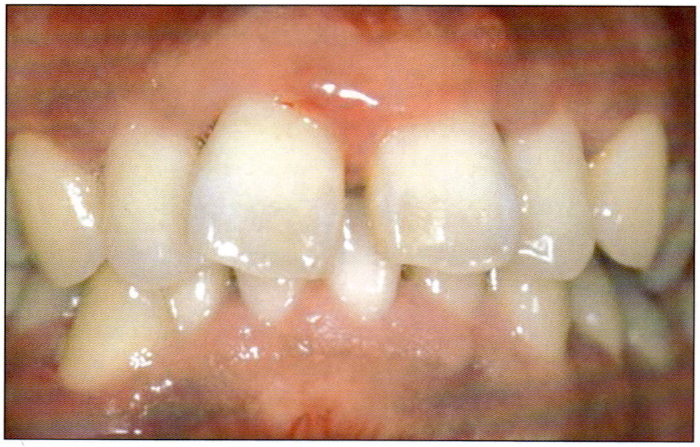

Fig 3-8a Scaling and root planing have been completed prior to a full arch gingivectomy to reduce residual 4 and 5 mm periodontal pockets.

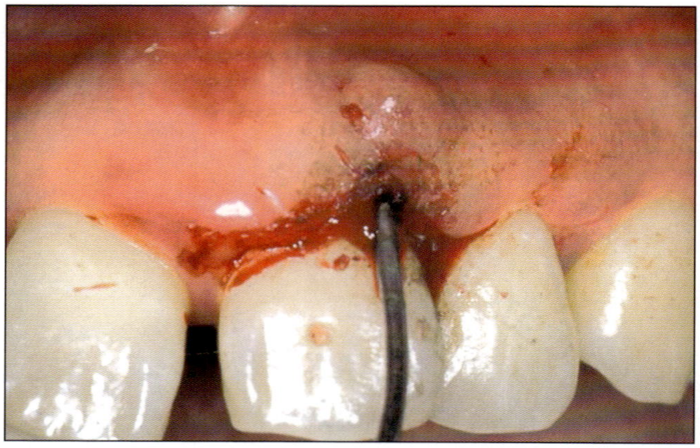

Fig 3-8b The laser recontours the gingival margin.

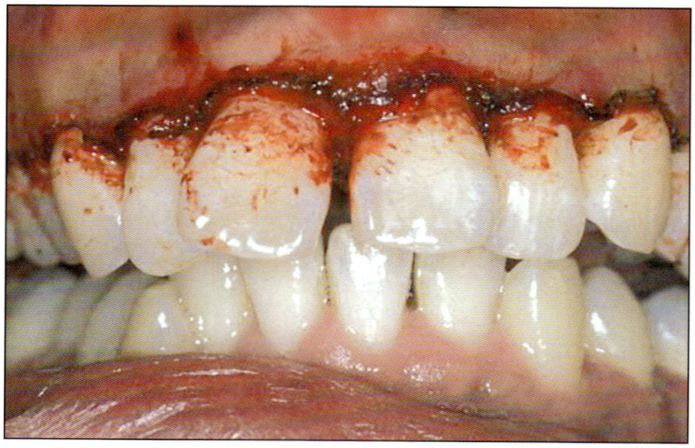

Fig 3-8c The immediate results of the maxillary gingivectomy.

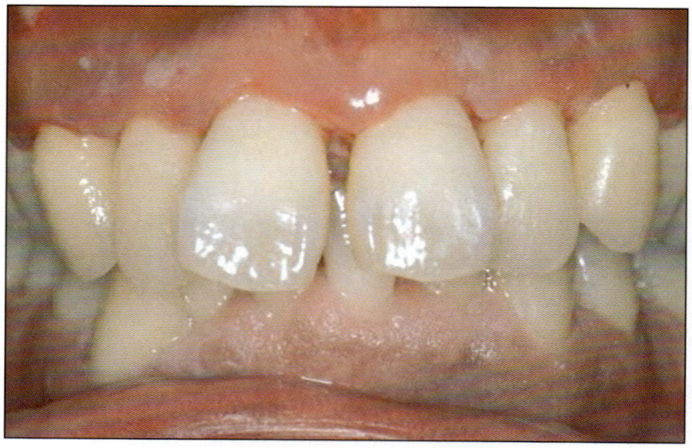

Fig 3-8d One-week postoperative view of the surgical site.

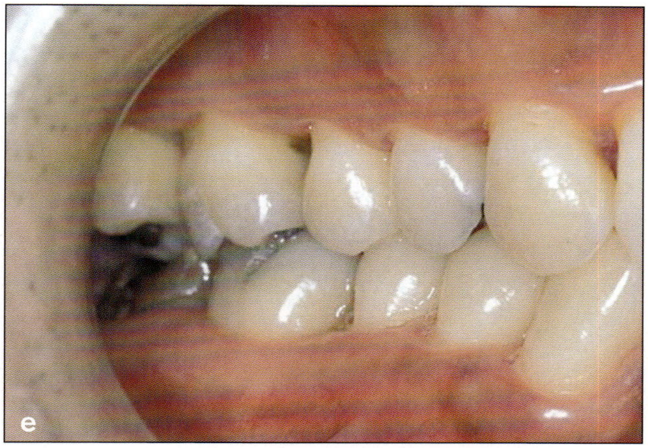

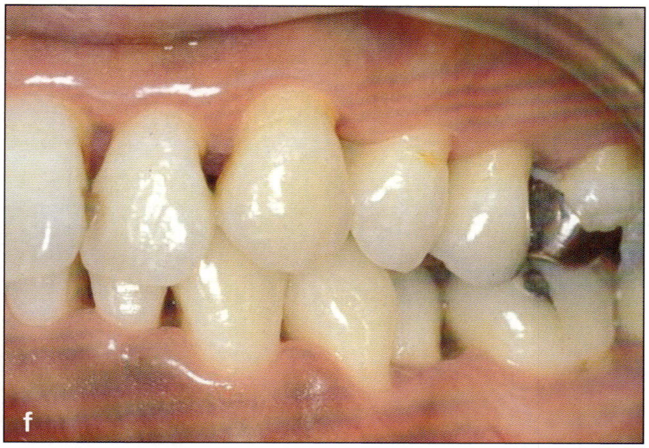

Figs 3-8e and 3-8f Close-ups of the right *(e)* and left *(f)* sides of the maxilla 6 months after treatment. The periodontal pockets have been reduced and the soft tissue has healed with excellent tissue tone and contours.

Purpose of the procedure	Reduction of residual periodontal pockets
After the scaling and root planing are completed for the maxillary dentition, residual periodontal pockets are reduced via laser gingivectomy.	

Wavelength and settings
Nd:YAG laser set to 2 W, 100 mJ, 20 Hz, with a 320 μm fiber.
Alternate wavelengths that may be used
Any laser can be used to perform this procedure.

Gingival Graft: Case 1

Recontouring a gingival graft in the maxilla in an adult patient.

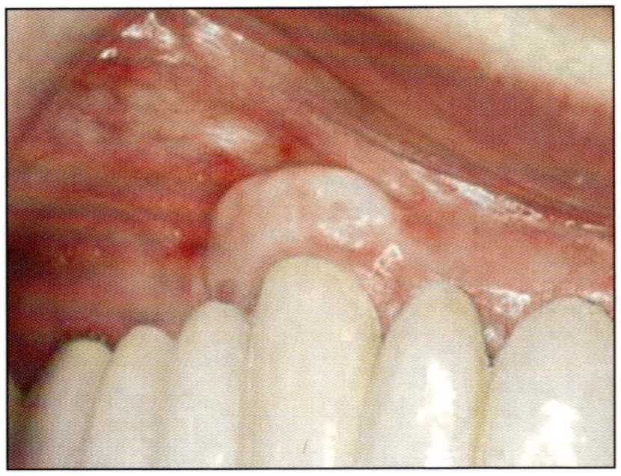

Fig 3-9a An integrated gingival graft with thickened fibrous tissue and unesthetic tissue contours.

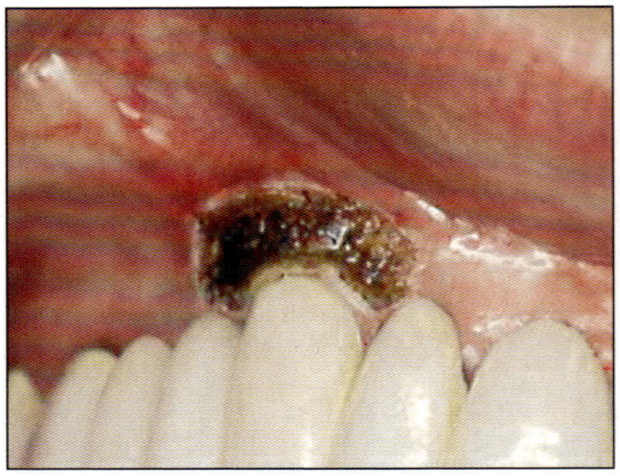

Fig 3-9b Immediate postoperative view of the surgical site. A laser was used to remove the tissue bulk and blend the graft into the surrounding gingiva.

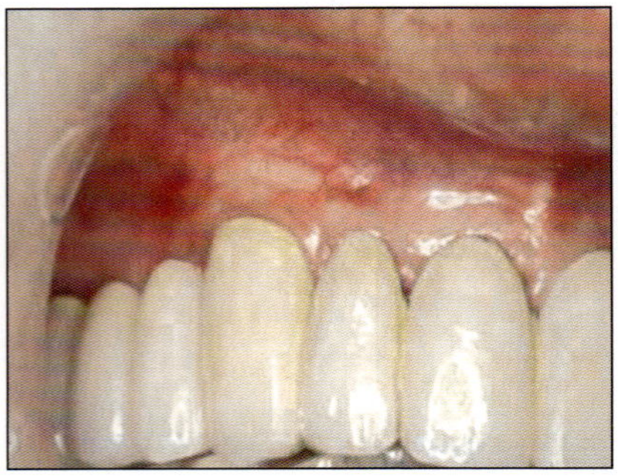

Fig 3-9c Three-week postoperative view shows excellent tissue contours and superior esthetics. (Case courtesy of Dr Stuart Coleton, White Plains, NY.)

Purpose of the procedure	Recontouring a gingival graft

After the thickened tissue is removed, the laser is used to recontour and blend in the graft with surrounding tissue.

Wavelength and settings

CO_2 laser set to 4 W, continuous wave.

Alternate wavelengths that may be used

Any laser can be used to perform this procedure.

Clinical tip

Some successful gingival grafts may look quite bulky. Since most grafts are taken from the palate, the tissue usually has different pigmentation than the host tissue. The combination of tissue bulk and varied pigmentation may lead to an unesthetic result. Laser energy can be used to thin out the bulky tissue, which often helps the remaining tissue to blend in with the surrounding gingiva (see Fig 3-9c). This procedure should not be performed until the graft has completely healed and successfully integrated with surrounding tissue.

Gingival Graft: Case 2

Graft placement in the anterior mandible in an adult patient.

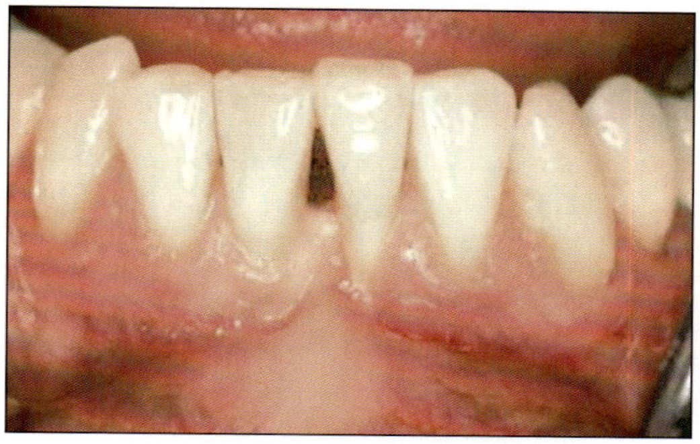

Fig 3-10a Preoperative view of the mandibular left central incisor with little attached gingiva.

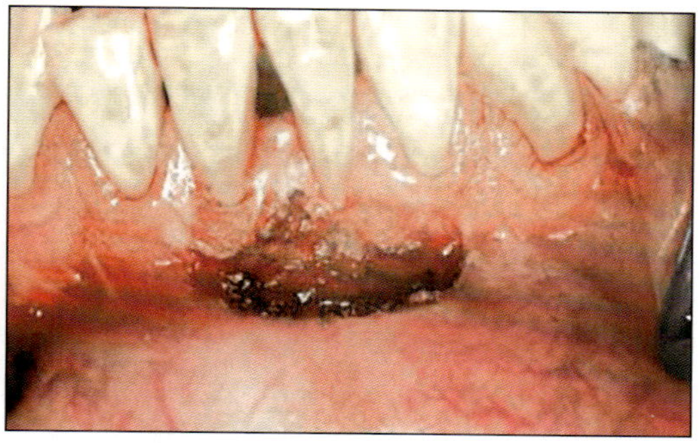

Fig 3-10b The graft site following the preparatory vestibuloplasty.

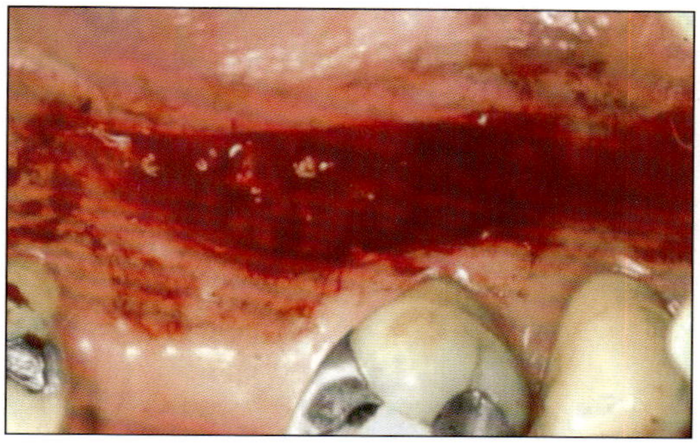

Fig 3-10c Tissue was harvested from the palatal donor site in the posterior maxilla.

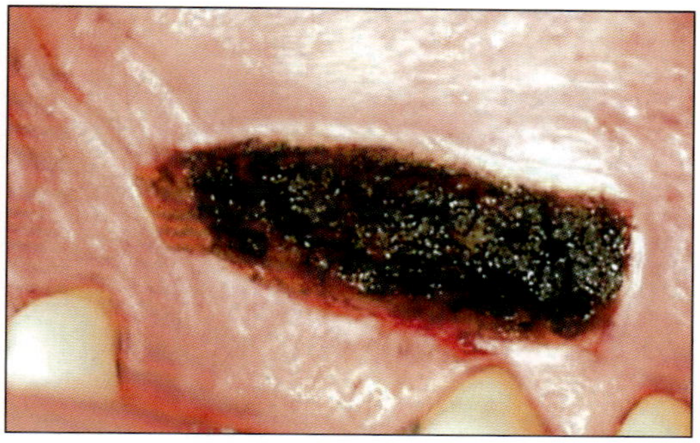

Fig 3-10d Laser hemostasis of the palatal donor site.

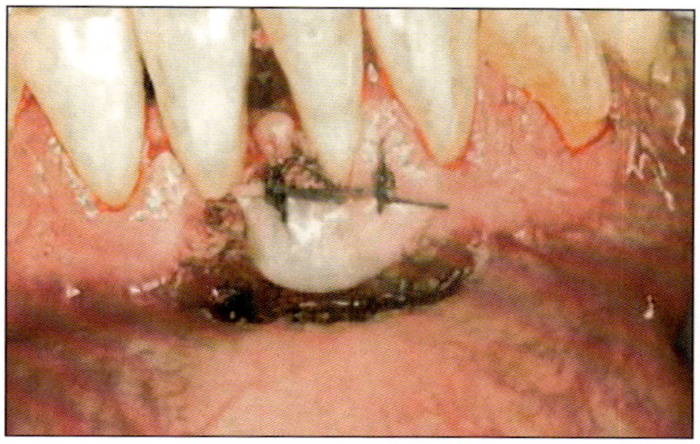

Fig 3-10e The palatal graft is sutured in place in the anterior mandible.

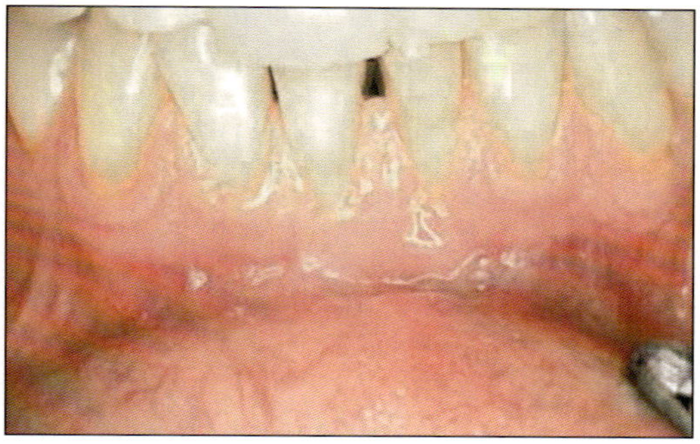

Fig 3-10f Four-week postoperative view showing the integrated gingival graft. (Case courtesy of Dr Stuart Coleton, White Plains, NY.)

Purpose of the procedure	Gingival graft

A gingival graft increases the amount of attached gingiva in the anterior region of the mandible.

Wavelength and settings

CO_2 laser; settings for vestibuloplasty: 4 W, continuous wave; settings for hemostasis of the donor site: 5 W, continuous wave, defocused.

Alternate wavelengths that may be used

Any laser can be used to perform the vestibuloplasty or hemostasis. The Er family of lasers, however, is least effective for coagulation, and the water spray must be shut off to achieve acceptable hemostasis.

Clinical tip

Due to the hemostatic ability of the CO_2 laser, there is minimal to no bleeding following the vestibuloplasty. When the palatal graft is ready to be sutured in place, a curette or similar instrument should be used to induce bleeding at the graft site. This will ensure that there is blood flowing to the site to properly perfuse the gingival graft.

Regenerative Periodontal Surgery: Case 1

Removal of diseased tissue in the furcation of a maxillary second molar in an adult male patient.

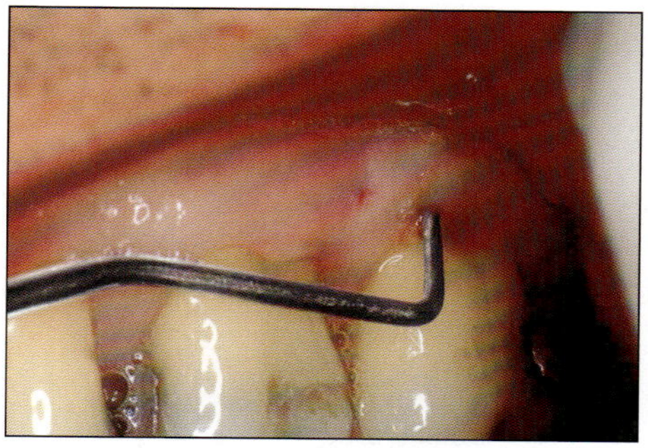

Fig 3-11a Extensive bone loss in the maxillary second molar in the furcation between the mesiobuccal and distobuccal roots.

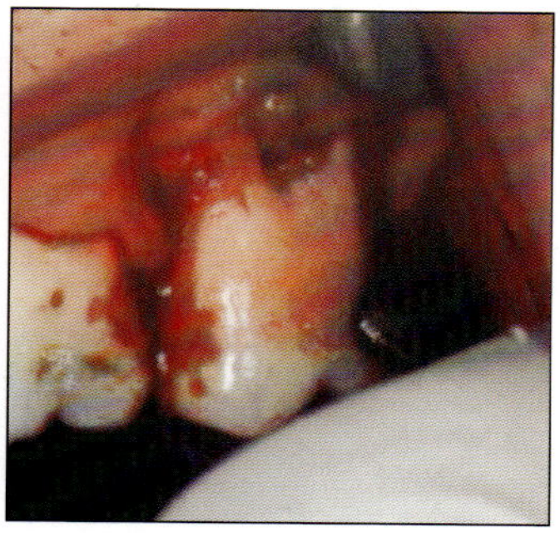

Fig 3-11b Intraoperative view of the exposed furcation following reflection of a soft tissue flap. A spherical area of diseased, granulomatous tissue is firmly attached to the furcation of the mesiobuccal and distobuccal roots.

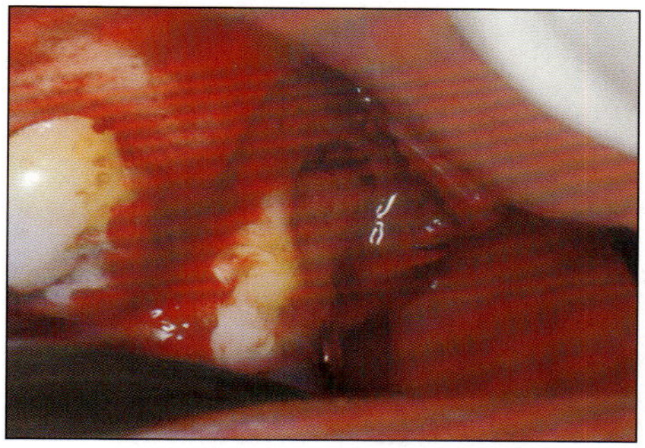

Fig 3-11c Immediate postoperative view of the laser-ablated furcation. The diseased tissue has been ablated, leaving a smooth root surface, free of debris and ready for reattachment of connective tissue.

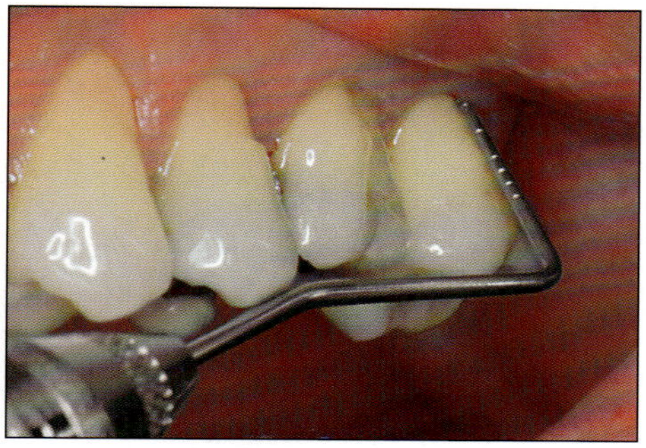

Fig 3-11d The 90-day postoperative view shows significant reduction of the probing depth.

Purpose of the procedure

Reduction of periodontal probing depth

Once the diseased tissue is removed from the furcation, the root surface is instrumented in preparation for gingival reattachment.

Wavelength and settings

CO_2 laser, 3 W, continuous wave, with an 800 μm ceramic tip in a contra-angle handpiece.

Alternate wavelengths that may be used

Any laser can be used to perform this procedure.

Regenerative Periodontal Surgery: Case 2

Removal of an infrabony defect followed by guided tissue regeneration in the anterior mandible in an adult female patient.

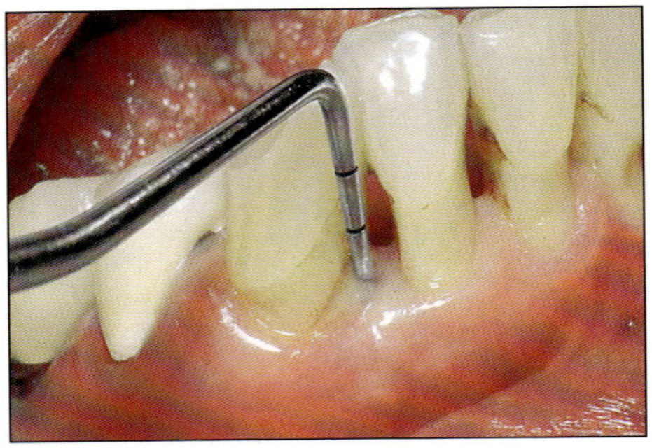

Fig 3-12a Periodontal probing of the mandibular right dentition between the lateral incisor and canine.

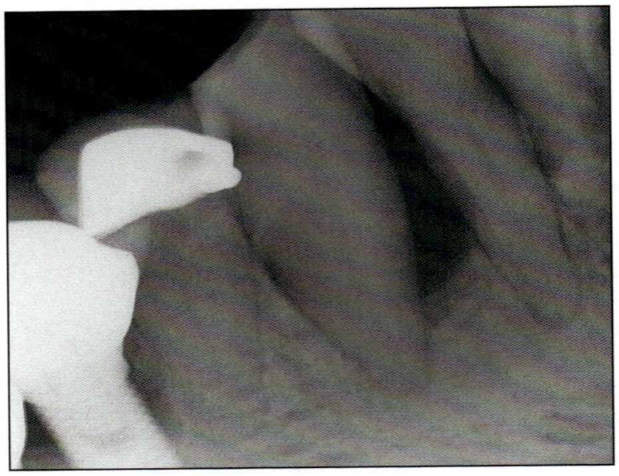

Fig 3-12b The mandibular right dentition shows radiographic evidence of extensive bone loss between the lateral incisor and canine.

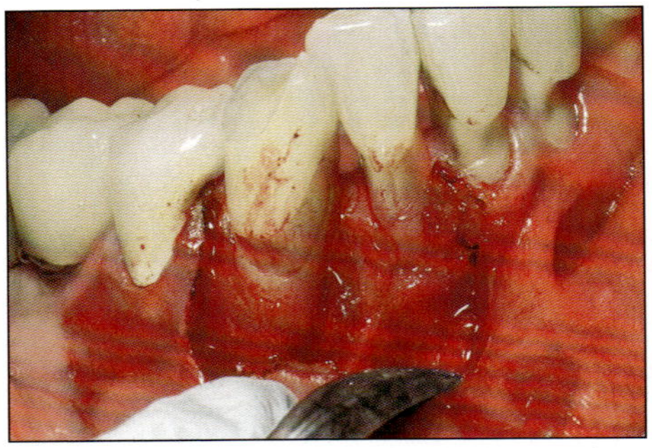

Fig 3-12c The granulomatous tissue in the infrabony defect is exposed by the reflection of a full-thickness flap.

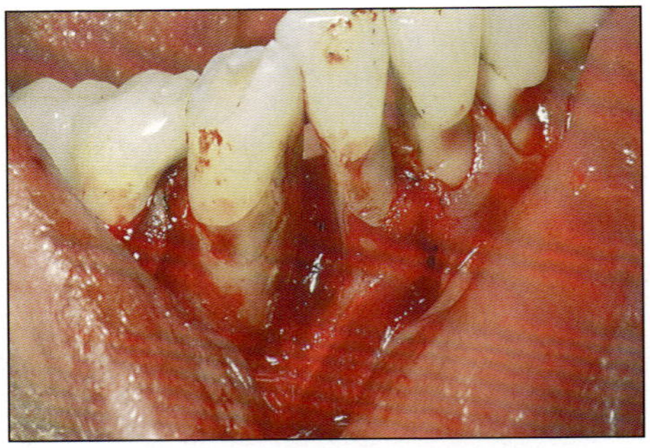

Fig 3-12d View of the surgical site after removal of the diseased tissue with the laser.

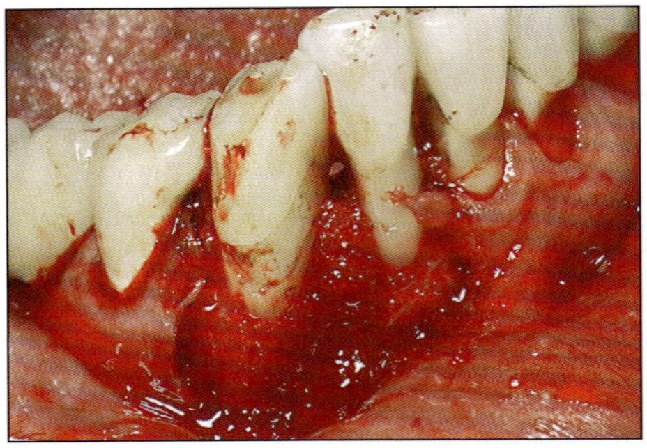

Fig 3-12e Freeze-dried demineralized bone material is packed into the infrabony defect.

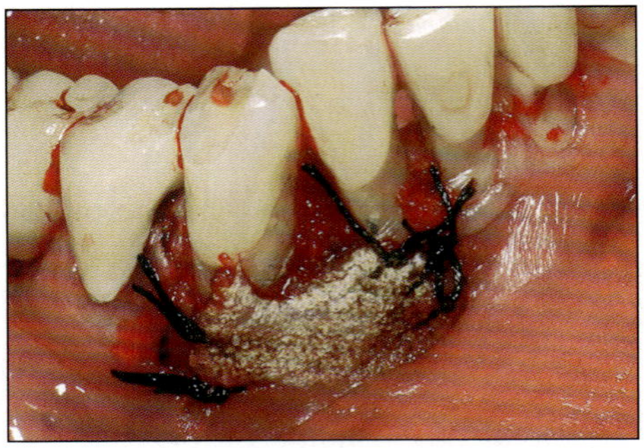

Fig 3-12f Postoperative view immediately following de-epithelialization of the soft tissue flap.

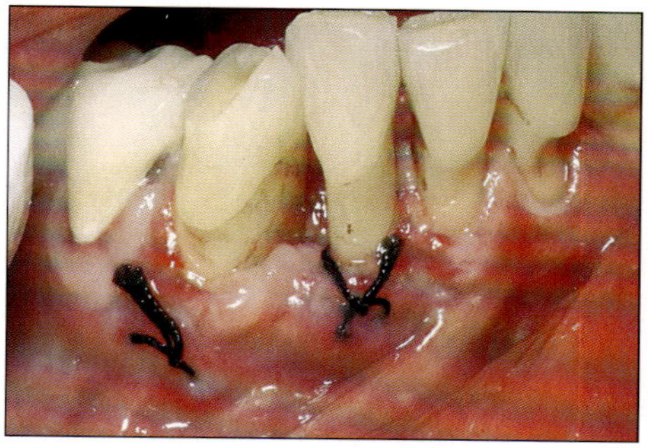

Fig 3-12g One-week postoperative view of surgical site prior to a second de-epithelialization procedure.

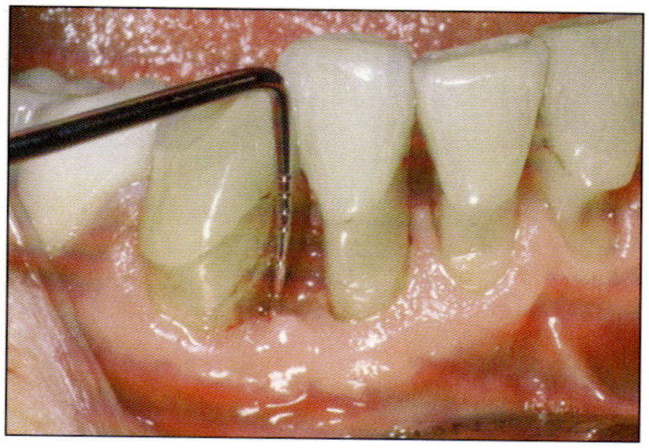

Fig 3-12h Periodontal probing 3 months following surgery.

Purpose of the procedure

Removal of diseased osseous tissue

Once the diseased tissue is removed from an infrabony defect, a new connective tissue attachment is created via guided tissue regeneration.

Wavelength and settings

CO_2 laser for the soft tissue ablation set to 3 W, continuous wave. Er:YAG laser for the hard tissue ablation set to 350 mJ and 10 Hz.

Alternate wavelengths that may be used

For the hard tissue procedure, both the Er:YAG and Er,Cr:YSGG lasers are able to perform the osseous surgery, but only the Er:YAG wavelength has been reported to alter the root surface for better adherence of periodontal fibroblasts than with conventional scaling and root planing.[28–31]

For soft tissue de-epithelialization, any laser can be used. However, the CO_2 wavelength has demonstrated histologic proof in three animal models (ie, beagles, monkeys, and humans) to safely and effectively de-epithelialize soft tissue flaps, thereby encouraging the growth of new connective tissue.[24–27]

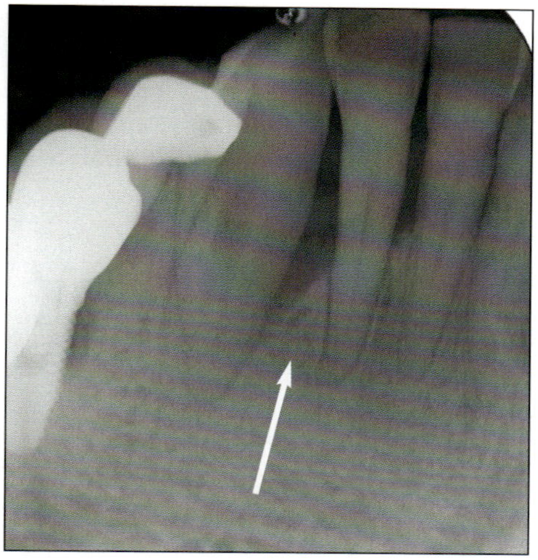

Fig 3-12i Three-month postoperative radiograph.

References

1. Pick RM, Pecaro BC, Silberman CJ. The laser gingivectomy. The use of the CO_2 laser for the removal of phenytoin hyperplasia. J Periodontol 1985;56:492–496.
2. Gopin BW, Cobb CM, Rapley JW, Killoy WJ. Histologic evaluation of soft tissue attachment to CO_2 laser-treated root surfaces: An in vivo study. Int J Periodontics Restorative Dent 1997;17:317–325.
3. Krause LS, Cob CM, Rapley JW, Killoy WJ, Spencer P. Laser irradiation of bone. 1. An in vitro study concerning the effects of the CO_2 laser on oral mucosa and subjacent bone. J Periodontol 1997;68:872–880.
4. Zambon JJ. Periodontal diseases: Microbial factors. Ann Periodontol 1996;1:879–925.
5. Kornman KS, Page RC, Tonetti MS. The host response to microbial challenge in periodontitis: Assembling the players. Periodontol 2000 1997;14:33–53.
6. Finkbeiner RL. The results of 1328 periodontal pockets treated with the argon laser: Selective pocket thermolysis. J Clin Laser Med Surg 1995;13:273–281.
7. Moritz A, Schoop U, Goharkhay K, et al. Treatment of periodontal pockets with a diode laser. Lasers Surg Med 1998;22:302–311.
8. Neill ME, Mellonig JT. Clinical efficacy of the Nd:YAG laser for combination periodontitis therapy. Pract Periodontics Aesthet Dent 1997;9:1–95.
9. Ando Y, Aoki A, Watanabe H, Ishikawa I. Bactericidal effects of Erbium YAG laser on periodontopathic bacteria. Lasers Surg Med 1996;19:190–200.
10. Walsh LJ. Utilization of a carbon dioxide laser for periodontal surgery: A three year longitudinal study. Periodontol 2000 1995;16:3–7.
11. Rowson JE. The contact diode laser—A useful instrument for excising oral lesions [abstract]. Br J Oral Maxillofac Surg 1995;33:123.
12. White JM, Goodis HE, Rose CL. Use of the pulsed Nd:YAG laser for intraoral soft tissue surgery. Lasers Surg Med 1991;11:455–461.
13. Pick RM, Pecaro BC. Use of the CO_2 laser in soft tissue dental surgery. Lasers Surg Med 1987;7:207–213.
14. Baraldi CE, Puricelli E, Kulkes S, Martins GL. Er:YAG laser in oral soft tissue surgery [abstract 59]. J Oral Laser Appl 2001;1:24.
15. Coluzzi DJ. Lasers and soft tissue curettage: An update. Compend Contin Educ Dent 2002;23:1104–1111.
16. Raffetto N, Gutierrez T. Lasers in periodontal therapy, a five year retrospective. J Calif Dent Hyg Assoc 2001;16:17–20.
17. Schwarz F, Sculean A, Georg T, Reich E. Periodontal treatment with an Er:YAG laser compared to scaling and root planing. A controlled clinical study. J Periodontol 2001;72:361–367.
18. Yukna RA, Evans GH, Vastardis S, Carr RF. Laser-assisted periodontal regeneration in humans. Presented at the 81st General Session of the International Association for Dental Research, Goteborg, Sweden, June 2003.
19. Kreisler M, Meyer C, Stender E, Daublander M, Willershausen-Zonnchen B, d'Hoedt B. Effect of diode laser irradiation on the attachment rate of periodontal ligament cells: An in vitro study. J Periodontol 2001;72:1312–1317.
20. Aoki A, Sasaki KM, Watanabe H, Ishikawa I. Lasers in nonsurgical periodontal therapy. Periodontol 2000 2004;36:59–97.
21. Frentzen M, Braun A, Aniol D. Er:YAG laser scaling of diseased root surfaces. J Periodontol 2002;73:524–530.
22. Ishikawa I, Aoki A, Takasaki AA. Potential applications of erbium:YAG laser in periodontics. J Periodont Res 2004;39:275–285.
23. Bader HI. Use of lasers in periodontics. Dent Clin North Am 2000;44:779–792.

24. Israel M, Rossmann JA. An epithelial exclusion technique using the CO_2 laser for the treatment of periodontal defects. Compend Contin Educ Dent 1998;19:86–95.
25. Rossmann JA, McQuade MJ, Turunen DE. Retardation of epithelial migration in monkeys using a carbon dioxide laser: An animal study. J Periodontol 1992;63:902–907.
26. Israel M, Rossmann JA, Froum SJ. Use of the carbon dioxide laser in retarding epithelial migration: A pilot histological human study utilizing case reports. J Periodontol 1995;66:197–204.
27. Rossmann JA, Parlar A, Adbel-Ghaffar KA, El-Khouli AM, Israel M. Use of the carbon dioxide laser in guided tissue-regeneration wound healing in the beagle dog [abstract]. J Dent Res 1996;75:31.
28. Schwarz F, Sculean A, Berakdar M, Szathmari L, Georg T, Becker J. In vivo and in vitro effects of an Er:YAG laser, a GaAlAs diode laser, and scaling and root planing on periodontally diseased root surfaces: A comparative histologic study Lasers Surg Med 2003;32:359–366.
29. Schwarz F, Putz N, Georg T, Reich E. Effects of an Er:YAG laser on periodontally involved root surfaces: An in vivo and in vitro SEM comparison. Lasers Surg Med 2001;29: 328–335.
30. Schwarz F, Sculean A, Berakdar M, Georg T, Reich E, Becker J. Clinical evaluation of an Er:YAG laser combined with scaling and root planing for non-surgical periodontal treatment: A controlled prospective clinical study. J Clin Periodontol 2003;30:26–34.
31. Schwarz F, Aoki A, Sculean A, Georg T, Scherbaum W, Becker J. In vivo effects of an Er:YAG laser, an ultrasonic system and scaling and root planing on the biocompatibility of periodontally diseased root surfaces in cultures of human PDL fibroblasts. Lasers Surg Med 2003;33:140–147.
32. Raffetto N. Lasers for initial periodontal therapy. Dent Clin North Am 2004;48:923–936.
33. Coleton S. Lasers in surgical periodontics and oral medicine. Dent Clin North Am 2004;48:937–962.

4

ADJUNCTIVE LASER SURGERY IN IMPLANT DENTISTRY

Lasers can be used in implant dentistry in a variety of ways.[1] Using lasers during soft tissue implant procedures offers the advantages of increased visibility due to hemostasis, greater ease in making incisions and contouring soft tissue, reduced bacteria at the surgical site, and increased patient comfort due to minimal postoperative swelling and pain.[2–5] Impressions for restorative procedures can be taken immediately after second-stage surgery because the surgical field will be clean and dry. Additionally, if the clinician employs the proper laser settings, the soft tissue margins shrink minimally after healing.[6] The erbium (Er) family of lasers, with its capacity for osseous ablation, can be used in osteotomy preparation and for removal of diseased osseous tissue around areas of inflammation.[7]

Numerous studies document the effect of different wavelengths on implant surfaces, including the potential for charring, pitting, or melting those surfaces and the possibility of transmitting laser-generated heat to the surrounding bone. Several studies indicate that neodymium-doped yttrium aluminum garnet (Nd:YAG) lasers are contraindicated for implant surgery,[8–10] whereas the diode, Er family, and carbon dioxide (CO_2) lasers can be used for specific procedures,[11] such as removing soft tissue covering the integrated implant.[12] Because Er and CO_2 laser wavelengths are reflected away from metal surfaces, they interact only minimally with the implant.[13,14] CO_2 and diode lasers facilitate hemostasis, and Er family lasers produce acceptable bleeding control when used without water spray. Er lasers can be used to remove and recontour bone safely and effectively and to help prepare edentulous sites for implant placement. The bactericidal properties of diode, Er, and CO_2 lasers successfully treat peri-implantitis.[15–19] These instruments remove diseased, granulomatous tissue from peri-implantitis sites as well as decontaminate implant surfaces and provide an environment favorable to osseous regeneration.

Implant Uncovering Surgery: Case 1

Second-stage surgery using a diode laser in a partially edentulous patient.

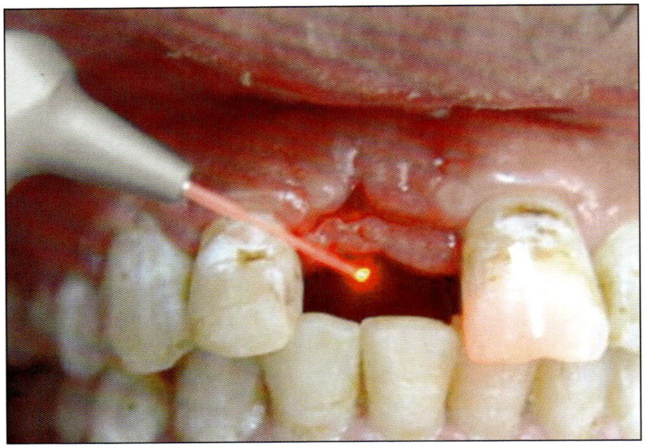

Fig 4-1a Intraoperative view of a diode laser at a maxillary central incisor implant site at the beginning of implant uncovering.

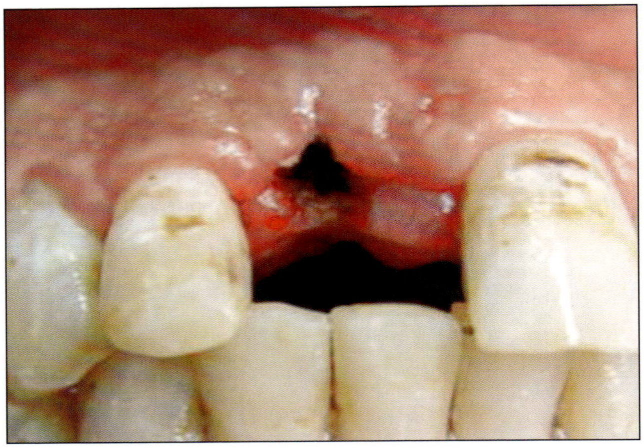

Fig 4-1b Immediate postoperative view of the implant site. The soft tissue that covered the implant has been ablated. The surgical field is clean and dry and requires no sutures.

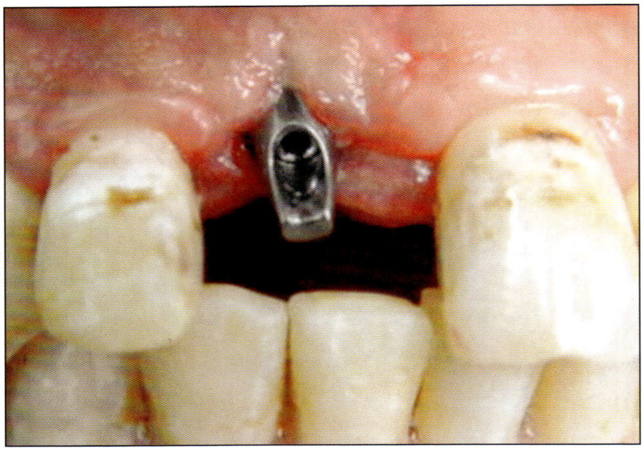

Fig 4-1c Postoperative view following placement of a standard abutment. The implant site is ready for taking the impression for the definitive prosthesis. (Case courtesy of Dr Avi Reyhanian, Natanya, Israel.)

Purpose of the procedure

Uncovering implants using a diode laser

After the implant is exposed, an impression can be taken for restoration.

Wavelength and settings

Diode, 810 nm, set to 3.5 W, continuous wave, with a 600 μm tip.

Alternate wavelengths that may be used

CO_2 and Er family lasers can be used to perform this procedure.

Implant Uncovering Surgery: Case 2

Second-stage surgery using a CO_2 laser in a partially edentulous patient.

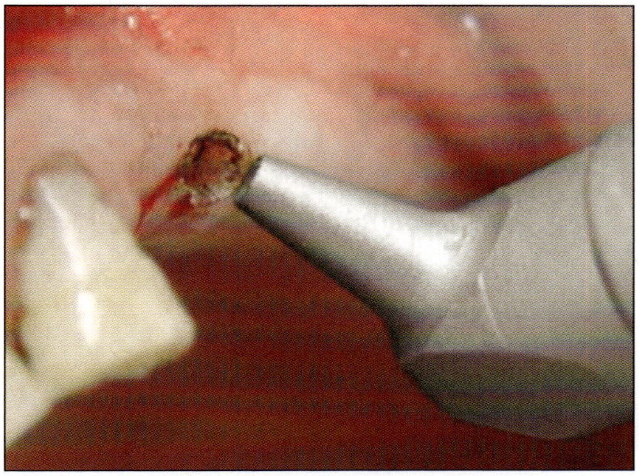

Fig 4-2a CO_2 laser removing soft tissue during second-stage implant surgery.

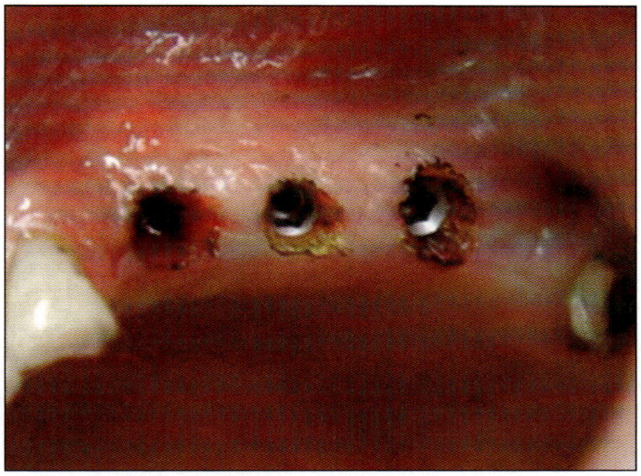

Fig 4-2b Immediate postoperative view showing three uncovered implants.

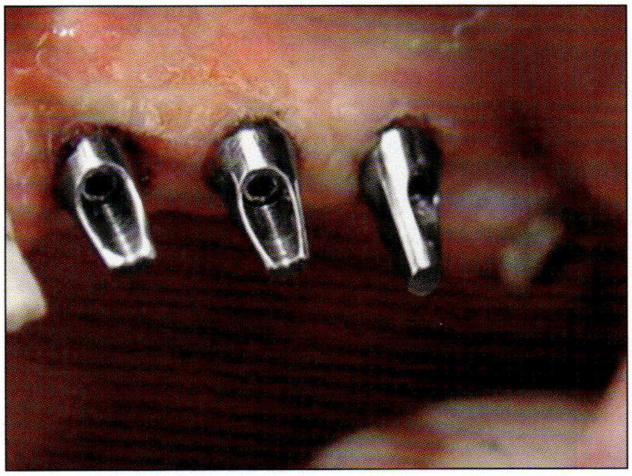

Fig 4-2c Three standard abutments have been placed.

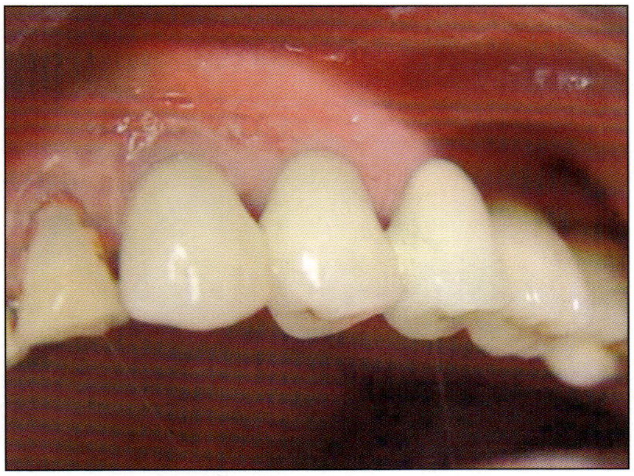

Fig 4-2d Definitive restorations in place over implant abutments. (Case courtesy of Dr Avi Reyhanian, Natanya, Israel.)

Purpose of the procedure

Uncovering implants using a CO_2 laser

Soft tissue ablation exposes implants in preparation for abutment placement and implant restoration.

Wavelength and settings

CO_2 laser set to 4.5 W, continuous wave, defocused.

Alternate wavelengths that may be used

Er family and diode lasers can be used to perform this procedure.

Implant Uncovering Surgery: Case 3

Second-stage surgery using an Er:YAG laser in a partially edentulous patient.

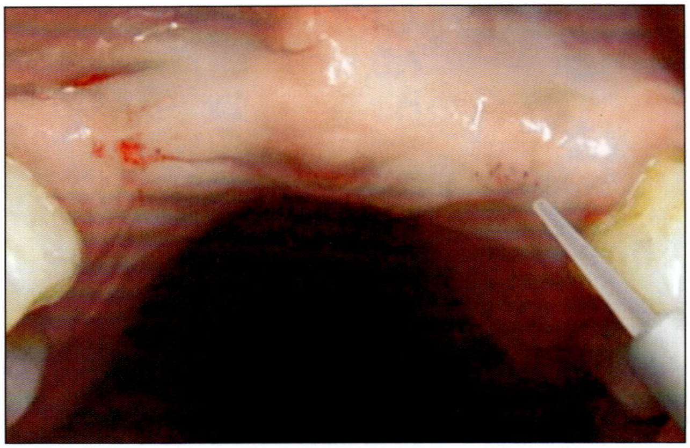

Fig 4-3a Er:YAG laser ablation of soft tissue in the maxillary anterior region.

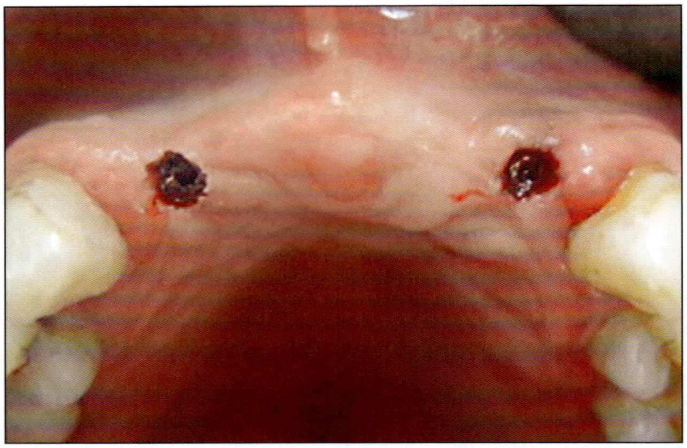

Fig 4-3b Immediate postoperative view showing the uncovered implants.

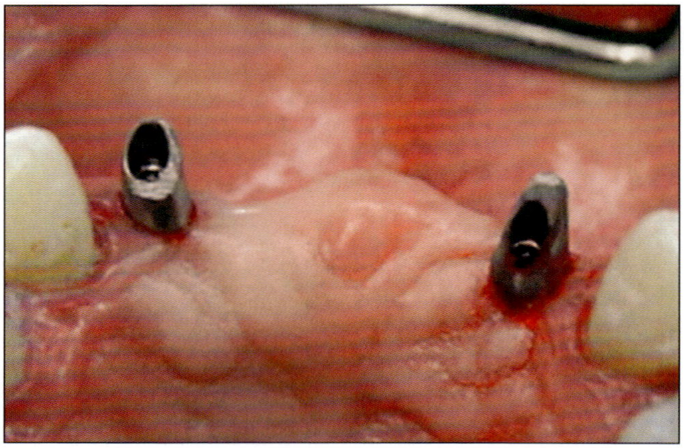

Fig 4-3c Postoperative palatal view following placement of standard abutments. (Case courtesy of Dr Avi Reyhanian, Natanya, Israel.)

Purpose of the procedure

Uncovering implants using an Er:YAG laser

Once implants are exposed, abutments can be placed for implant restoration.

Wavelength and settings

Er:YAG laser set to 9 W, 450 mJ, 20 Hz, with a 200 µm sapphire tip with water spray.

Alternate wavelengths that may be used

CO_2 and diode lasers can be used to perform this procedure.

Implant Uncovering Surgery: Case 4

Second-stage surgery using an Er:YAG laser in a partially edentulous patient.

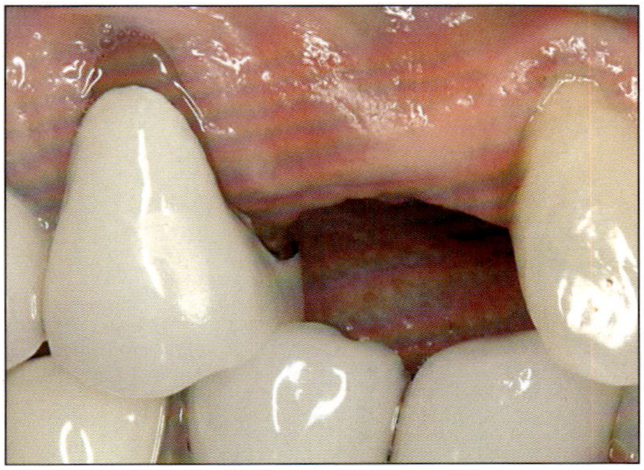

Fig 4-4a The maxillary right canine site is prepared for second-stage surgery.

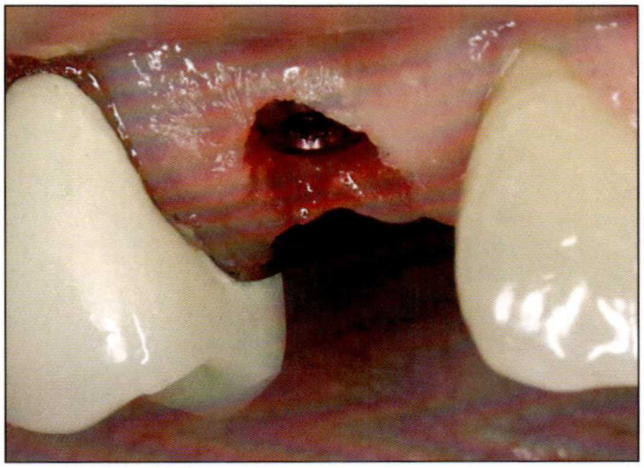

Fig 4-4b Immediate postoperative view following implant uncovering.

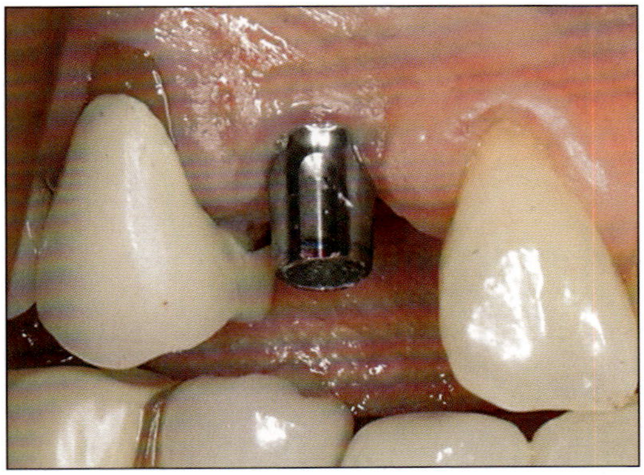

Fig 4-4c Three-week postoperative view of a standard implant abutment.

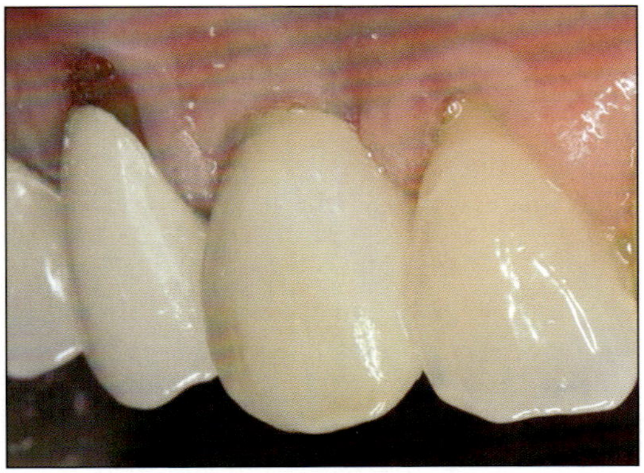

Fig 4-4d Four-week postoperative view following implant restoration. (Case courtesy of Dr Grace Sun, Los Angeles, CA.)

Purpose of the procedure

Uncovering implants using an Er:YAG laser

Soft tissue ablation exposes implants in preparation for abutment placement and implant restoration.

Wavelength and settings

Er:YAG laser set to 2.7 W, 90 mJ, 30 Hz, with a 600 μm tip with no water spray.

Alternate wavelengths that may be used

CO_2 and diode lasers can be used to perform this procedure.

Implant Uncovering Surgery: Case 5

Second-stage surgery using an Er:YAG laser in a partially edentulous patient.

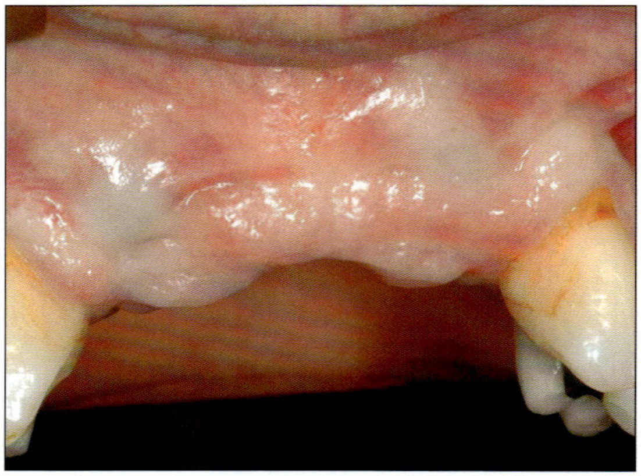

Fig 4-5a Implants have been placed in the anterior maxilla in this partially edentulous patient.

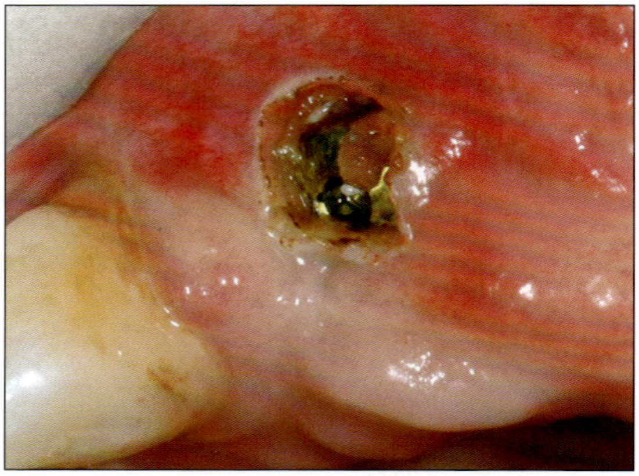

Fig 4-5b The laser begins to uncover the right implant.

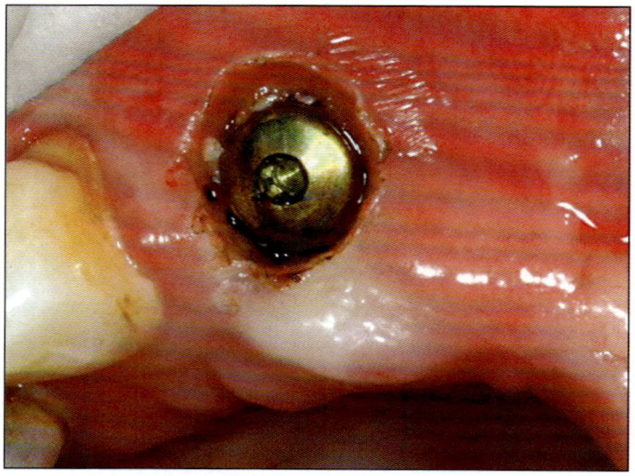

Fig 4-5c Exposed right implant.

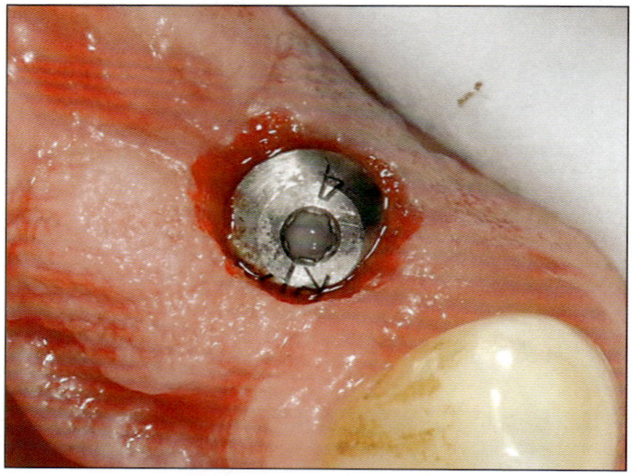

Fig 4-5d Exposed left implant.

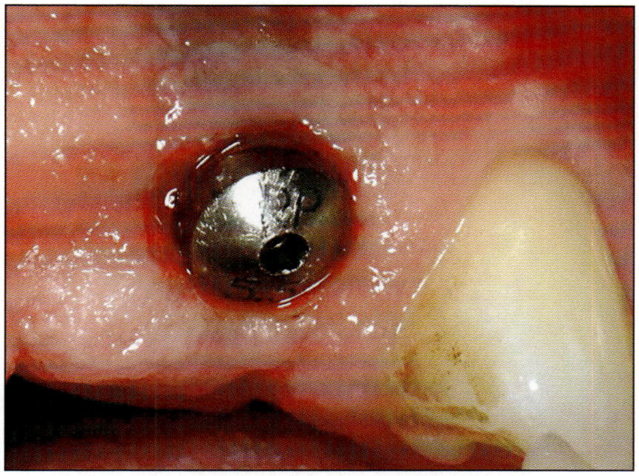

Fig 4-5e Healing cap placed on left implant.

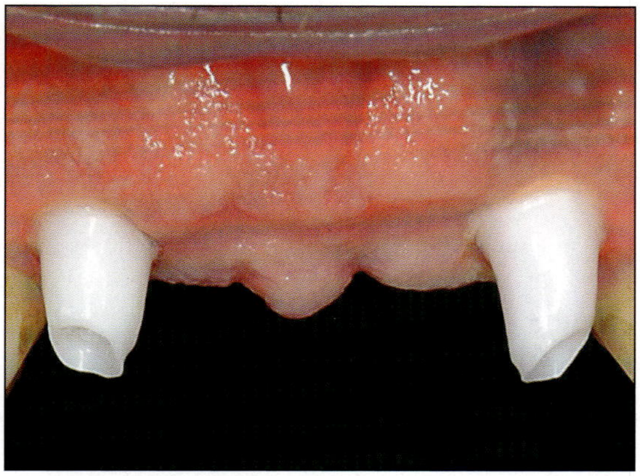

Fig 4-5f Two-week postoperative view immediately following abutment placement.

Purpose of the procedure	Uncovering implants using an Er:YAG laser
Once implants are exposed, abutments can be placed in preparation for implant restoration.	

Wavelength and settings
Er:YAG laser set to 50 Hz, 30 mJ, with no water spray.
Alternate wavelengths that may be used
CO_2 and diode lasers can be used to perform this procedure.

Implant Uncovering Surgery: Case 6

Second-stage surgery using a mucoperiosteal flap in a partially edentulous patient.

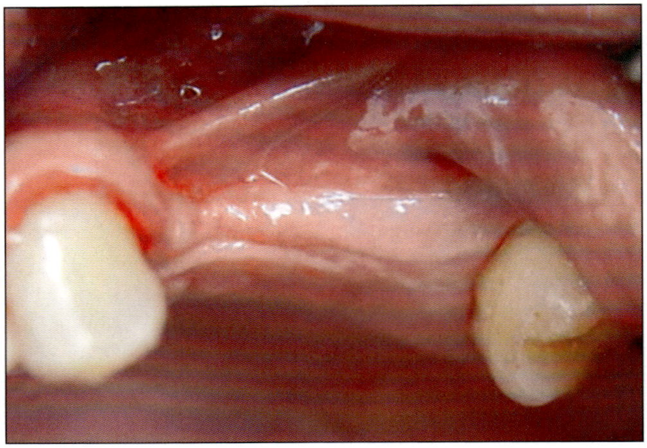

Fig 4-6a Preoperative view showing the implant site prior to second-stage surgery.

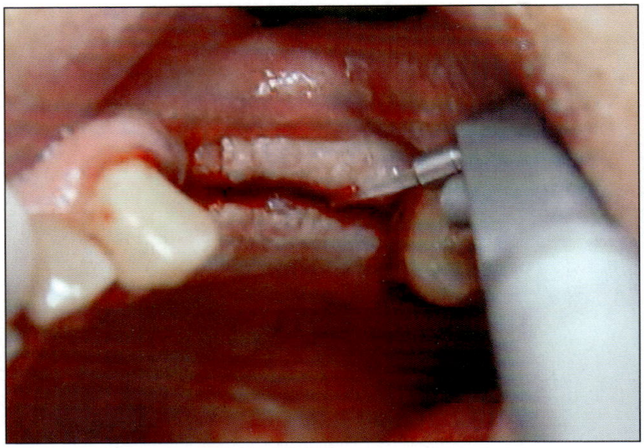

Fig 4-6b A crestal incision is made for a soft tissue flap using an Er:YAG laser.

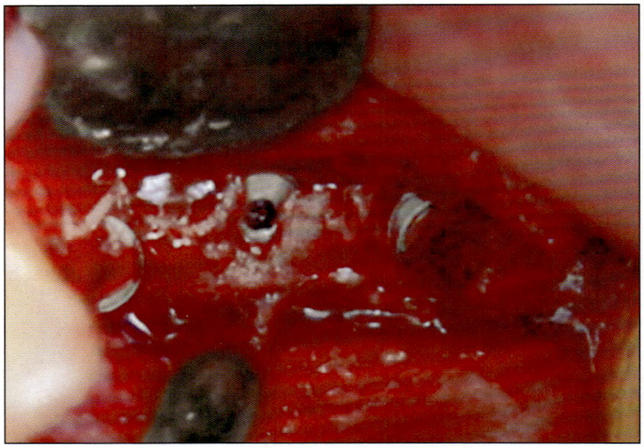

Fig 4-6c Exposed implants.

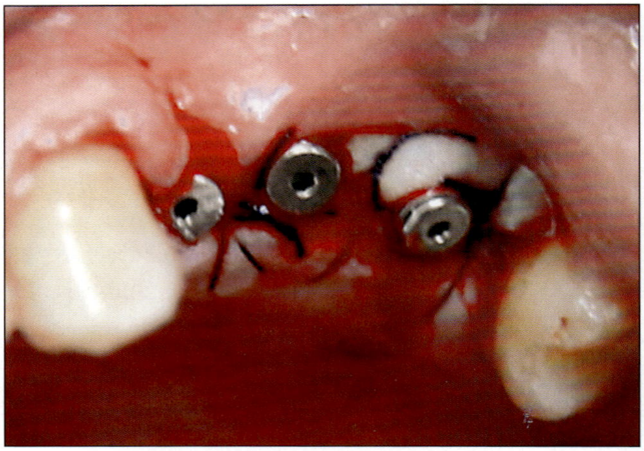

Fig 4-6d Immediate postoperative view of the exposed implants with the soft tissue flap repositioned and sutured in place.

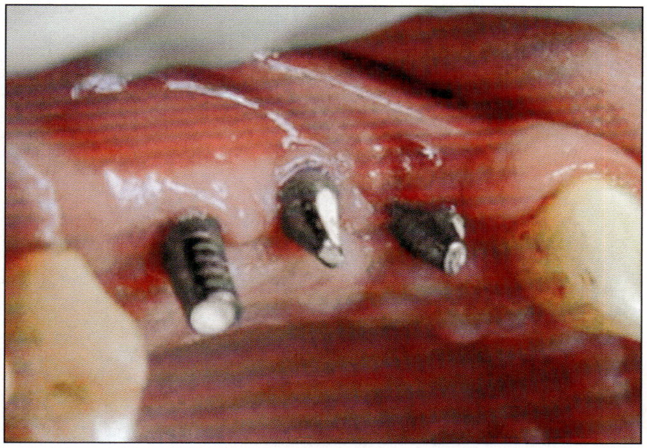

Fig 4-6e Five-week postoperative view with the abutments in place.

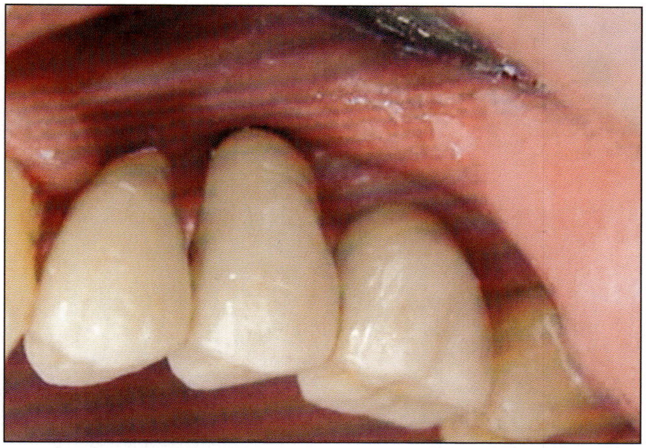

Fig 4-6f Definitive implant restorations 7 weeks following second-stage surgery. (Case courtesy of Dr Avi Reyhanian, Natanya, Israel.)

Purpose of the procedure

Uncovering implants using an Er:YAG laser

Reflection of a mucoperiosteal flap exposes implants in preparation for abutment placement and implant restoration.

Wavelength and settings

Er:YAG laser set to 9 W, 450 mJ, 20 Hz, with a 200 µm sapphire tip with water spray.

Alternate wavelengths that may be used

Diode and CO_2 lasers can be used to perform this procedure.

Clinical discussion

In the six cases of implant uncovering surgery, three different laser wavelengths were used to uncover integrated implants. Because laser instruments can provide precise soft tissue removal as well as good hemostasis, the definitive impression can be taken immediately following the uncovering surgery.

Implant Placement: Case 1

Implant placement in the anterior maxilla in a young patient.

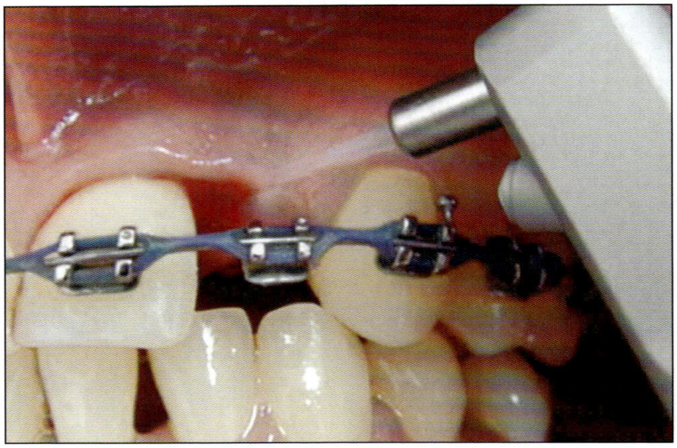

Fig 4-7a An Er:YAG laser can be used to make an incision for a soft tissue flap prior to implant placement at the maxillary left lateral incisor site.

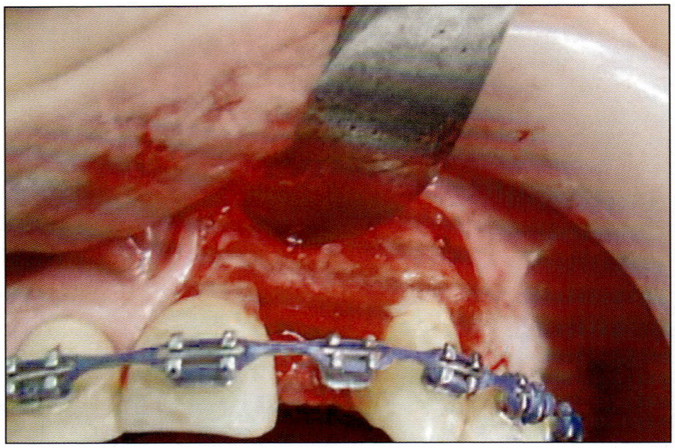

Fig 4-7b Reflected soft tissue flap.

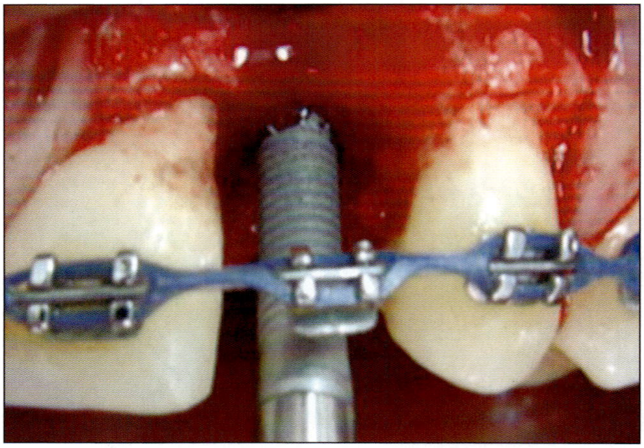

Fig 4-7c Implant placement. The Er:YAG laser was used to make a pilot hole in the alveolar bone before a conventional handpiece was used to complete the osseous preparation.

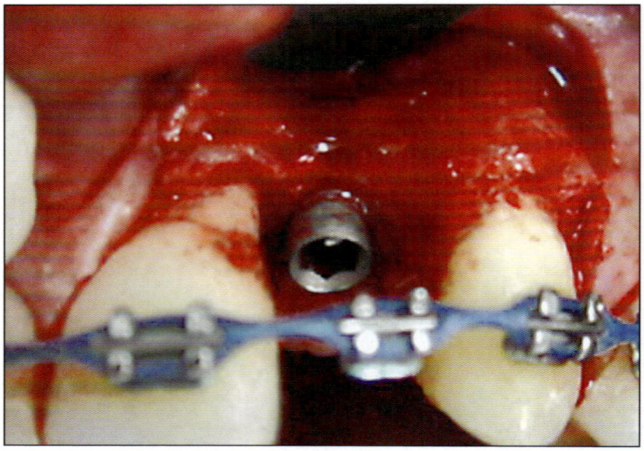

Fig 4-7d Immediate postoperative view of the implant in the maxillary left lateral incisor site.

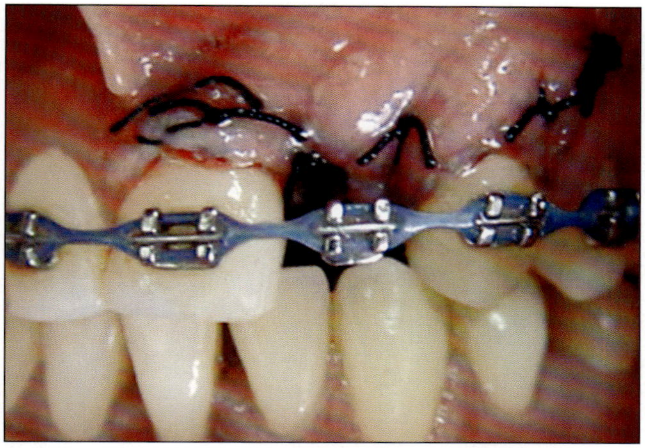

Fig 4-7e The soft tissue flap has been sutured in position.

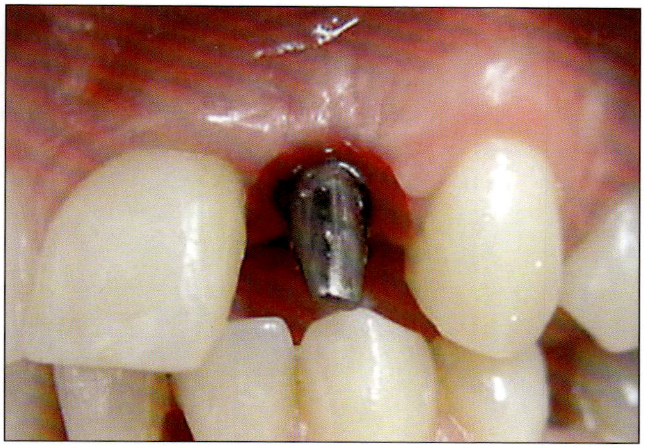

Fig 4-7f Eight-month postoperative view with an abutment in place. (Case courtesy of Dr Avi Reyhanian, Natanya, Israel.)

Purpose of the procedure	Implant placement using an Er:YAG laser

After the Er:YAG laser has been used to create a soft tissue flap and a pilot hole in the alveolar bone, the site preparation and implant placement can be completed with conventional instruments.

Wavelength and settings

Er:YAG laser; settings for soft tissue incision: 9 W, 450 mJ, 20 Hz, with a 200 µm sapphire tip with water spray; settings for osseous preparation: 8.5 W, 500 mJ, 17.5 Hz, with a 1,300 µm sapphire tip with water spray.

Alternate wavelengths that may be used

CO_2 and diode lasers can be used for soft tissue preparation. However, only the Er family of lasers can be used for osseous preparation.

Implant Placement: Case 2

Implant placement in the posterior maxilla in an adult patient.

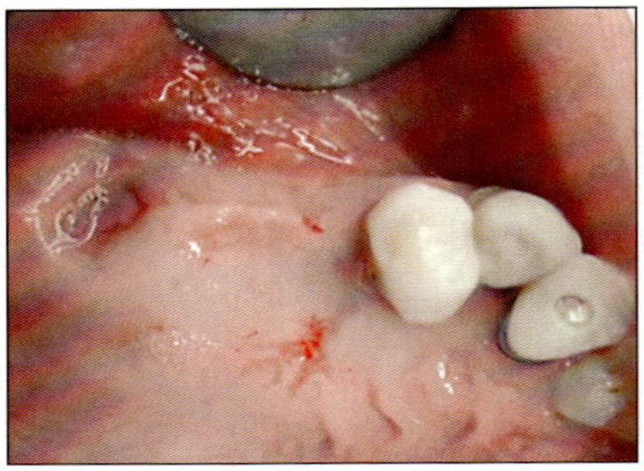

Fig 4-8a Partially edentulous posterior maxilla.

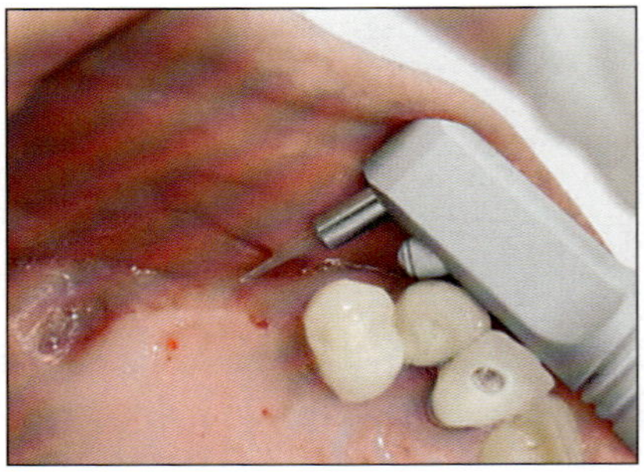

Fig 4-8b The Er:YAG laser begins soft tissue preparation.

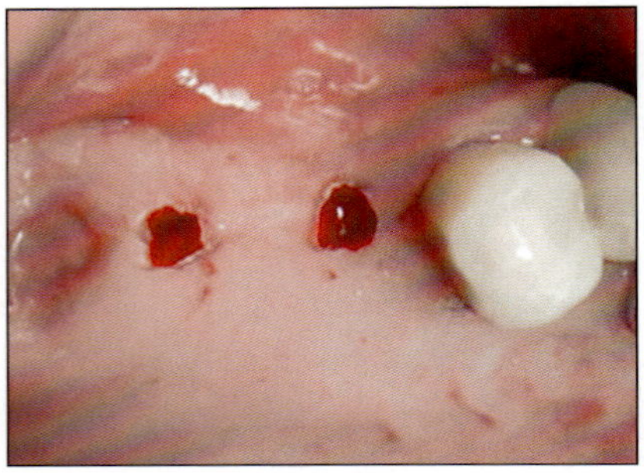

Fig 4-8c After soft tissue ablation is completed, the surgical site is ready for pilot holes.

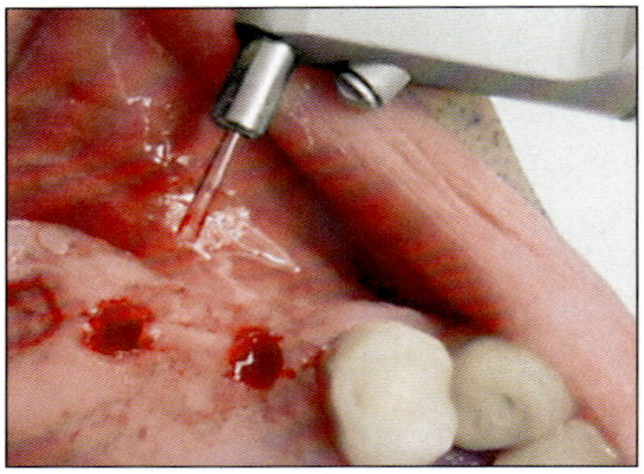

Fig 4-8d The Er:YAG laser begins osseous preparation.

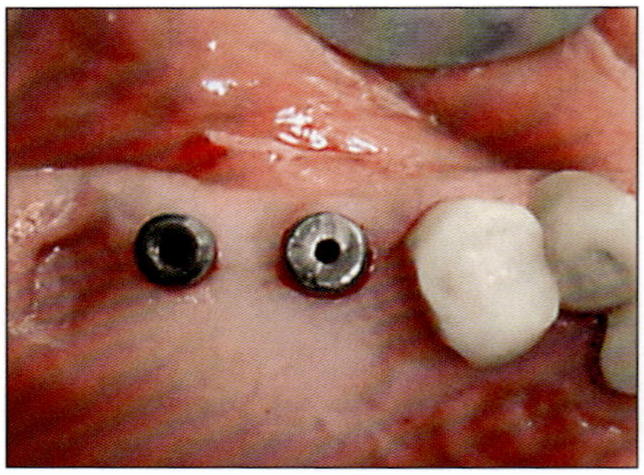

Fig 4-8e Implant placement with supragingival healing caps.

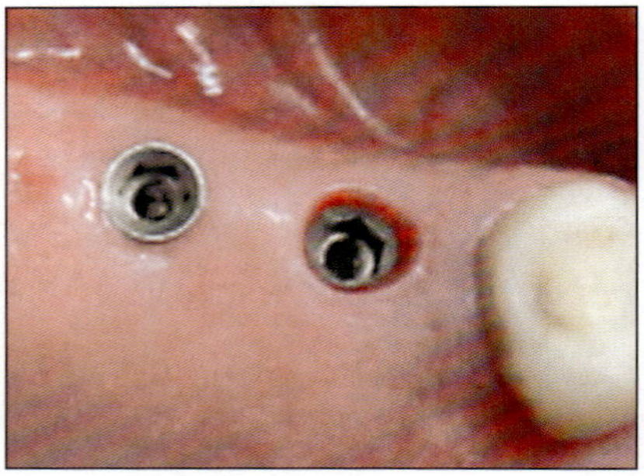

Fig 4-8f Three-month postoperative view of implants.

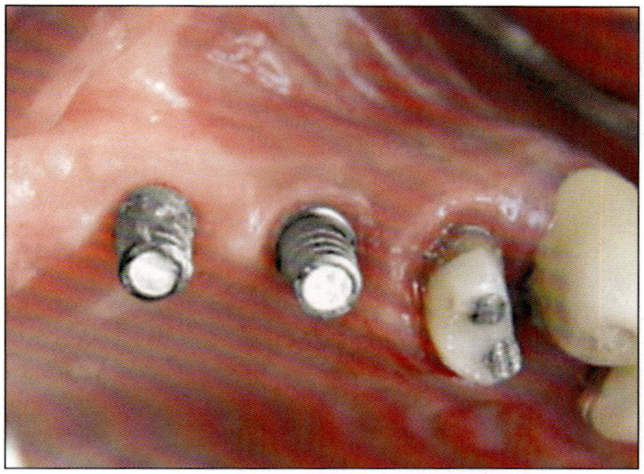

Fig 4-8g Three-month postoperative view following abutment placement.

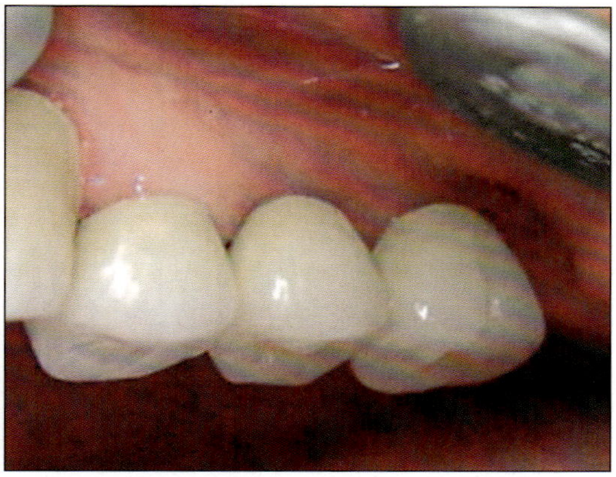

Fig 4-8h Definitive restorations, 6 months following implant placement. (Case courtesy of Dr Gabi Kesler, Petach Tiqva, Israel.)

Purpose of the procedure

Implant placement using an Er:YAG laser

After the Er:YAG laser has been used to ablate soft tissue and create pilot holes in the alveolar bone, the site preparation and implant placement can be completed with conventional instruments.

Wavelength and settings

Er:YAG laser; settings for soft tissue ablation: 9 W, 450 mJ, 20 Hz, with a 200 µm sapphire tip with water spray; settings for osseous preparation: 8.5 W, 500 mJ, 17.5 Hz, with a 1,300 µm sapphire tip with water spray.

Alternate wavelengths that may be used

CO_2 and diode lasers can be used for soft tissue preparation. However, for osseous preparation, only the Er family of lasers may be used.

Implant Placement: Case 3

Implant placement in the posterior mandible in a male patient.

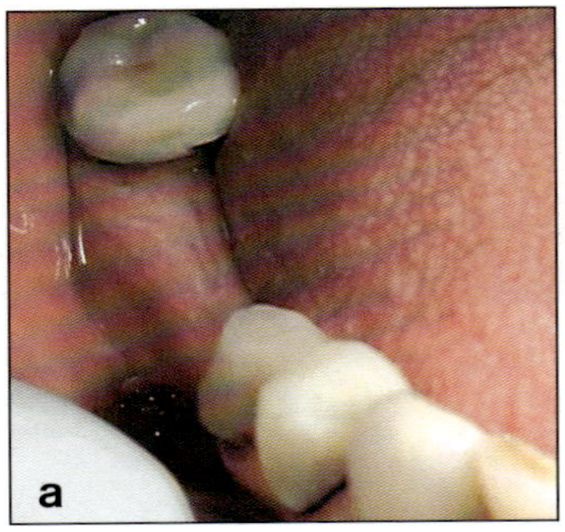

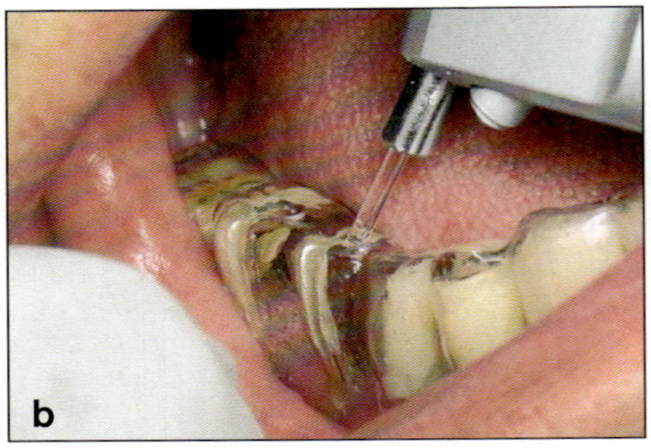

Fig 4-9a Preoperative view of an edentulous gap in the posterior mandible.

Fig 4-9b An Er:YAG laser is positioned on a surgical stent.

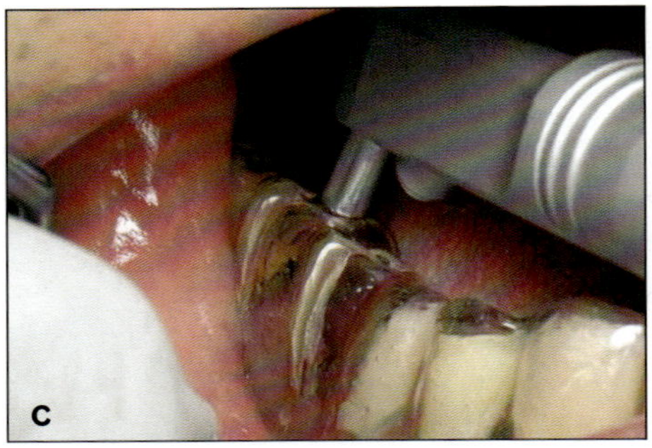

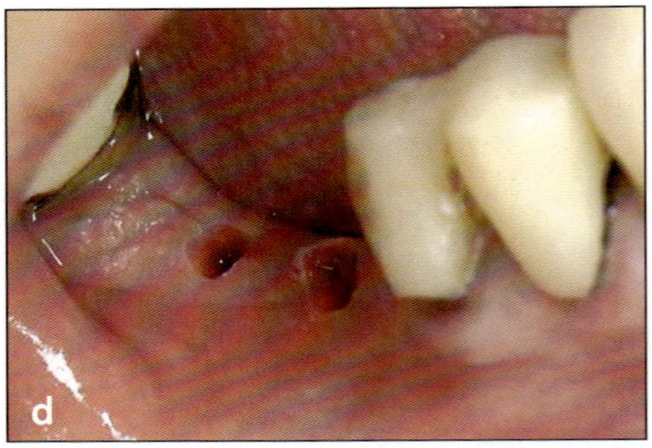

Fig 4-9c The laser ablates the soft tissue prior to preparing a pilot hole in the alveolar bone.

Fig 4-9d Postoperative view immediately following laser preparation. Note the precision of the soft tissue laser ablation.

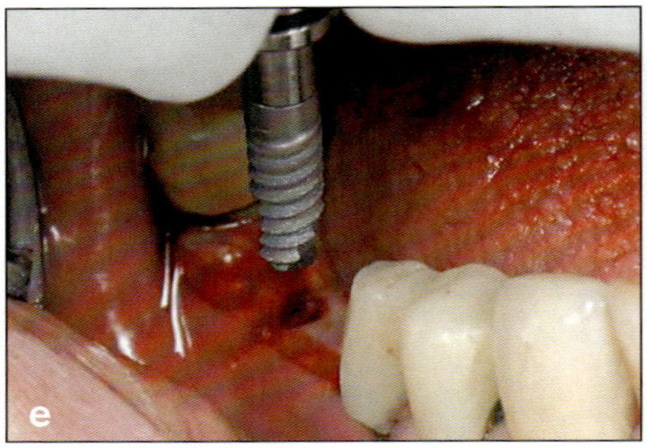

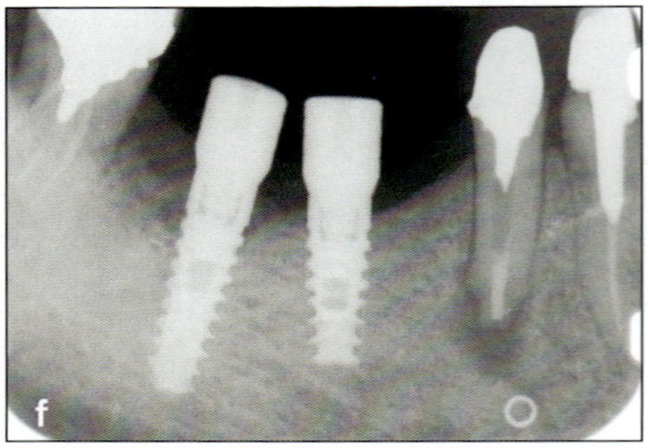

Fig 4-9e Implant placement.

Fig 4-9f Six-month postoperative radiograph demonstrates complete osseointegration. (Case courtesy of Dr Pablo Schilman, Ramat Hasavon, Israel.)

Purpose of the procedure	Implant placement using an Er:YAG laser

After the Er:YAG laser has been used to ablate soft tissue and create pilot holes in the alveolar bone, the site preparation and implant placement can be completed with conventional instruments.

Wavelength and settings

Er:YAG laser; settings for soft tissue ablation: 350 mJ, 10 Hz, with an 800 μm tip with water spray; settings for osseous preparation: 100 mJ, 10 Hz, with a 200 μm tip with water spray.

Alternate wavelengths that may be used

CO_2 and diode lasers can be used for soft tissue preparation. However, for osseous preparation, only the Er family of lasers may be used.

Clinical discussion

The three cases of implant placement demonstrate the use of an Er:YAG laser in both soft tissue and osseous preparation for implant placement. After the laser ablates a precise area of soft tissue, a pilot hole is made in the alveolar bone for the osteotomy, which is subsequently prepared using conventional surgical burs. In case 3, a surgical stent was used to guide the laser in implant positioning on the edentulous ridge. In general, in order to achieve adequate hemostasis, water spray is not used when Er:YAG lasers ablate soft tissue. In the three cases presented here, however, water spray was used during the soft tissue ablation because the laser continued to ablate through the periosteum and cortical plate. Use of the water spray ensured that laser ablation would not char the osseous tissue.

Alternate techniques

A CO_2, Nd:YAG, or diode laser can be used to remove soft tissue. However, the surgeon must keep the laser ablation limited to soft tissue, since CO_2, diode, and Nd:YAG wavelengths could potentially cause thermal damage to the periosteum and/or bone. The osseous pilot hole can be prepared using either an Er family laser or conventional surgical burs. Even if an Er family laser is used to prepare the pilot hole, enlarging the osteotomy requires conventional implant instrumentation.

Peri-implantitis Treatment: Case 1

Treatment of peri-implantitis involving an osseous defect in the posterior maxilla in an adult patient.

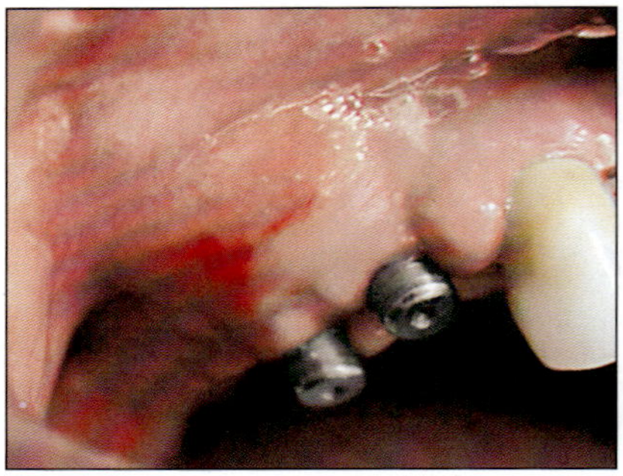

Fig 4-10a Preoperative swelling around implants.

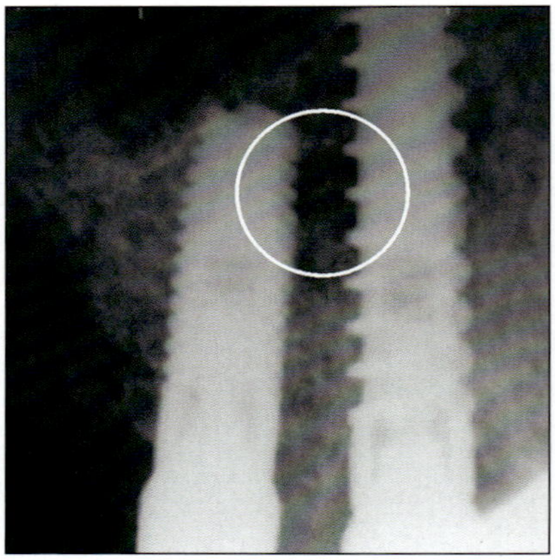

Fig 4-10b Radiographic view showing radiolucency between implants.

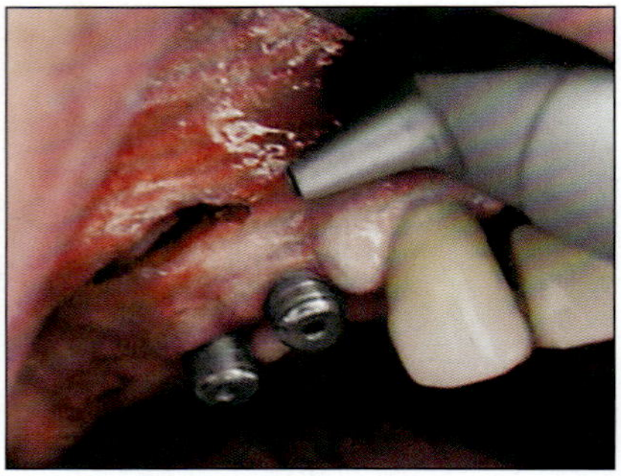

Fig 4-10c Intraoperative view of a CO_2 laser making an incision in the soft tissue for drainage.

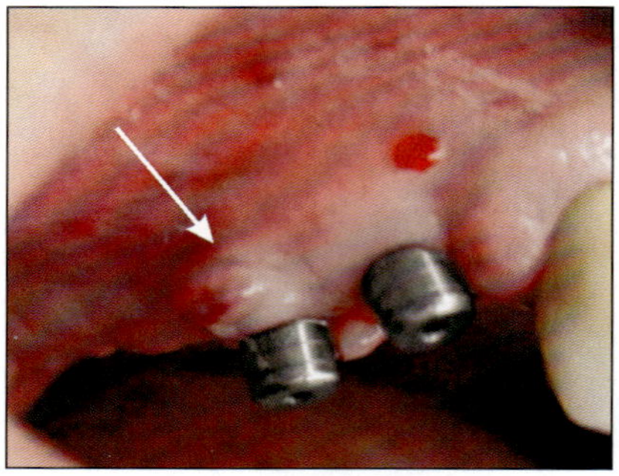

Fig 4-10d Two months postsurgery, drainage occurs in the infected area (*white arrow*).

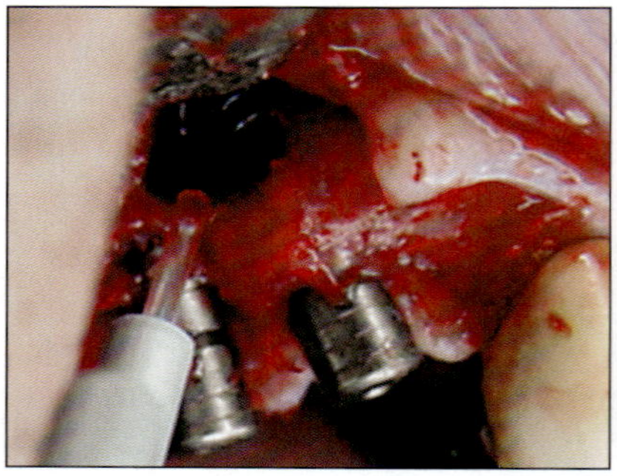

Fig 4-10e After a soft tissue flap is reflected, an Er:YAG laser ablates granulomatous tissue.

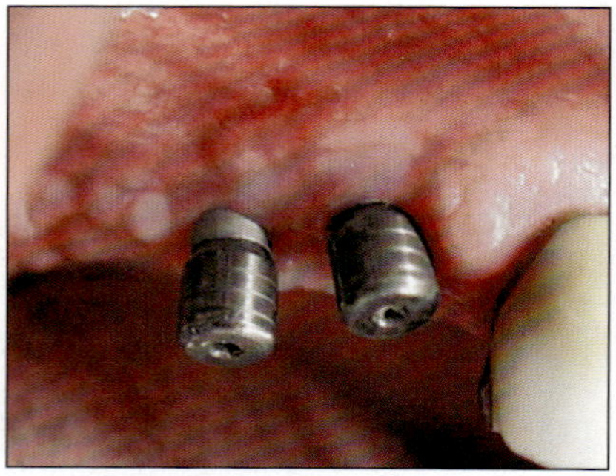

Fig 4-10f Two-month postoperative view of healthy soft tissue.

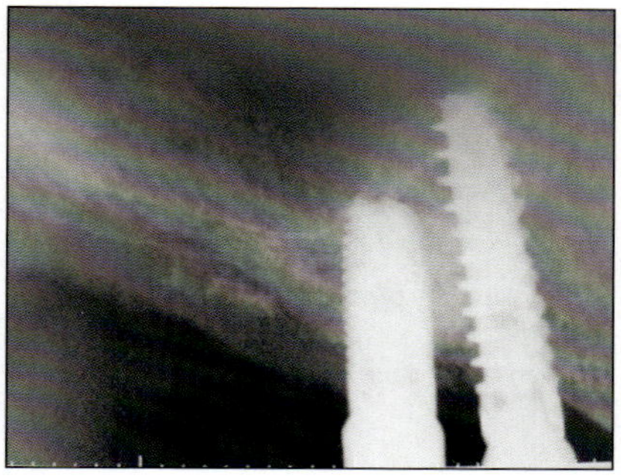

Fig 4-10g Radiographic view 2 months following peri-implantitis treatment.

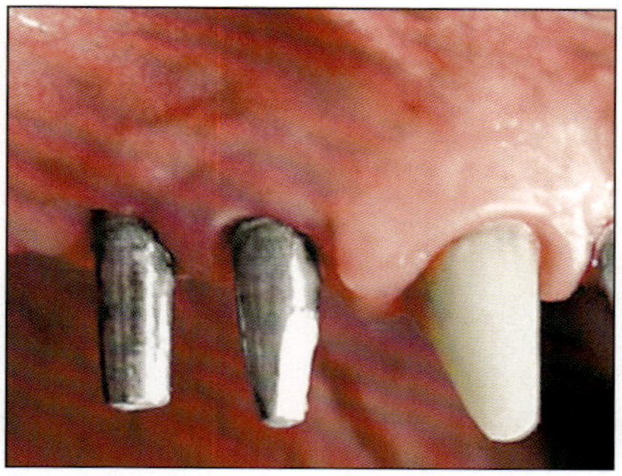

Fig 4-10h Two-year postoperative view.

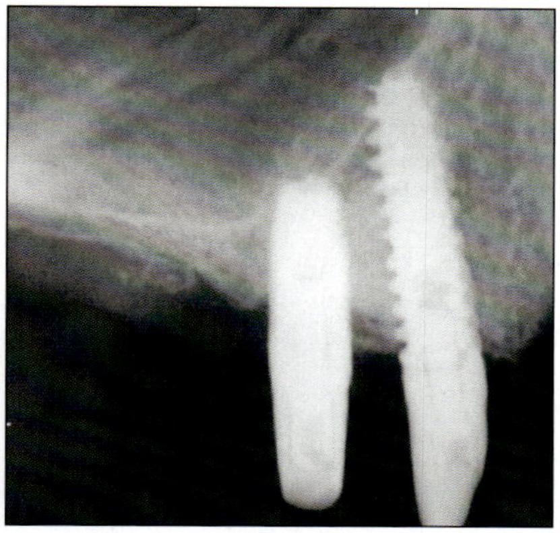

Fig 4-10i Two-year postoperative radiograph. (Case courtesy of Dr Avi Reyhanian, Natanya, Israel.)

Purpose of the procedure	Treatment of peri-implantitis
Once the infected site is drained and a soft tissue flap is reflected, a laser can be used to ablate granulomatous tissue.	

Wavelength and settings

CO_2 laser in a 110-degree curved handpeice set to average power at 3.5 W, superpulsed mode for 5 seconds. Er:YAG laser set to 8.4 W, 700 mJ, with a 1,300 μm noncontact sapphire tip with water spray.

Alternate wavelengths that may be used

A diode laser can be used for soft tissue preparation. However, only the Er family of lasers can be used for osseous ablation.

Peri-implantitis Treatment: Case 2

Treatment of peri-implantitis involving an osseous defect in the posterior mandible in an adult patient.

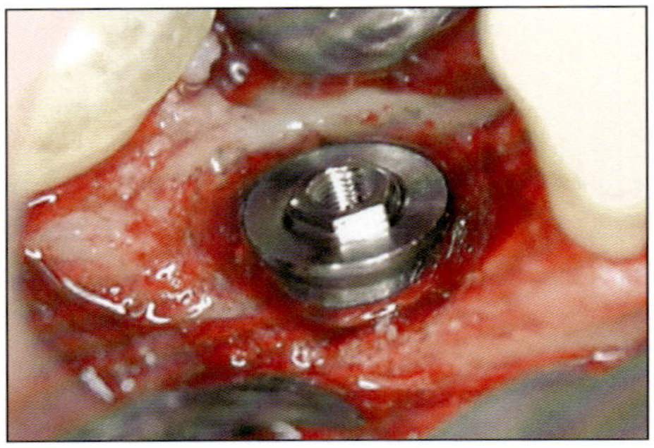

Fig 4-11a After a soft tissue flap is reflected, the preoperative view reveals granulomatous tissue and exudate around the implant head.

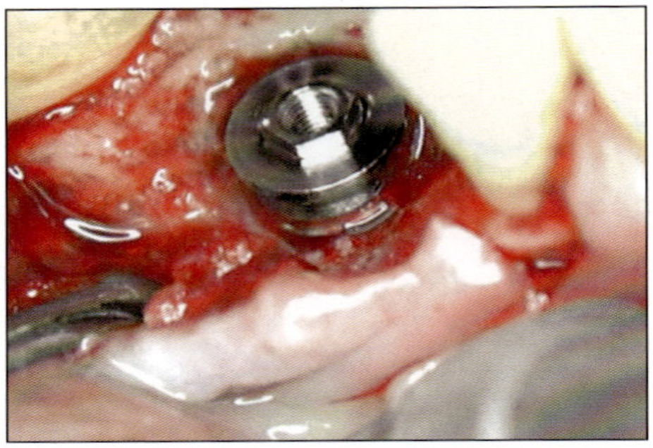

Fig 4-11b Immediate postoperative view following removal of diseased tissue via laser ablation.

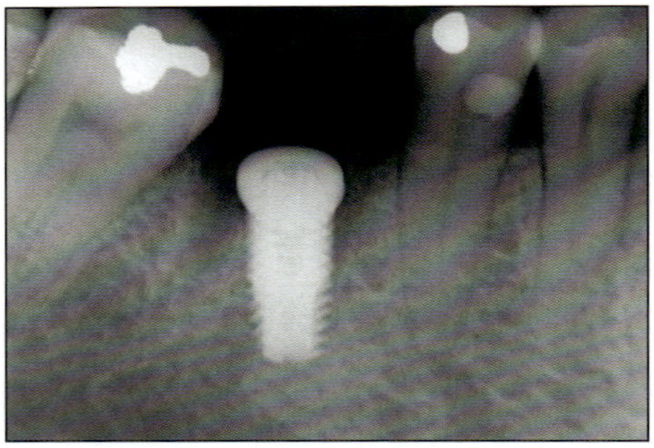

Fig 4-11c The 6-month postoperative radiograph confirms the healing. (Case courtesy of Dr Kenneth Luk, Hong Kong, China.)

Purpose of the procedure	Treatment of peri-implantitis

Once a soft tissue flap is reflected, a laser can be used to ablate granulomatous tissue and exudate from around the implant head.

Wavelength and settings

Diode laser, 980 nm, in an irrigating handpiece set to 8 W, gated mode of 0.05 seconds on and 0.05 seconds off, with a 400 µm fiber with a copious flow of sterile saline solution.

Alternate wavelengths that may be used

CO_2 and Er family lasers can be used to perform this procedure.

Peri-implantitis Treatment: Case 3

Treatment of peri-implantitis involving an osseous defect in the posterior mandible in an adult patient.

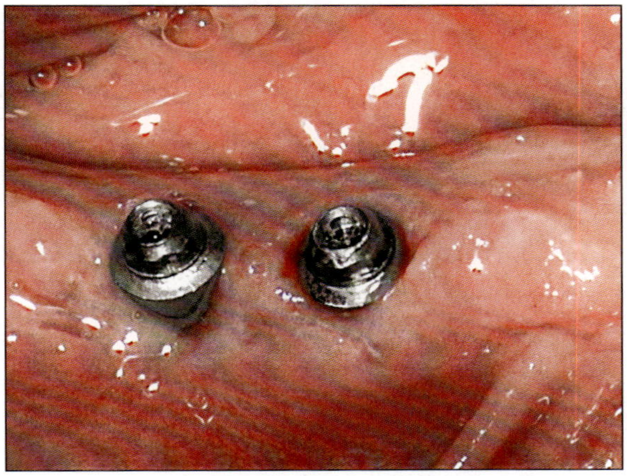

Fig 4-12a Preoperative peri-implantitis around a mandibular right second premolar implant.

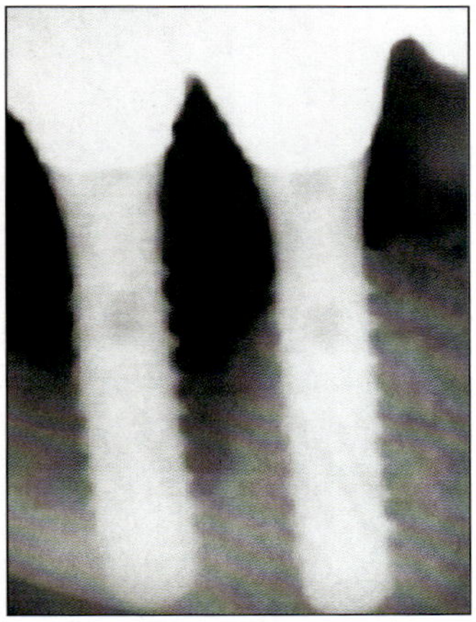

Fig 4-12b An extensive bony defect around the implant is visible radiographically.

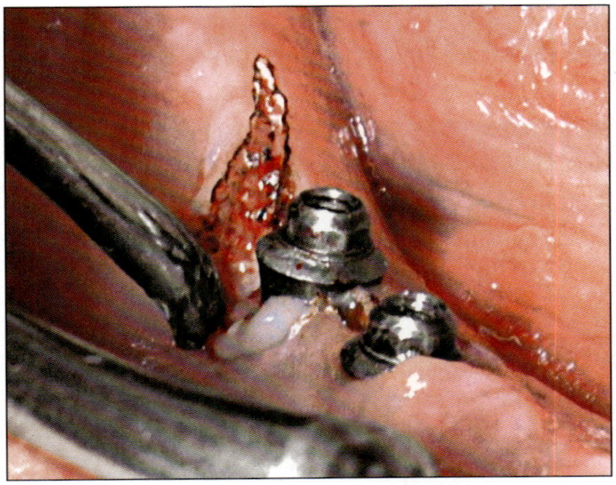

Fig 4-12c Flap reflection around the infected site.

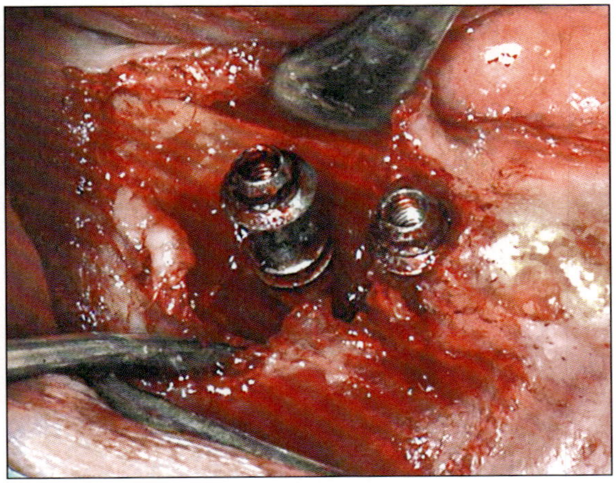

Fig 4-12d The soft tissue flap is reflected to expose the osseous defect.

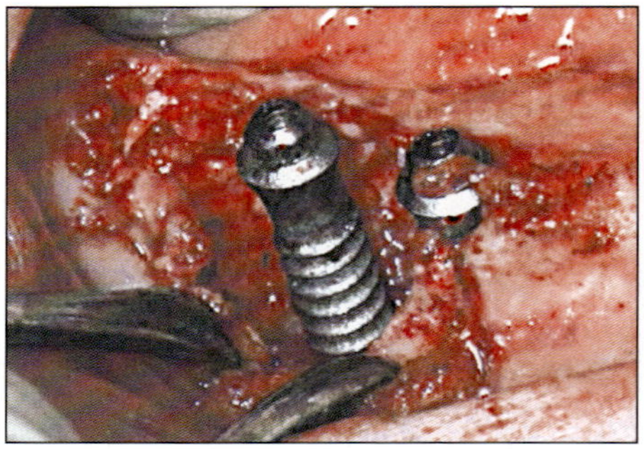

Fig 4-12e Removal of diseased tissue and debridement of the implant surface via laser instrumentation.

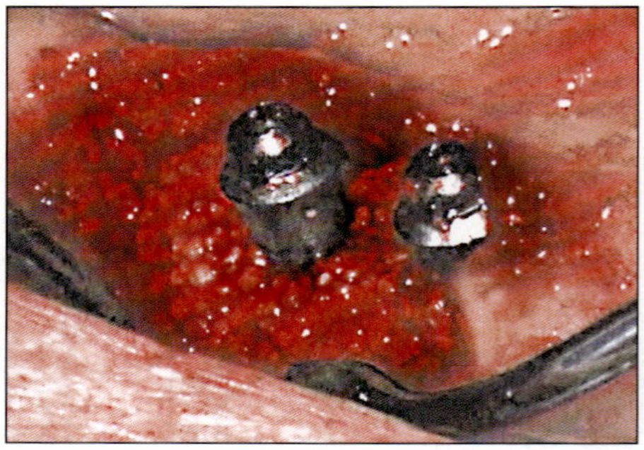

Fig 4-12f Placement of bone-grafting material to fill the osseous defect.

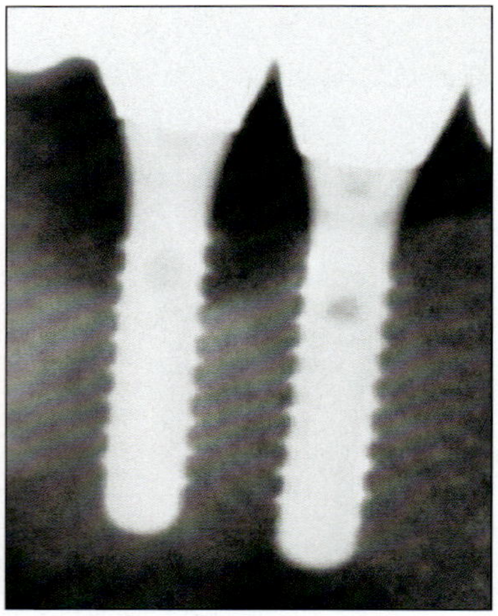

Fig 4-12g Two-year follow-up radiograph showing excellent healing and bone fill. (Case courtesy of Dr Manfred Wittschier, Landshut, Germany.)

Purpose of the procedure	Treatment of peri-implantitis

Once a soft tissue flap is reflected, the diseased tissue can be removed and the osseous defect filled with a bone graft.

Wavelength and settings

CO_2 laser set to 3 W and 100 Hz.

Alternate wavelengths that may be used

Diode and Er family lasers can be used to perform this procedure.

Clinical discussion

Three different wavelengths were used for treatment of peri-implantitis involving an osseous defect. The laser provides an excellent environment for healing because of its ability to remove diseased tissue, reduce bacteria, and decontaminate the implant surface with negligible surface defects. As with all laser procedures, the laser cannot replace conventional instruments but rather should be used in conjunction with conventional instruments. Plastic implant scalers are used in combination with laser ablation to debride the surgical site. The surgical site must be irrigated with saline before the soft tissue flap is sutured in position.

Peri-implantitis Treatment: Case 4

Treatment of soft tissue peri-implantitis in the anterior mandible in an adult patient.

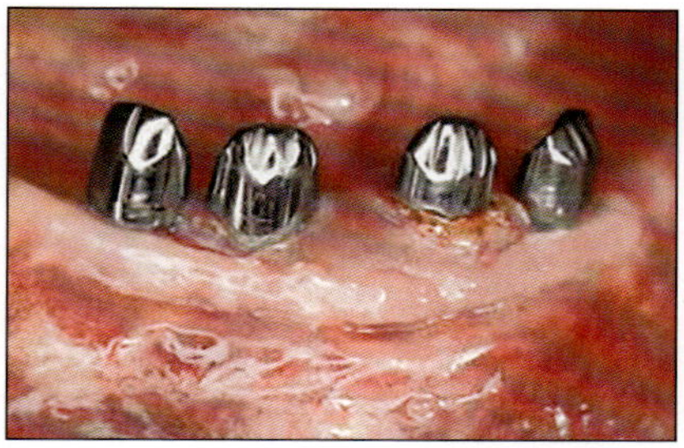

Fig 4-13a Inflamed hyperplastic tissue surrounding implant abutments.

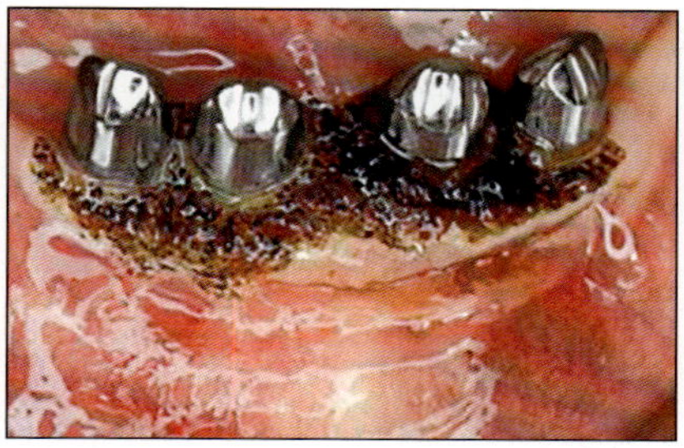

Fig 4-13b Immediate postoperative view following laser ablation.

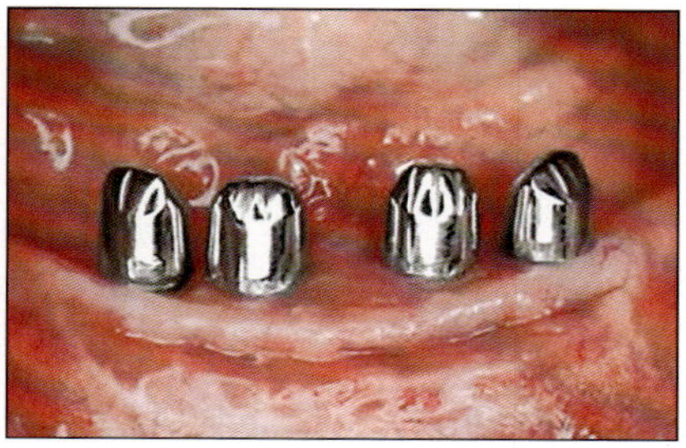

Fig 4-13c Excellent soft tissue tone, contour, and health are restored 6 months after laser treatment. (Case courtesy of Dr George Romanos, Fort Lauderdale, FL.)

Purpose of the procedure

Treatment of soft tissue peri-implantitis

Ablation of infected soft tissue effectively treats the peri-implantitis.

Wavelength and settings

CO_2 laser set to 6 W, continuous wave, with an 800 μm ceramic tip.

Alternate wavelengths that may be used

Diode and CO_2 lasers can be used to perform the procedure.

Clinical tip

In this case, the dentist applied a thin layer of petroleum jelly over the implant abutments to ensure that no laser energy would be absorbed by the implants.

Implant Problem Solving: Case 1

Soft tissue growth around implant threads in the mandible in an adult male patient.

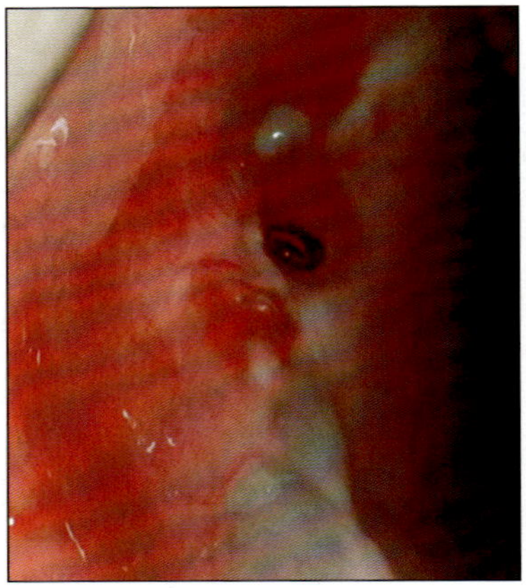

Fig 4-14a This patient lost the implant healing cap several weeks before returning to the clinic. Removing soft tissue growth around implant threads is difficult when conventional instruments are used. Care must be taken to ensure that the implant threads are not damaged because such damage cannot be restored.

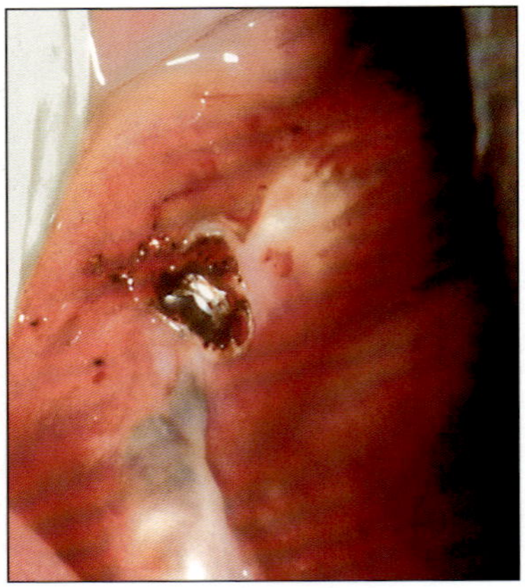

Fig 4-14b Immediate postoperative view of implant site following tissue ablation with a CO_2 laser. Laser energy removed the soft tissue to leave a clean implant surface without risking damage to the implant threads.

Purpose of the procedure	Ablation of soft tissue growth around implant threads
Once soft tissue growth around the implant threads is ablated, the implant can be restored.	

Wavelength and settings

CO_2 laser; settings for bulk tissue removal: 3 W, continuous wave, with an 800 μm ceramic tip; settings for fine tissue removal: 2 W, continuous wave, with a 250 μm metal tip.

Alternate wavelengths that may be used

Diode and Er family lasers can be used to perform this procedure.

Implant Problem Solving: Case 2

Soft tissue growth over an implant in the posterior maxilla in an adult patient.

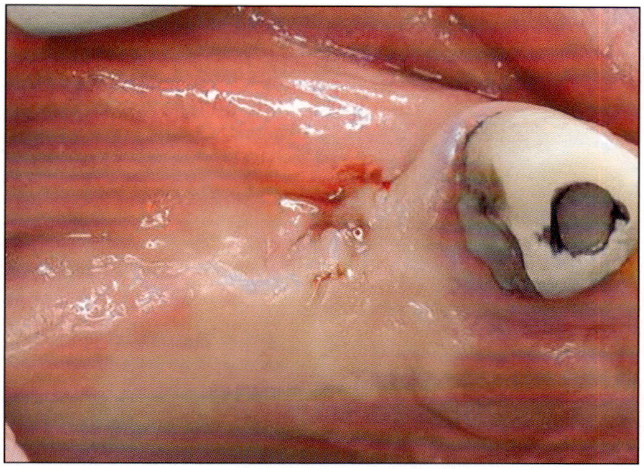

Fig 4-15a Preoperative view of a covered implant in a patient who lost his healing cap several months before returning to the clinic. Soft tissue completely covers the implant.

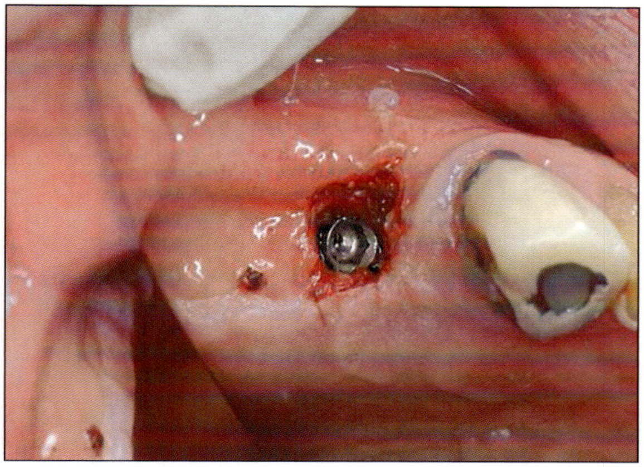

Fig 4-15b Immediate postoperative view of the uncovered implant. The soft tissue was ablated with a CO_2 laser, and the implant sustained no damage, despite the removal of a large amount of soft tissue.

Purpose of the procedure	Ablation of soft tissue growth over an implant
Once soft tissue is ablated around the implant head, the implant can be restored.	

Wavelength and settings

CO_2 laser; settings for bulk tissue removal: 3 W, continuous wave, with an 800 μm ceramic tip; settings for fine tissue removal: 2 W, continuous wave, with a 250 μm metal tip.

Alternate wavelengths that may be used

Diode and Er family lasers can be used to perform this procedure.

Implant Problem Solving: Case 3

Soft tissue growth over an implant in the anterior mandible in an elderly female patient.

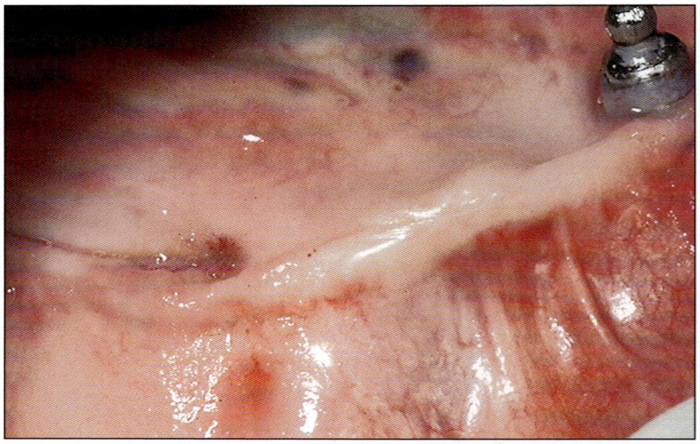

Fig 4-16a Preoperative view of a covered implant in an elderly patient who lost an abutment for her implant-supported overdenture and was unable to return to the office for 3 months.

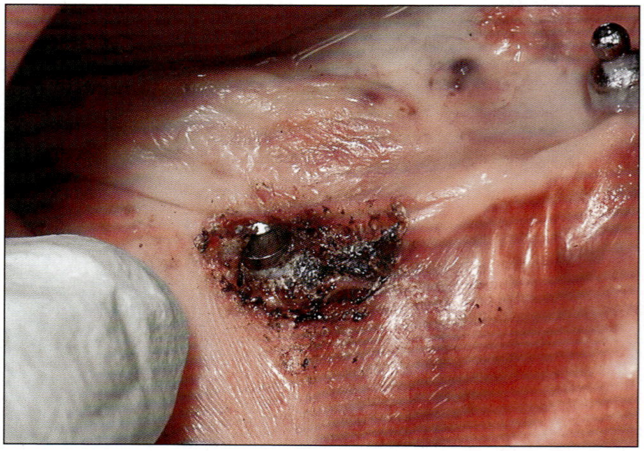

Fig 4-16b Immediate postoperative view of the exposed implant following CO_2 soft tissue ablation.

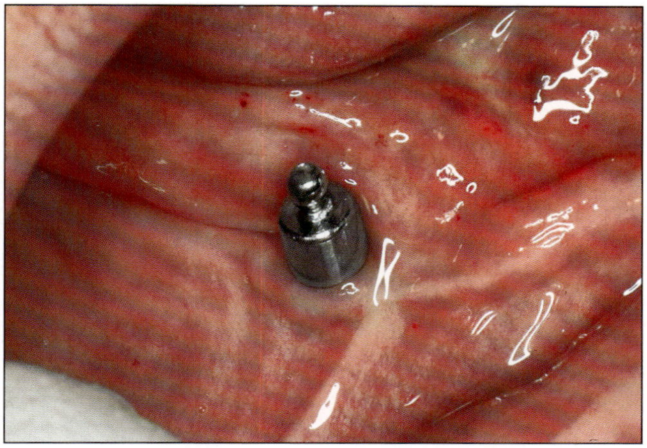

Fig 4-16c Three-week postoperative view of the overdenture abutment back in place.

Purpose of the procedure	Ablation of soft tissue growth over an implant
Once soft tissue is ablated around the implant head, an abutment can be placed to support an overdenture.	

Wavelength and settings
CO_2 laser; settings for bulk tissue removal: 4 W, continuous wave, with an 800 µm ceramic tip; settings for fine tissue removal: 3 W, continuous wave, with a 250 µm metal tip.
Alternate wavelengths that may be used
Diode and Er family lasers can be used to perform this procedure.

References

1. Martin E. Lasers in dental implantology. Dent Clin North Am 2004;48:999–1015.
2. Rowson JE. The contact diode laser—A useful instrument for excising oral lesions [abstract]. Br J Oral Maxillofac Surg 1995; 33:123.
3. White JM, Goodis HE, Rose CL. Use of the pulsed Nd:YAG laser for intraoral soft tissue surgery. Lasers Surg Med 1991;11:455–461.
4. Baraldi CE, Puricelli E, Kulkes S, Martins GL. Er:YAG laser in oral soft tissue surgery [abstract 59]. J Oral Laser Appl 2001;1: 24.
5. Wilder-Smith P, Arrastia AM, Liaw LH, Berns M. Incision properties and thermal effects of three CO_2 lasers in soft tissue. Oral Surg Oral Med Oral Pathol Radiol Endod 1995;79:685–691.
6. Manni JG. Dental Applications of Advanced Lasers. Burlington, MA: JGM Associates, 2005.
7. Ishikawa I, Aoki A, Takasaki AA. Potential applications of erbium:YAG laser in periodontics. J Periodont Res 2004;39:275–285.
8. Walsh LJ. The use of lasers in implantology: An overview. J Oral Implantol 1992;18:335–340.
9. Block CM, Mayo JA, Evans GH. Effects of the Nd:YAG dental laser on plasma-sprayed and hydroxyapatite-coated titanium dental implants: Surface alteration and attempted sterilization. Int J Oral Maxillofac Implants. 1992;7:441–449.
10. Chu RT, Watanabe L, White JM, Marshal GW, Marshal SJ, Hutton JE. Temperature rises and surface modification of lased titanium cylinders. J Dent Res 1992;71(special issue):144.
11. Kreisler M, Gotz H, Duschner H. Effect of Nd:YAG, Ho:YAG, Er:YAG, CO_2, and GaAIAs laser irradiation on surface properties of endosseous dental implants. Int J Oral Maxillofac Implants 2002;17:202–211.
12. Yeh S, Jain K, Andreana S. Using a diode laser to uncover dental implants in second-stage surgery. Gen Dent 2005;53:414–417.
13. Park CY, Kim SG, Kim MD, Eom TG, Yoon JH, Ahn SG. Surface properties of endosseous dental implants after NdYAG and CO_2 laser treatment at various energies. J Oral Maxillofac Surg 2005;63:1522–1527.
14. Schwarz F, Rothamel D, Becker J. Influence of an Er:YAG laser on the surface structure of titanium implants [in German]. Schweiz Monatsschr Zahnmed 2003;13:660–671.
15. Bach G, Neckel C, Mall C, Krekeler G. Conventional versus laser-assisted therapy of periimplantitis: A five-year comparative study. Implant Dent 2000;9:247–251.
16. Kreisler M, Kohnen W, Marinello C, et al. Bactericidal effect of the Er:YAG laser on dental implant surfaces: An in vitro study. J Periodontol 2002;73:1292–1298.
17. Deppe H, Horch HH, Henke J, Donath K. Peri-implant care of ailing implants with the carbon dioxide laser. Int J Oral Maxillofac Implants 2001;16:659–667.
18. Deppe H, Greim H, Brill T, Wagenpfeil S. Titanium deposition after peri-implant care with the carbon dioxide laser. Int J Oral Maxilofac Implants 2002;17:707–714.
19. Stubinger S, Henke J, Donath K, Deppe H. Bone regeneration after peri-implant care with the CO_2 laser: A fluorescence microscopy study. Int J Oral Maxillofac Implants 2005;20:203–210.

5

LASER USE IN OPERATIVE DENTISTRY

The erbium (Er) family of lasers is safe and efficient for caries removal and tooth preparation for direct restorations.[1,2] Water, which is present in all dental tissues in varying amounts, readily absorbs Er wavelengths.[3] Since carious tooth structure contains more water than healthy tooth structure, a lower amount of laser energy can be used to ablate carious tooth structure.[3,4] The natural selectivity of Er wavelengths offers a significant advantage over conventional rotary and hand instruments.

The basic rule for any laser procedure is to begin with the minimum power necessary to accomplish the treatment objective. Of the three hard tissues composing tooth structure, cementum has the highest water content, followed by dentin, then enamel. Since the water in the hard tissues absorbs the wavelength of the Er family lasers, healthy enamel requires the highest amount of laser energy per pulse to produce an average power of 6 W for ablation to occur. However, lasers can remove caries using less than half of that power. Er lasers also readily remove nonmetallic fillings, such as composite restorations, glass-ionomer restorations, compomer restorations, and resin sealants.[5]

Lasers cannot always effectively prepare the tooth surface for bonding. Although using a laser to prepare the surface minimizes surface cracking and crazing, the general conclusion is that the tooth surface must be prepared using conventional etching to achieve adequate bond strength and marginal seal.[6] After finishing the laser treatment, the clinician should use a hand instrument or an abrasive disk around the preparation margins to remove any ablation products prior to applying primer or bonding agents.[7]

Studies have shown that laser tooth preparation can provide a number of advantages over using the traditional rotary handpiece. Lasers significantly reduce the bacteria on the walls of the cavity preparation, eliminate the smear layer on the dentinal surface, and provide pulpal benefits,[8–14] which can facilitate patient comfort and minimize postoperative sensitivity.[15] In addition, the laser is much safer when unexpected patient movement occurs.[16,17]

Each Er laser device has unique operating variables; therefore no settings will be listed for the restoration cases. No alternative wavelengths are listed because the Er family of lasers offers the only wavelengths that are safe and effective for caries removal and tooth preparation. The Nd:YAG laser has an indication for removal of first degree caries in enamel[18]; however, the wavelength is inefficient for cutting dentin or cementum and is now obsolete in operative dentistry. Other wavelengths are currently under investigation for hard tissue procedures.[19]

Clinical tip

The nature of laser light makes the technique for using Er devices for cavity preparation very different from using high-speed rotary handpieces. Although both kinds of instruments require adequate water spray, too much water can reduce the efficiency of a laser because water absorbs laser energy. In addition, lasers only cut at the point of their tip, while most rotary burs produce the greatest abrasion from their sides. In order to deepen a cavity preparation, the laser must be used in an up-and-down, pumping motion with minimal side-brushing action. Finally, with each pulse of laser energy, an outward microexplosion occurs in the hard tissue. There must be at least 1 mm of clearance between the end of the laser tip and the tooth structure to allow dehydrated ablation products to exit the preparation. If there is not enough clearance, the pulse of laser energy will strike the ablation product rather than the carious tooth structure, and the lasing action will cease. Clearance room must also must be sufficient for the water spray to reach the target tissue. If there is too much space between the end of the laser tip and the caries, the laser beam will not be in focus, and the ablation will proceed slowly and inefficiently.

Class I Restoration: Case 1

Restoration of a molar in an adult male patient.

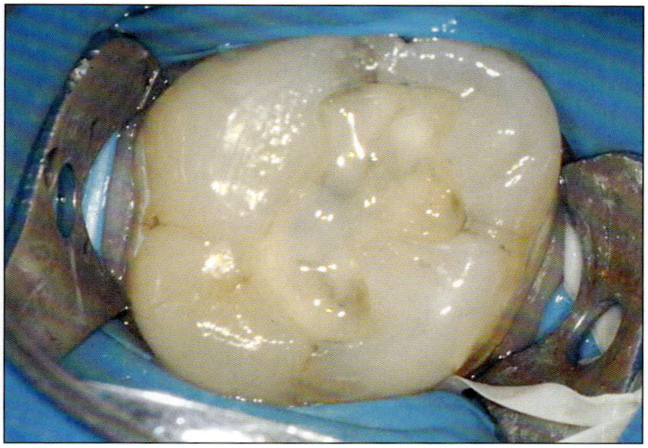

Fig 5-1a Preoperative view of a leaking composite restoration in a molar.

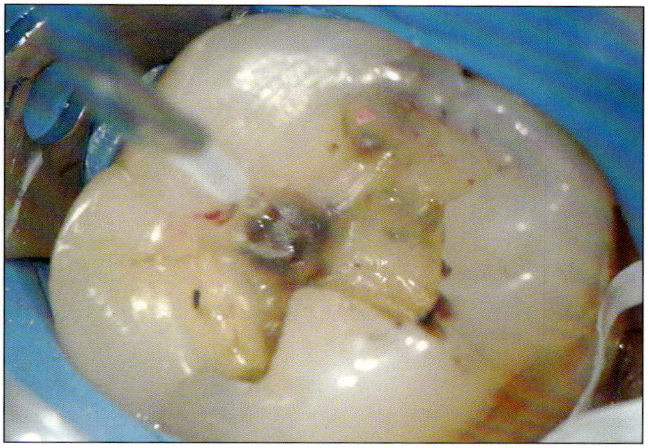

Fig 5-1b Intraoperative view showing removal of the defective composite restoration.

Purpose of the procedure

Class I restoration

A defective composite restoration is removed to restore a molar.

Wavelength

Er laser.

Alternate wavelength that may be used

Only the Er family of lasers can be used for tooth preparation.

Clinical tip

The Er wavelengths easily ablate resin composite and similar restorative materials. The laser was used on high power to remove the defective restoration and then on reduced power for caries removal. As with any good clinical technique, the finished tooth preparation should be as conservative as possible.

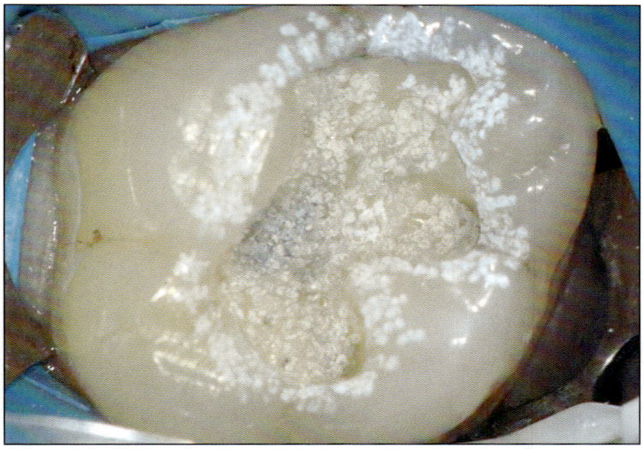

Fig 5-1c Postoperative view showing completed tooth preparation. (Case courtesy of Dr Glenn van As, North Vancouver, BC, Canada.)

Class I Restoration: Case 2

Restoration of a molar in a teenaged female patient.

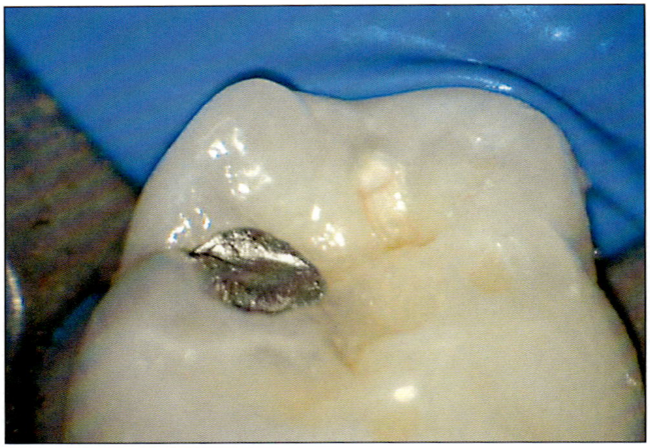

Fig 5-2a Preoperative view showing a molar with caries and a faulty amalgam filling.

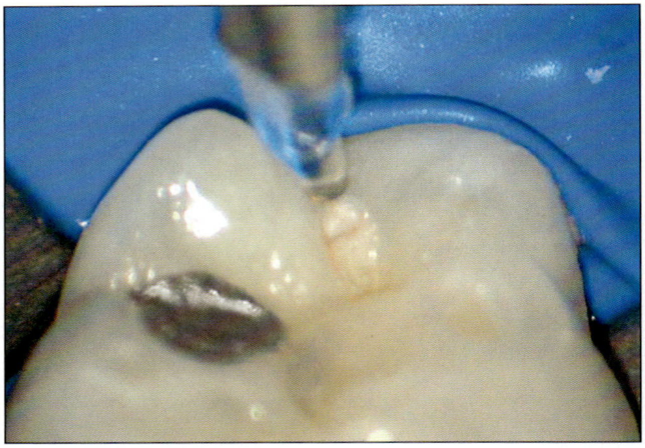

Fig 5-2b Intraoperative view of the laser beginning to remove caries.

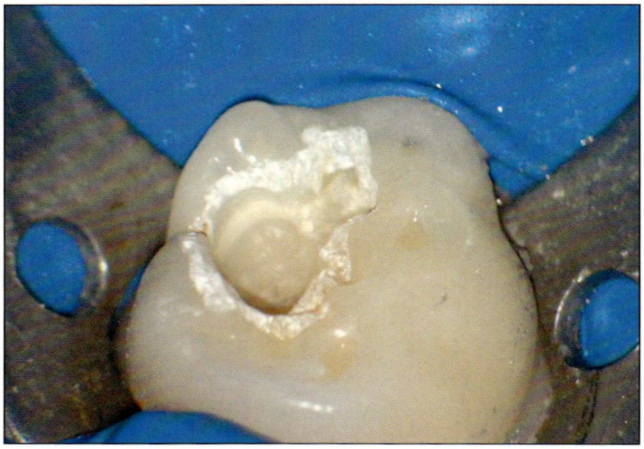

Fig 5-2c Completed tooth preparation with a laser-created bevel. The defective amalgam filling was first outlined with the laser before being removed with a rotary bur.

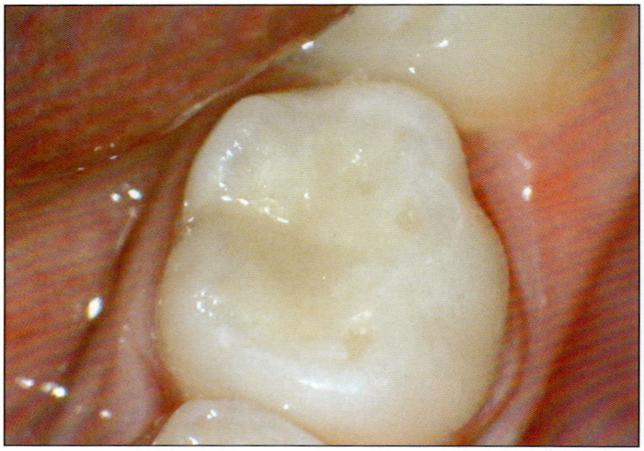

Fig 5-2d Definitive restoration. (Case courtesy of Dr Glenn van As, North Vancouver, BC, Canada.)

Purpose of the procedure	Class I restoration

Once the carious tooth structure is ablated and the defective filling outlined by the laser, the amalgam filling is removed with a rotary bur to complete the tooth preparation.

Wavelength

Er laser.

Alternate wavelength that may be used

Only the Er family of lasers can be used for tooth preparation.

Clinical tip

The laser tip must be properly positioned (see Fig 5-2b) for maximum interaction with the carious tooth structure. Lasers are not indicated to remove amalgam; attempting to remove an amalgam filling with a laser could damage or pit the laser tip with amalgam ablation products. Some clinicians use a laser instrument to outline and undermine the amalgam before removing it with conventional instruments. Fig 5-2c shows a completed preparation in which the amalgam was first outlined with a low-power laser before conventional instruments were used to remove the amalgam.

Class II Restoration: Case 1

Restoration of a maxillary primary first and second molars with adjacent caries in a teenaged female patient.

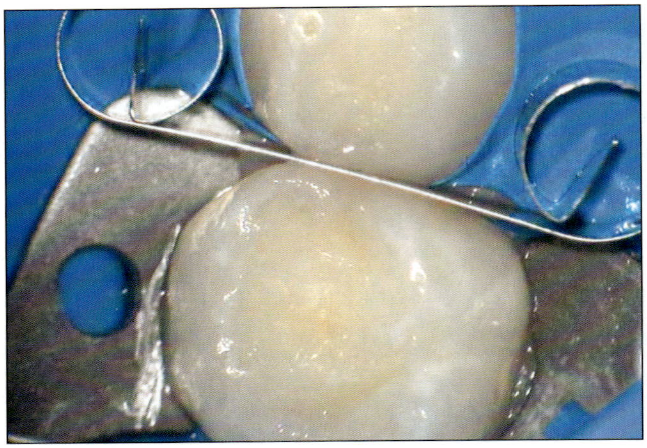

Fig 5-3a Preoperative view of adjacent caries.

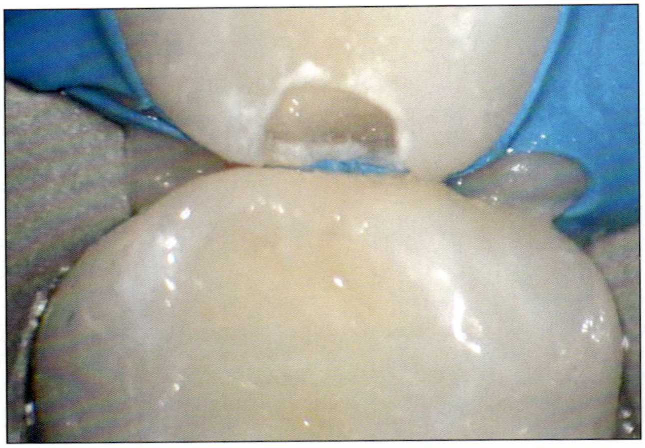

Fig 5-3b Completion of laser preparation on the distal surface of the first molar.

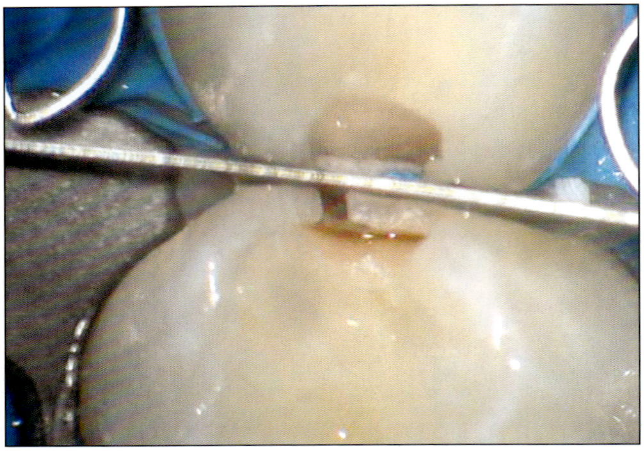

Fig 5-3c Beginning of laser preparation on the mesial surface of the second molar.

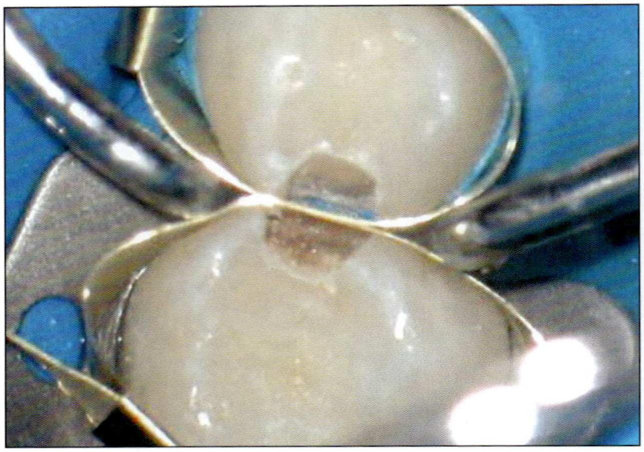

Fig 5-3d Completion of laser ablation on adjacent caries.

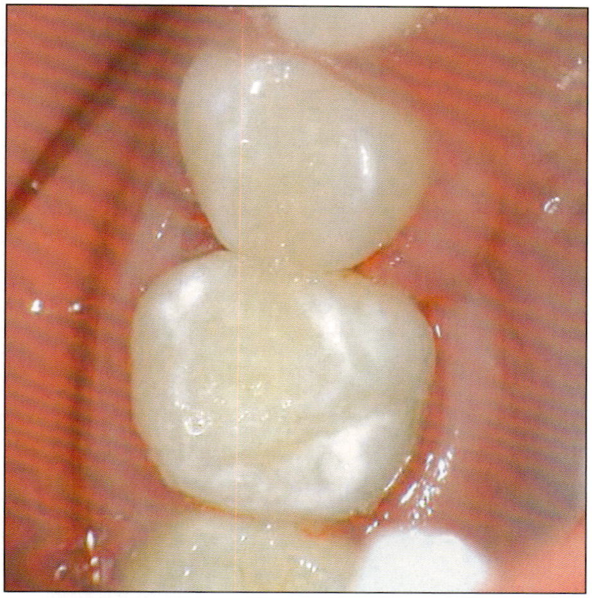

Fig 5-3e Definitive restorations. (Case courtesy of Dr Glenn van As, North Vancouver, BC, Canada.)

Purpose of the procedure	Class II restoration
After the adjacent carious tooth structure is removed, the maxillary primary first and second molars are restored.	

Wavelength

Er laser.

Alternate wavelength that may be used

Only the Er family of lasers can be used for tooth preparation.

Clinical tip

After completion of the preparation on the first molar, a matrix band was placed to separate the adjacent preparation surfaces. The end-cutting nature of laser instruments is ideal for interproximal restorations because it minimizes the possibility of damaging the tooth surface adjacent to the preparation.

Class II Restoration: Case 2

Restoration of caries on mesial and occlusal surfaces of a premolar in an adult female patient.

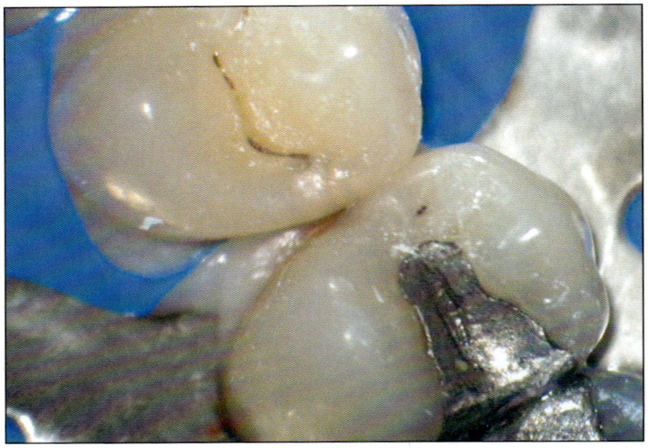

Fig 5-4a Preoperative view showing a premolar with new mesial and occlusal caries.

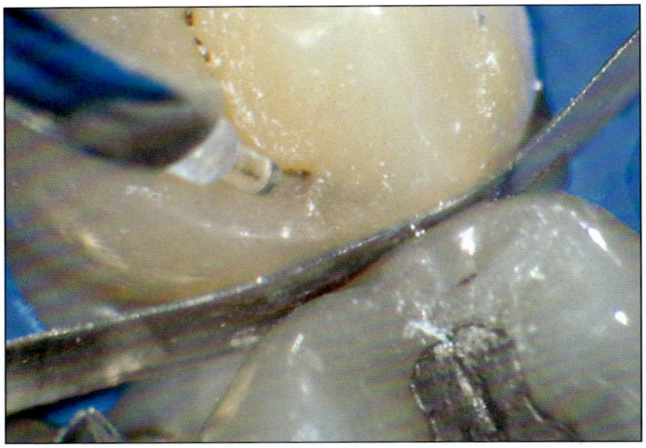

Fig 5-4b Intraoperative view of the beginning of tooth preparation. Despite the end-cutting nature of lasers, the adjacent tooth is shielded from the interproximal preparations.

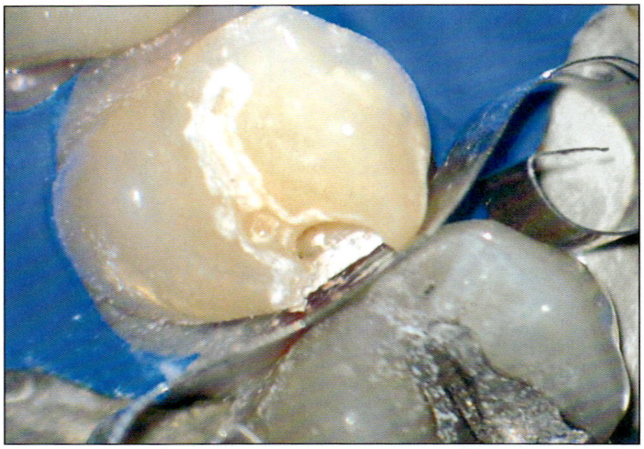

Fig 5-4c Completion of tooth preparation. (Case courtesy of Dr Glenn van As, North Vancouver, BC, Canada.)

Purpose of the procedure

Class II restoration

Once new caries is ablated on the mesial and occlusal surfaces of the premolar, the tooth is restored.

Wavelength

Er laser.

Alternate wavelength that may be used

Only the Er family of lasers can be used for tooth preparation.

Class III Restoration: Case 1

Restoration of a maxillary canine in an adult female patient.

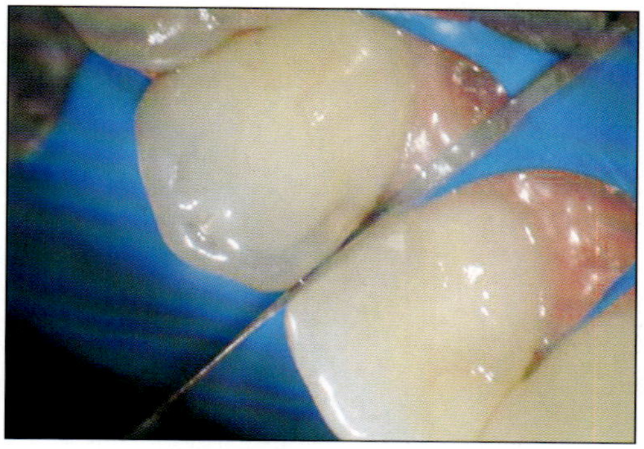

Fig 5-5a Preoperative view of caries on the mesial surface of a maxillary canine.

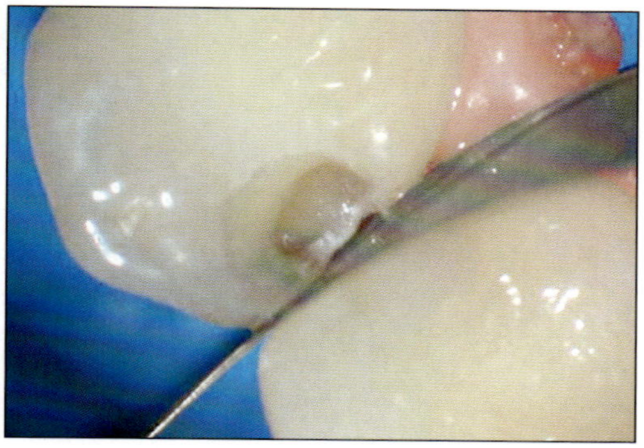

Fig 5-5b Tooth preparation is completed following ablation of carious tooth structure.

Fig 5-5c Definitive restoration of the maxillary canine. (Case courtesy of Dr Glenn van As, North Vancouver, BC, Canada.)

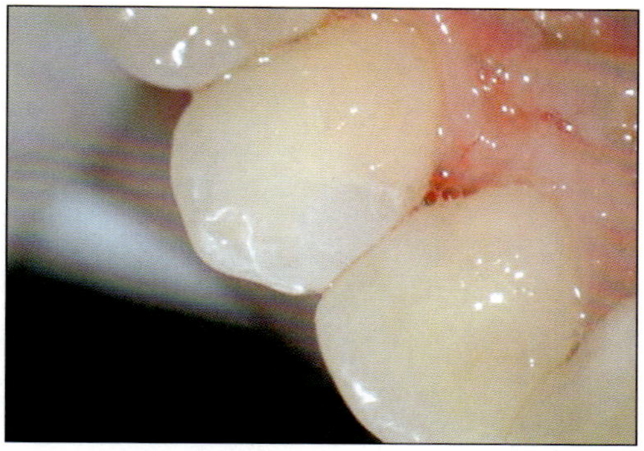

Purpose of the procedure	Class III restoration
Once the caries is removed, the maxillary canine is restored.	

Wavelength
Er laser.
Alternate wavelength that may be used
Only the Er family of lasers can be used for tooth preparation.

Class III Restoration: Case 2

Removal of caries and restoration of a mandibular incisor.

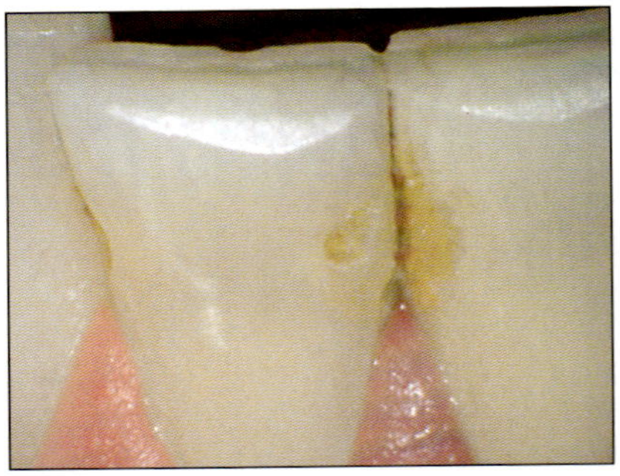

Fig 5-6a Preoperative view of caries on a mandibular incisor.

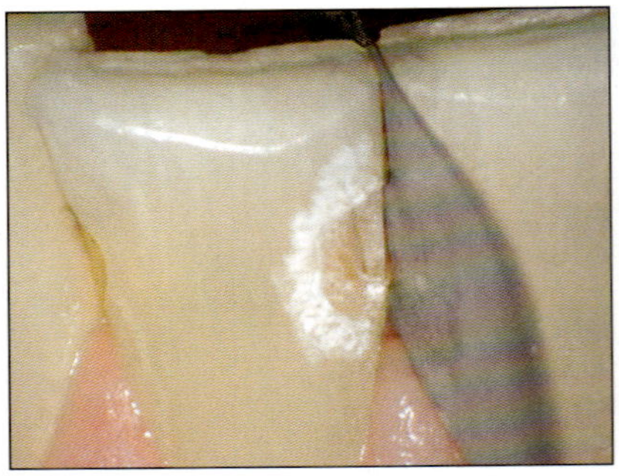

Fig 5-6b Completed tooth preparation.

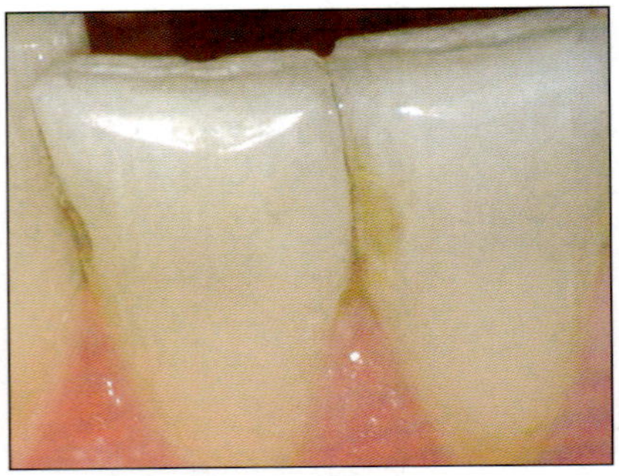

Fig 5-6c Definitive restoration. (Case courtesy of Dr Glenn van As, North Vancouver, BC, Canada.)

Purpose of the procedure

Class III restoration

The mandibular incisor is restored after the caries is removed.

Wavelength

Er laser.

Alternate wavelength that may be used

Only the Er family of lasers can be used for tooth preparation.

Clinical tip

Since the caries is visible in this case, and the clinician did not have to ablate healthy enamel, as in the previous case, or remove a faulty restoration to access the decay, a low-power setting was used to complete the preparation.

Class IV Restoration: Case 1

Restoration of a maxillary central incisor in an adult male patient.

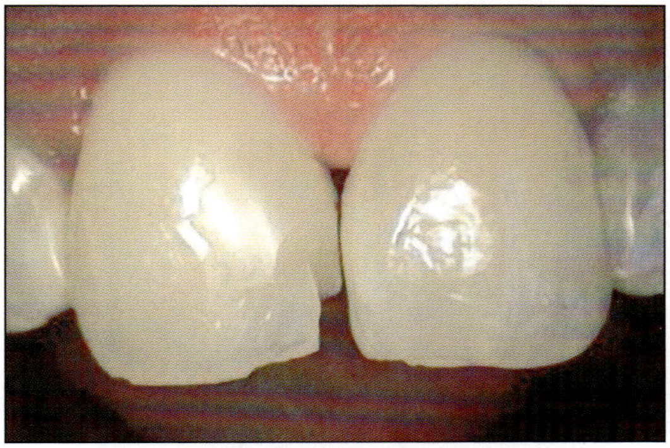

Fig 5-7a Preoperative view of the fractured incisal edge of a central incisor.

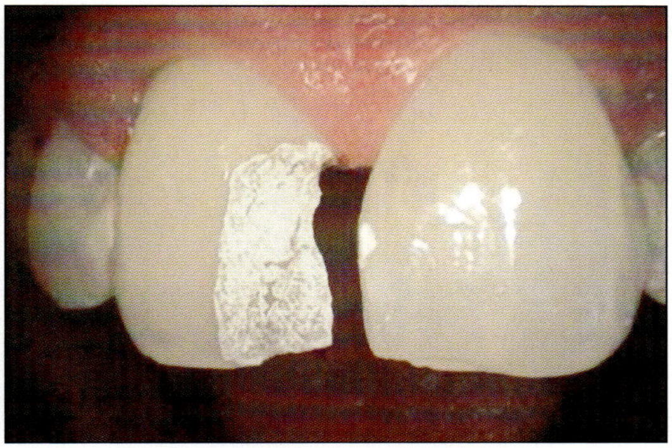

Fig 5-7b Completed laser preparation of the central incisor.

Fig 5-7c Definitive restoration. (Case courtesy of Dr Philip Hudson, Spokane, WA.)

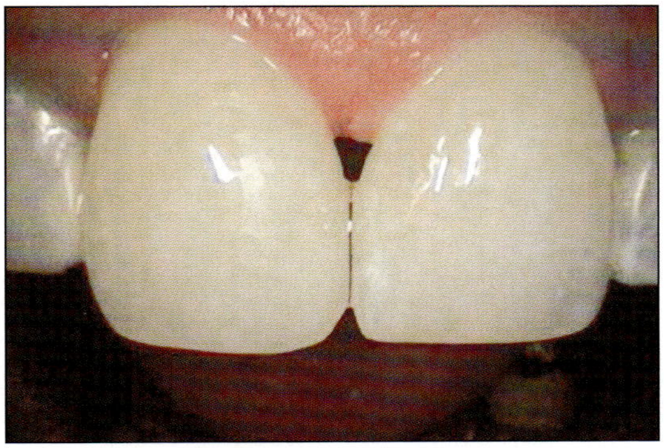

Purpose of the procedure	Class IV restoration
The fractured incisal edge of a maxillary central incisor is prepared for restoration.	

Wavelength

Er laser.

Alternate wavelength that may be used

Only the Er family of lasers can be used for tooth preparation.

Class IV Restoration: Case 2

Restoration of chipped enamel on a maxillary lateral incisor in an adult female patient.

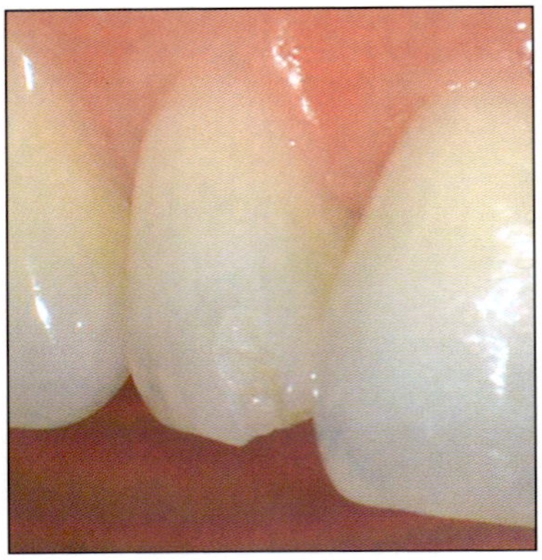

Fig 5-8a Preoperative view of chipped enamel on a maxillary lateral incisor.

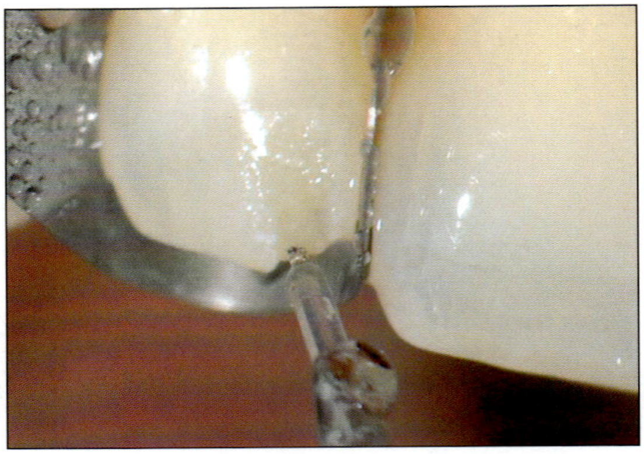

Fig 5-8b Completed tooth preparation.

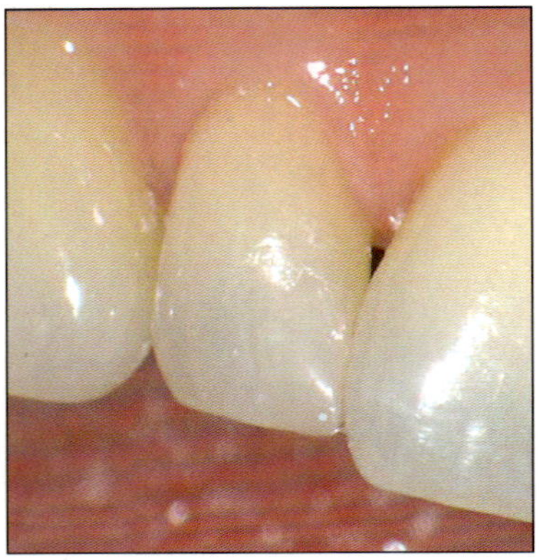

Fig 5-8c Definitive restoration. (Case courtesy of Dr Glenn van As, North Vancouver, BC, Canada.)

Purpose of the procedure	Class IV restoration
The chipped enamel on a maxillary lateral incisor is prepared for restoration.	

Wavelength

Er laser.

Alternate wavelength that may be used

Only the Er family of lasers can be used for tooth preparation.

Class IV Restoration: Case 3

Restoration of fractured edges on maxillary central incisors in a teenaged male patient.

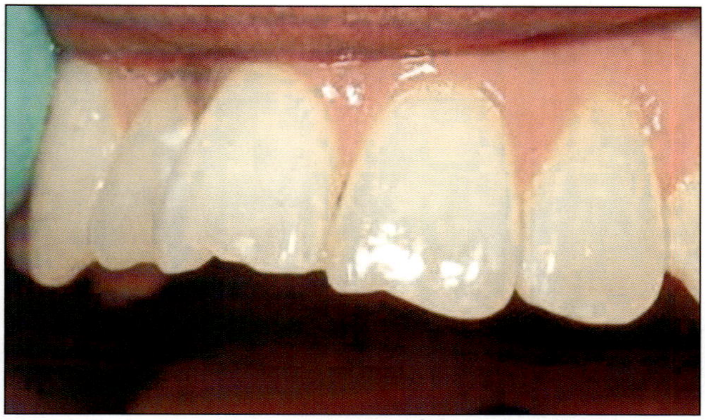

Fig 5-9a Preoperative view of fractured incisal edges.

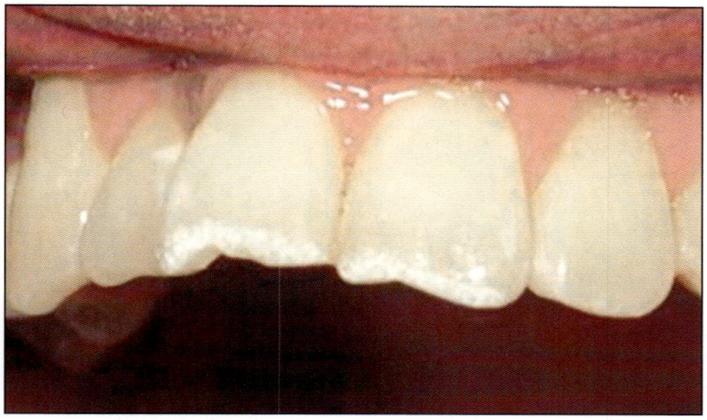

Fig 5-9b Completed tooth preparations.

Purpose of the procedure

Class IV restoration

The fractured incisal edges of maxillary central incisors are prepared for restoration.

Wavelength

Er laser.

Alternate wavelength that may be used

Only the Er family of lasers can be used for tooth preparation.

Clinical tip

The laser was used at low power to remove undermined enamel. After the incisal edges were prepared with the laser, chemical etchant was applied to the surface of the preparation to ensure adequate bonding strength.

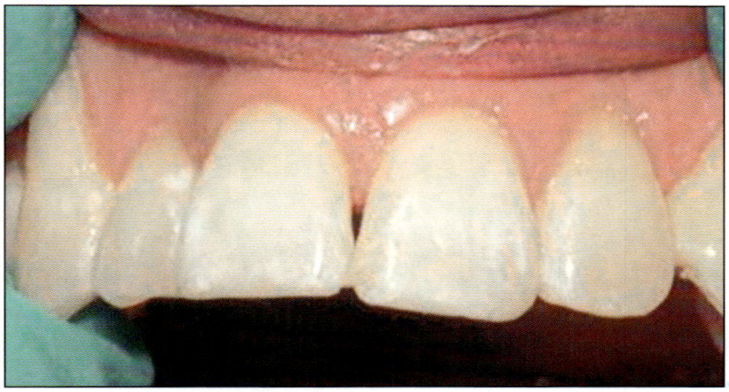

Fig 5-9c Definitive restorations.

Class IV Restoration: Case 4

Restoration of broken mandibular incisors in an adult male patient.

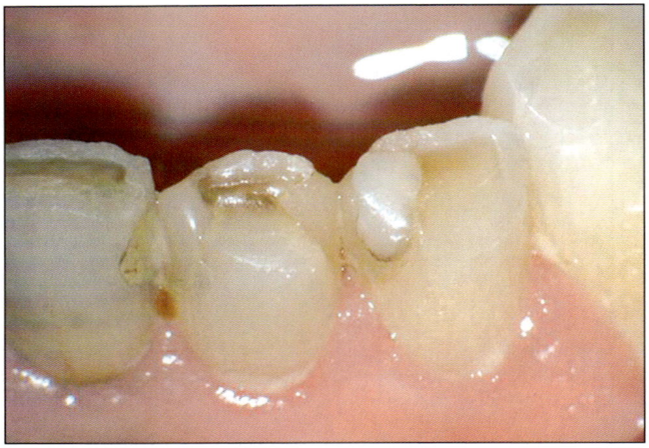

Fig 5-10a Preoperative view of broken incisal edges of mandibular central and lateral incisors with failing composite restorations.

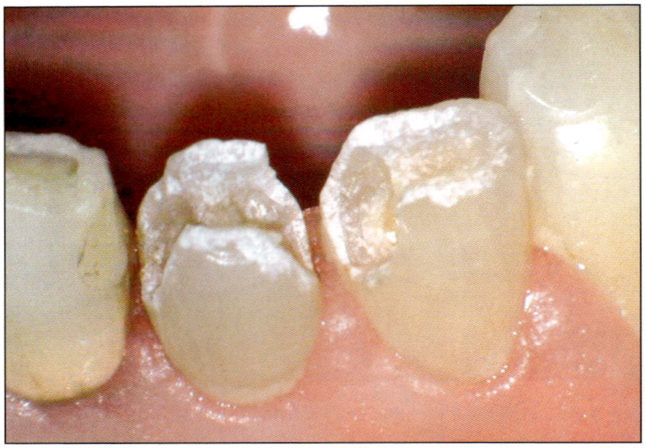

Fig 5-10b Completed tooth preparations.

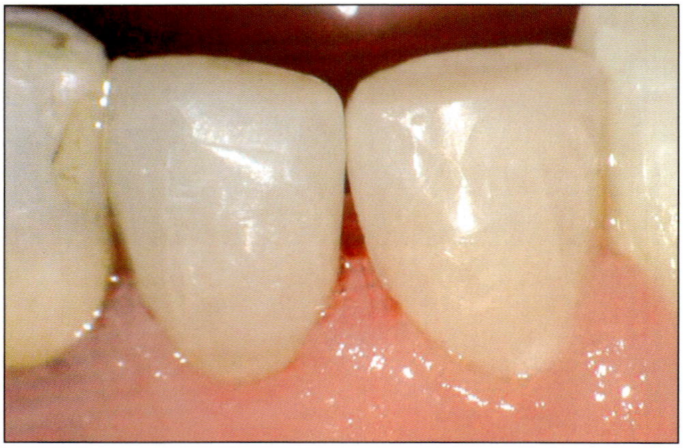

Fig 5-10c Definitive restorations.

Purpose of the procedure

Class IV restoration

Once the failing composite fillings are removed, the broken incisal edges are prepared and the mandibular incisors are restored.

Wavelength

Er laser.

Alternate wavelength that may be used

Only the Er family of lasers can be used for tooth preparation.

Clinical tip

An alternative treatment would involve crown restorations, but the laser preparation has the advantage of preserving healthy tooth structure with minimal surface disruption.

Class V Restoration: Case 1

Restoration of a maxillary canine in a teenaged female patient.

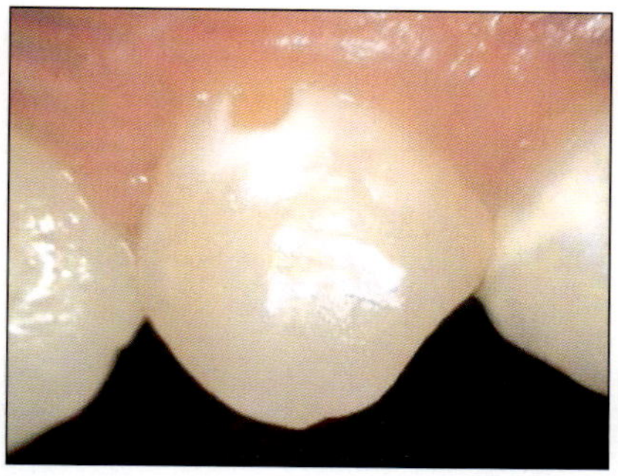

Fig 5-11a Preoperative view of caries on a maxillary canine.

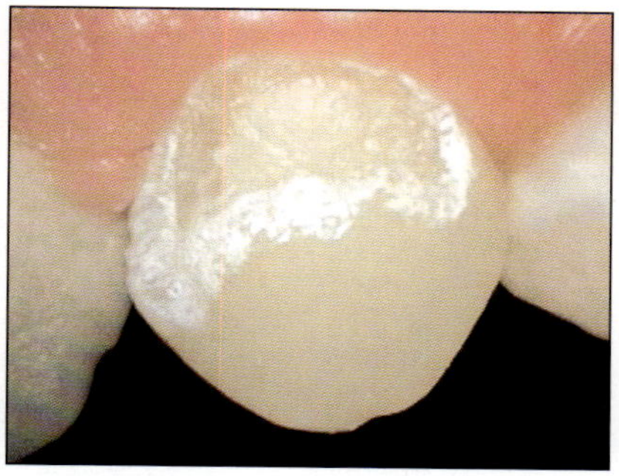

Fig 5-11b Completed laser tooth preparation.

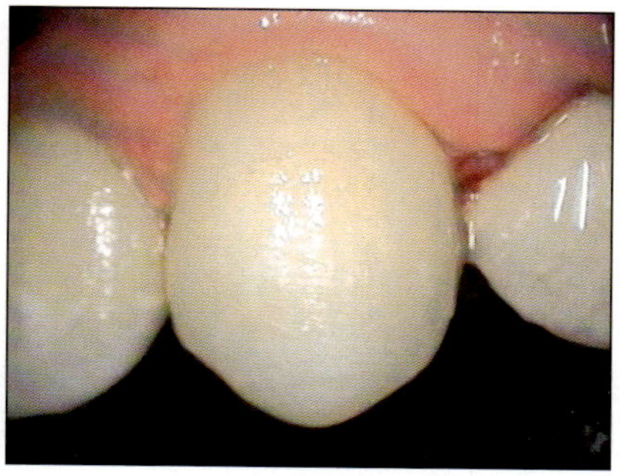

Fig 5-11c Definitive restoration. (Case courtesy of Dr Philip Hudson, Spokane, WA.)

Purpose of the procedure	Class V restoration
The maxillary canine is restored after caries is removed.	

Wavelength

Er laser.

Alternate wavelength that may be used

Only the Er family of lasers can be used for tooth preparation.

Clinical tip

The precision of using a laser during tooth preparation allows for a clean, dry field of operation.

Class V Restoration: Case 2

Restoration of abfraction lesions on a mandibular premolar in an adult male patient.

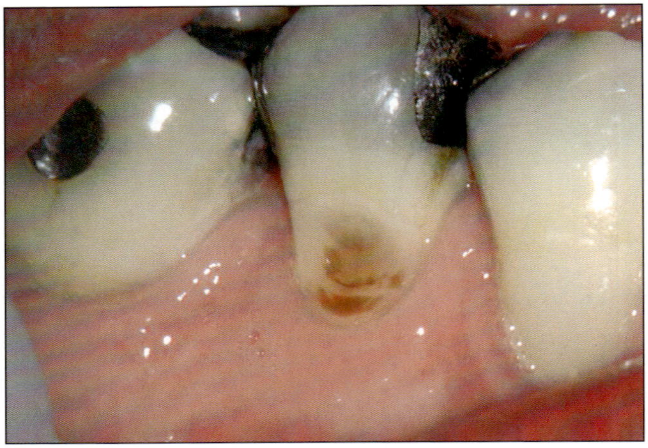

Fig 5-12a Preoperative view showing caries in a mandibular premolar.

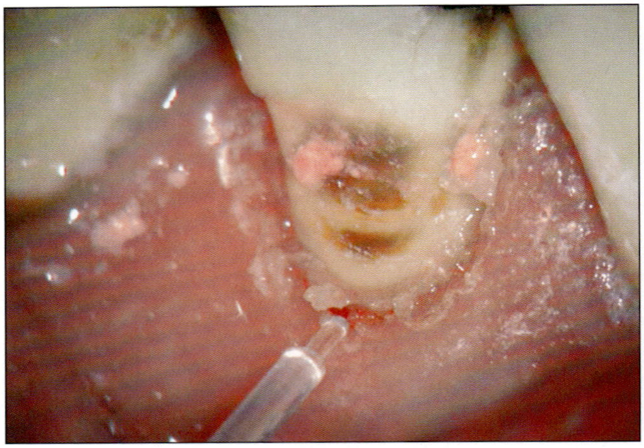

Fig 5-12b Intraoperative view showing laser removal of soft tissue at the gingival margin to reveal the extent of the caries. To increase hemostasis, water spray is not used during gingival ablation.

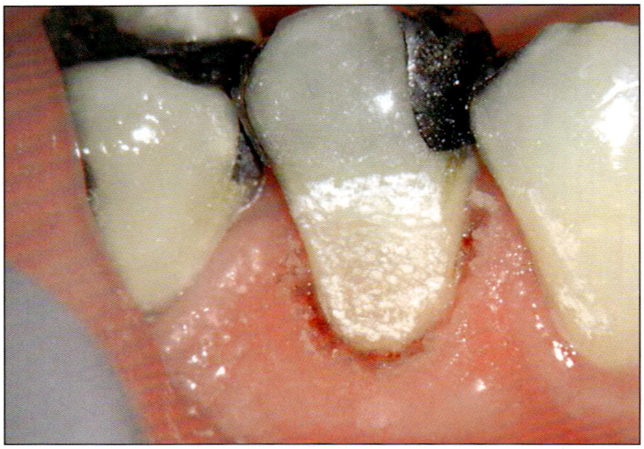

Fig 5-12c Completed tooth preparation.

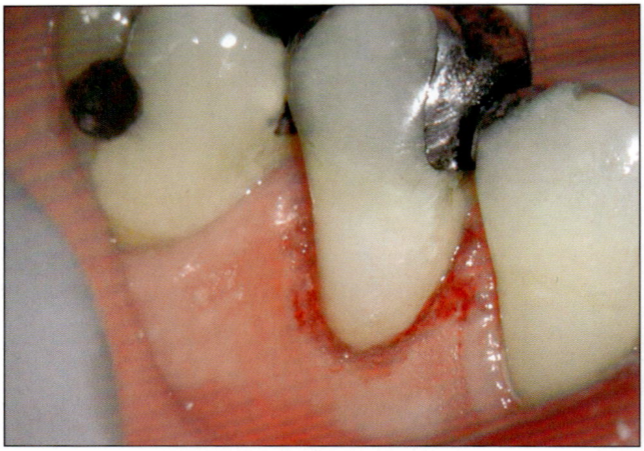

Fig 5-12d Definitive restoration immediately following the tooth preparation.

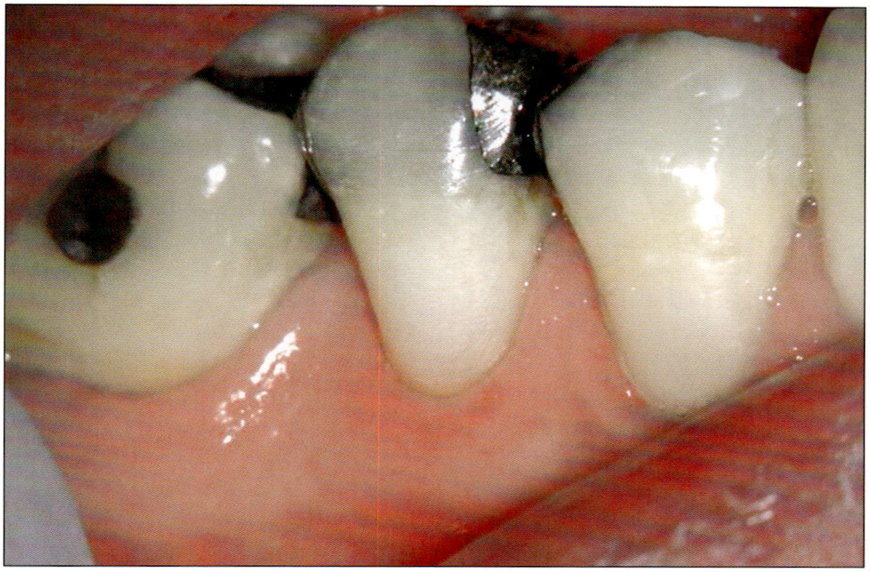

Fig 5-12e Two-week postoperative view showing that the gingiva has completely healed. (Case courtesy of Dr Glenn van As, North Vancouver, BC, Canada.)

Purpose of the procedure	Class V restoration
Restoration requires removal of tissue at the gingival margin to gain access to caries.	

Wavelength

Er laser.

Alternate wavelength that may be used

Only the Er family of lasers can be used for tooth preparation.

Clinical tip

In order to achieve acceptable hemostasis, the Er laser was used without water spray when the gingiva covering the abfraction lesion was ablated (see Fig 5-12b). During preparation of the tooth, the water spray was turned on.

References

1. Gimbel CB. Hard tissue laser procedures. Dent Clin North Am 2000;44:931–953.
2. Eversole LR, Rizoiu IM. Preliminary investigations on the utility of an erbium, chromium YSGG laser. J Calif Dent Assoc 1995; 23:41–47.
3. Coluzzi DJ. Fundamentals of dental lasers: Science and instruments. Dent Clin North Am 2004;48:751–770.
4. Featherstone JB, Fried D. Fundamental interactions of lasers with dental hard tissue. Med Laser Appl 2001;16:181–194.
5. van As G. Erbium lasers in dentistry. Dent Clin North Am 2004;48:1017–1059.
6. Rechmann P, Goldin DS, Hennig T. Changes in surface morphology of enamel after Er:YAG laser irradiation. In: Featherstone JD, Rechmann P, Fried D (eds). Lasers in Dentistry IV. San Jose, CA: International Society of Optical Engineering, 1998:62–68.
7. Hibst R. Lasers for caries removal and cavity preparation: State of the art and future directions. J Oral Laser Applic 2002;4: 203–212.
8. Hibst R, Stock K, Gall R, Keller U. Controlled tooth surface heating and sterilization by Er:YAG laser radiation. In: Altshuler GB, Chiesa F, Geschwind HJ, et al (eds). Laser Applications in Medicine and Dentistry. San Jose, CA: International Society of Optical Engineering, 1996:119–126.
9. Sharon-Buller A, Block C, Savion I, Sela M. Reduced bacteria levels in cavities prepared by Er:YAG laser. J Oral Laser Applic 2003; 3:153–155.
10. Lee BS, Lin CP, Hung YL, Lan WH. Structural changes of Er:YAG laser-irradiated human dentin. Photomed Laser Surg 2004; 22:330–334.
11. Glockner K, Rumpler J, Ebeleseder K, Stadtler P. Intrapulpal temperature during preparation with the Er:YAG laser compared to the conventional bur: An in vitro study. J Clin Laser Med Surg 1998;16:153–157.
12. Oelgiesser D, Blasbalg J, Ben-Amar A. Cavity preparation by Er-YAG laser on pulpal temperature rise. Am J Dent 2003;16:96–98.
13. Cavalcanti BN, Lage-Marques JL, Rode SM. Pulpal temperature increases with Er:YAG laser and high-speed handpieces. J Prosthet Dent 2003;90:447–451.
14. Eversole LR, Rizoiu I, Kimmel AI. Pulpal response to cavity preparation by an erbium, chromium:YSGG laser-powered hydrokinetic system. J Am Dent Assoc 1997;128: 1099–1106.
15. Keller U, Hibst R, Geurtsen W, Schilke R, Heidemann D, Klaiber B. Erbium:YAG laser application in caries therapy. Evaluation of patient perception and acceptance. J Dent 1998;26:649–656.
16. Kotlow LA. Lasers in pediatric dentistry. Dent Clin North Am 2004;48:889–922.
17. Parkins FM, Miller RL, Furnish GM, O'Toole TJ. A preliminary report: YAG laser treatment in pediatric dentistry. J Calif Dent Assoc 1991;19:43–50.
18. White JM, Goodis HE, Setcos JC, Eakle S, Hulscher BE, Rose CL. Effects of pulsed Nd:YAG laser energy on human teeth: A three-year follow-up study. J Am Dent Assoc 1993;124:45–51.
19. Fried D, Ragadio J, Akrivou M, Featherstone JD, Murray MW, Dickenson KM. Dental hard tissue modification and removal using sealed transverse excited atmospheric-pressure lasers operating at λ 9.6 and 10.6 μm. J Biomed Opt 2001;6: 231–238.

6

LASER APPLICATIONS IN FIXED PROSTHODONTICS

Dental lasers may be used adjunctively for many fixed prosthodontic procedures.[1] Management and surgical treatment of gingival tissues involve procedures that may be accomplished with laser instruments, such as removing intrusive or excessive tissue around the margins of tooth preparations, increasing the length of clinical crowns, or contouring edentulous sites for fixed partial dentures. It is essential that the clinician employ the proper laser parameters and technique. Laser instruments provide excellent surgical precision, hemostasis, and tissue healing when correct laser technique is followed in selecting the size of laser fiber or tip, adapting the parameters to the clinical situation, and positioning the laser tip toward the target tissue.[2–7]

The guiding principle of successful restorative dentistry is maintenance of the biologic width. This zone consists of the gingival sulcus, junctional epithelium, and connective tissue attachment[8] and must measure approximately 3 mm.[9] Encroaching on the biologic width can result in chronic inflammation of the gingiva, periodontal disease, or even a compromised restoration and tooth loss.[10]

All dental lasers may be used for soft tissue procedures, but only the erbium (Er) family of lasers is effective in removing and recontouring bone. Laser technology has not yet completely replaced conventional modalities for tooth preparation. A few clinicians have used Er lasers for complete tooth preparation for a crown or veneer[11]; however, because laser instruments are end cutting, the capacity for axial shaping is limited. Removal of amalgam is not presently indicated for use with laser instruments, and laser energy will not interact with restorations of either cast gold or porcelain. Successful fixed prosthodontics ensure excellent esthetics, improved occlusion, and healthy periodontium, and dental lasers can be used to achieve these results.[12]

Gingival Retraction for Impressions

The goal of gingival retraction is the same whether lasers or more conventional methods are used. Precision impression taking requires a clean, dry field, free of contaminants like blood and saliva, to accurately record the restoration margins. All dental lasers can be used for soft tissue retraction. The shorter wavelength lasers, such as diode and neodymium-doped yttrium aluminum garnet (Nd:YAG), have virtually no interaction with healthy tooth structure and can easily achieve hemostasis to facilitate visualization of the tooth preparations. The longer wavelengths of Er and carbon dioxide (CO_2) more readily ablate hard tissue and must therefore be used with care during gingival retraction. If proper parameters are used, gingiva will remain healthy and stable. Knowing that gingival margins will remain where they are placed helps to ensure the success of the definitive restoration.

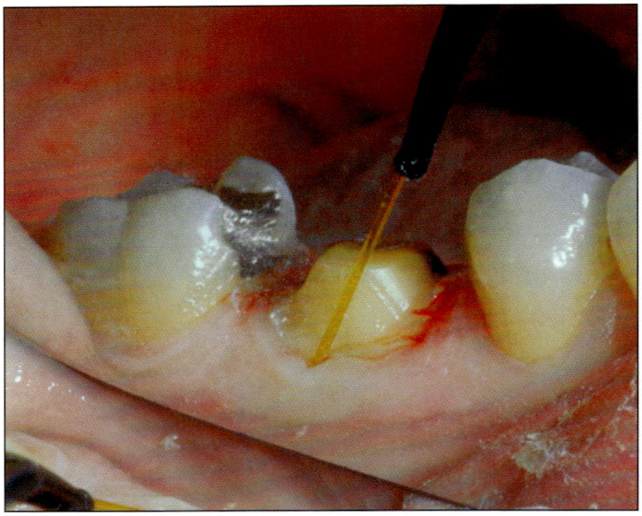

Fig 6-1 Correct instrument positioning for gingival retraction. The laser fiber is within the gingival sulcus and held parallel to the long axis of the tooth.

Clinical tip

Gingival laser retraction is a low-power procedure that dehydrates the sulcus and gingival cuff to create sufficient room for the impression material (Fig 6-1). Always keep the laser fiber or tip parallel to the long axis of the tooth. Move the laser slowly around the circumference of the tooth, keeping the fiber or tip just barely within the sulcus. The laser should smoothly glide around the tooth. If the tip starts to drag through the soft tissue, examine the fiber or tip to make certain that it is clean and has a sharp cleave. Remove any debris from the fiber or tip and recleave if necessary. Gingival laser retraction should not cut the tissue.

Gingival Retraction: Case 1

Subgingival retraction around four maxillary incisors prepared for full crown restorations.

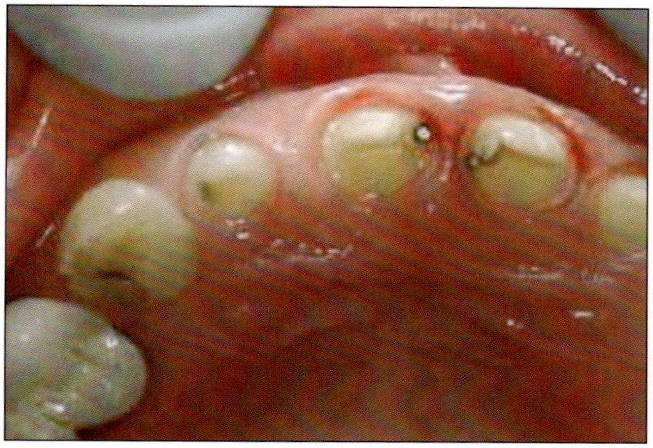

Fig 6-2a Postoperative occlusal view immediately following the gingival laser retraction around four maxillary incisors that have been prepared for full crown restorations.

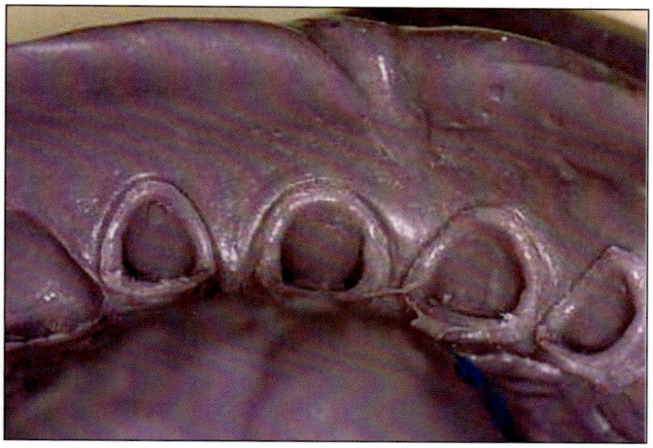

Fig 6-2b Impression taken following the gingival laser retraction. The definitive impression exhibits clear preparation margins. (Case courtesy of Dr Steven Parker, North Yorkshire, Harrogate, England.)

Purpose of the procedure	Subgingival retraction
Once the gingiva is retracted, a definitive impression can be taken for full crown restorations.	

Wavelength and settings
Nd:YAG laser set to 20 Hz, 100 mJ, with a 320 µm fiber.
Alternate wavelengths that may be used
Any laser can be used to perform this procedure.

Gingival Retraction: Case 2

Subgingival retraction around two maxillary central incisors in a young adult female patient.

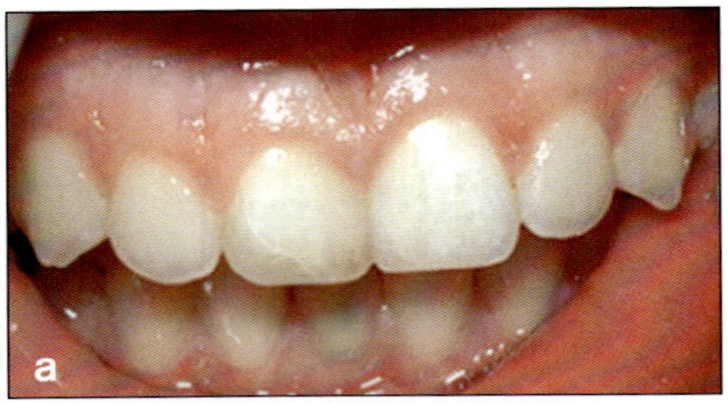

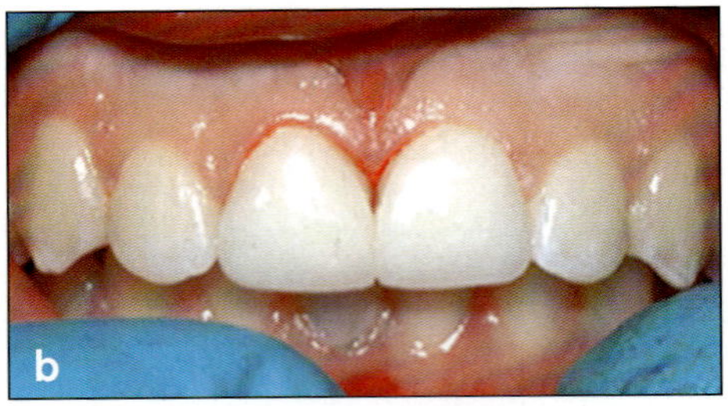

Figs 6-3a and 6-3b *(a)* Preoperative view of two maxillary central incisors prior to preparation for porcelain veneers. *(b)* Immediate postoperative view showing provisional restorations in place. A diode laser was used for minor gingival recontouring and retraction prior to placing the restoration margins, taking the impression, and fabricating the provisional restoration. The laser was used on low power because the gingiva was thin.

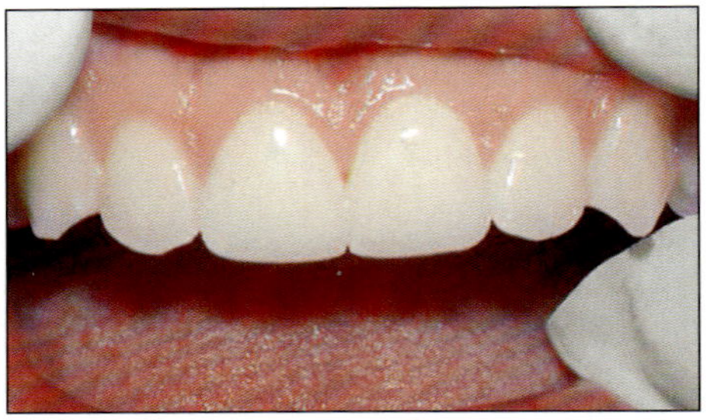

Fig 6-3c Two-week postoperative view showing the definitive porcelain restorations in place. The soft tissue has healed.

Purpose of the procedure	Subgingival retraction
A precision impression for two porcelain laminate veneers can be taken only after the gingiva is retracted.	

Wavelength and settings

Diode laser set to 0.6 W, continuous wave, with a 400 μm fiber.

Alternate wavelengths that may be used

Any laser can be used to perform this procedure.

Gingival Retraction: Case 3

Subgingival retraction around an implant abutment.

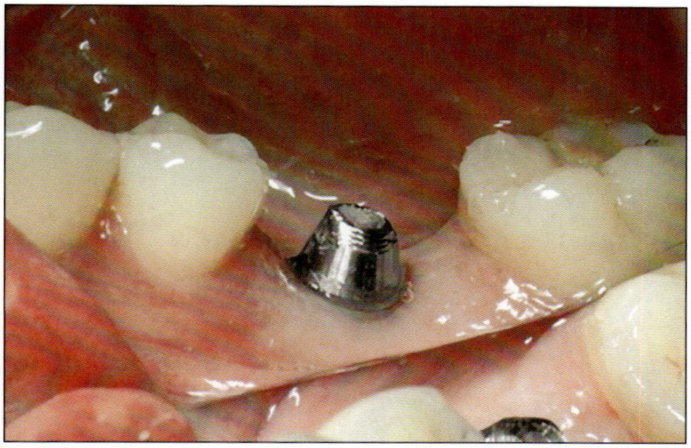

Fig 6-4a Preoperative view of implant abutment placed during second-stage surgery.

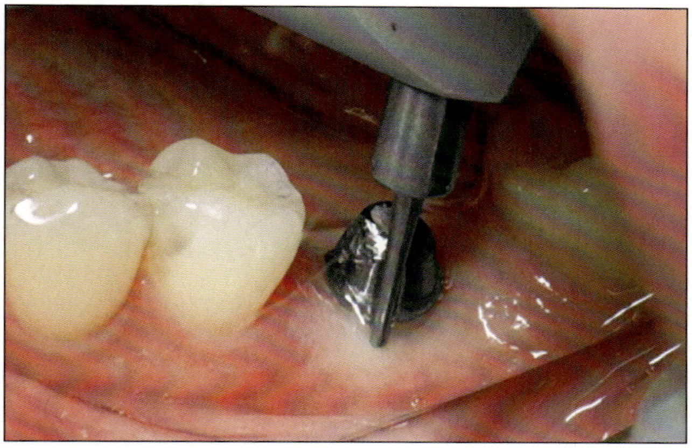

Fig 6-4b Laser tip in position for gingival retraction around an implant abutment prior to taking the definitive impression.

Purpose of the procedure

Subgingival retraction

Once the gingiva is retracted, a definitive impression can be taken to restore an implant with a crown.

Wavelength and settings

CO_2 laser set to 2.6 W, 50 Hz, with a 250 μm tip.

Alternate wavelengths that may be used

Diode lasers may be used for gingival retraction around implant abutments. The Er family of lasers may also be used with the water spray turned off. The Nd:YAG wavelength, however, is unsuitable for use around implants.

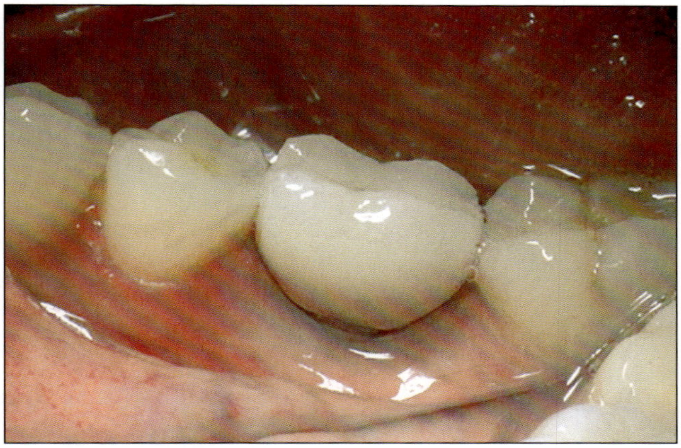

Fig 6-4c Definitive restoration in place over the implant abutment.

Gingival Retraction: Case 4

Subgingival retraction around an indirect onlay preparation in an adult female patient.

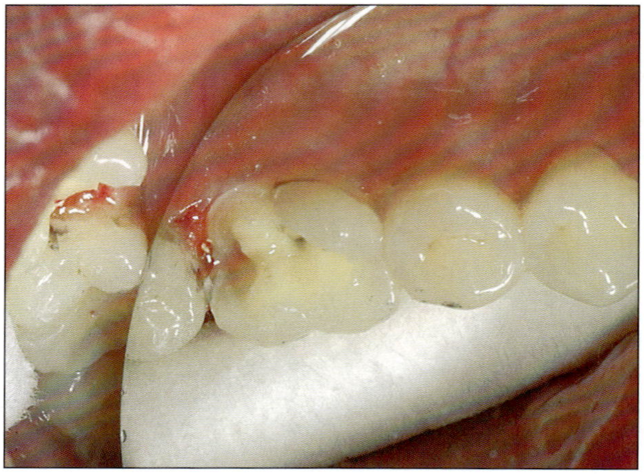

Fig 6-5a Clinical view of onlay preparation prior to impression taking.

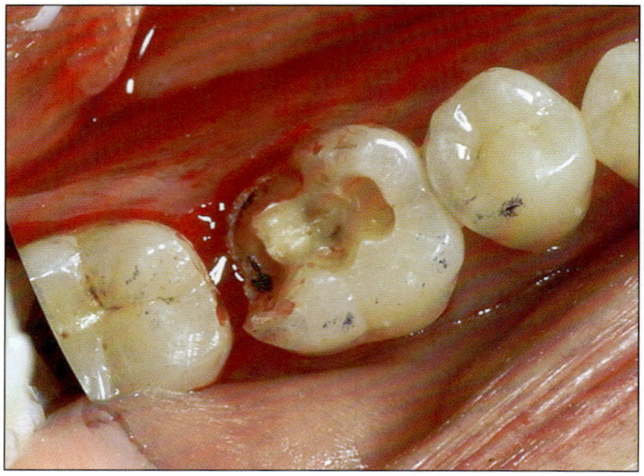

Fig 6-5b Postoperative view immediately following subgingival retraction around the onlay preparation. The visibility of the margins around the entire preparation ensures that soft tissue will not interfere with the recording of preparation margins and that the definitive impression will reproduce all details.

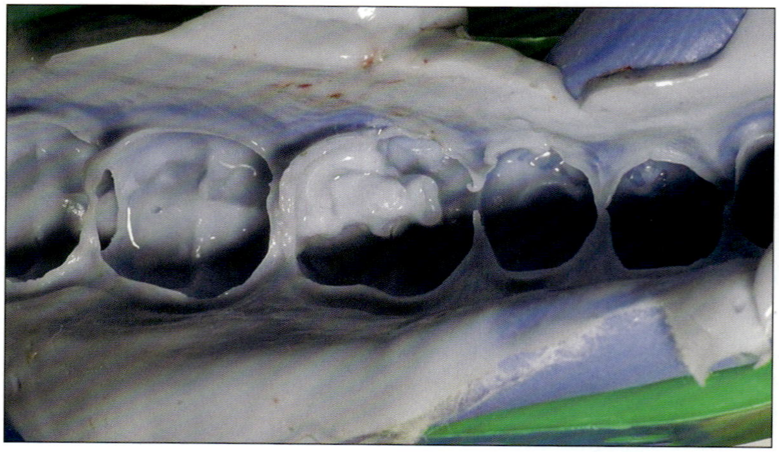

Fig 6-5c Definitive impression of the onlay preparation. Note the extension of the impression material apical to the gingival seat of the preparation and the clarity of the margins around the entire preparation.

Purpose of the procedure	Subgingival retraction
Once the gingiva is retracted, a definitive impression can be taken for an indirect onlay restoration.	

Wavelength and settings
CO_2 laser set to 2.6 W, 50 Hz, ultrapulsed, with a 250 μm tip.
Alternate wavelengths that may be used
Any laser can be used to perform this procedure.

Clinical tip
This technique can be used for all types of inlay and onlay preparations—cast gold, porcelain, or resin composite. Users of computer-assisted–design and/or computer-assisted–manufacture technology find this technique useful prior to imaging preparations.

Recontouring of the Gingival Margin for Crown Lengthening

The clinician must understand the relationship between the final position of the restoration margin and the biologic width of the periodontium. The dental laser can be used to reestablish biologic width when tooth preparation must encroach on this area. Gingival recontouring may be performed with all dental laser wavelengths.

Clinical tip

When crown lengthening is performed, a complete periodontal and radiographic examination must be performed, including measurement of probling depth. Maintenance of a viable biologic width is imperative because its violation will lead to restoration failure. The clinical cases in this section follow the established protocol of pre- and postoperative measurement of the biologic width.

Recontouring of the Gingival Margin for Crown Lengthening: Case 1

Crown lengthening in an adult male patient.

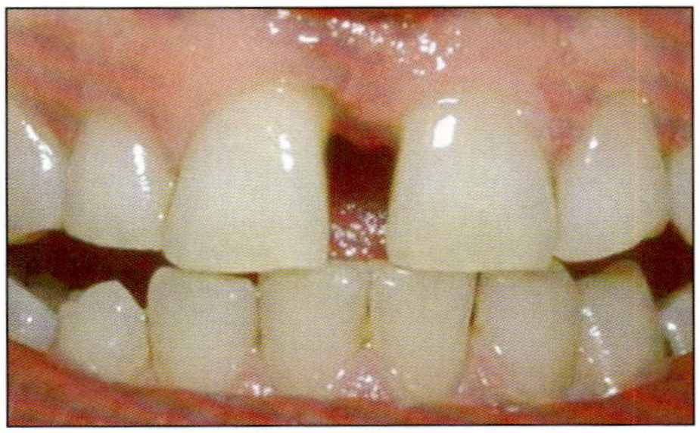

Fig 6-6a Preoperative view of the maxillary central and lateral incisors prior to tooth preparation for porcelain laminate veneers. Note the asymmetric and irregular gingival contour of the maxillary incisors.

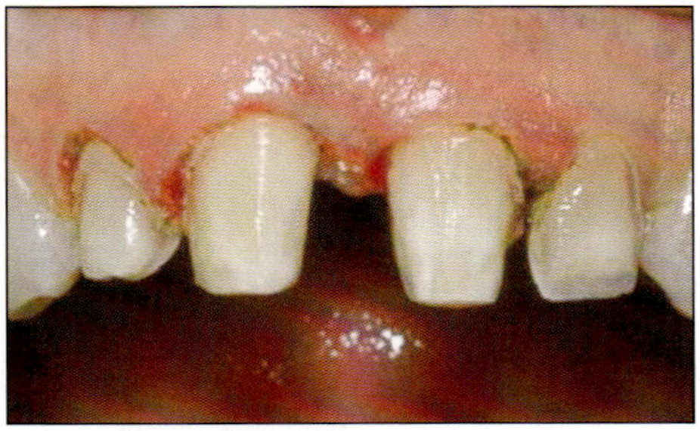

Fig 6-6b Postoperative view immediately following tooth preparation and crown lengthening. A more acceptable gingival contour has been obtained with laser surgery.

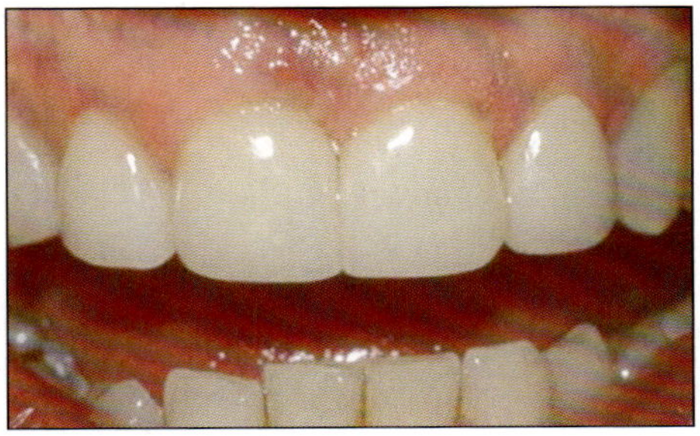

Fig 6-6c Postoperative view of the definitive restorations cemented in place 2 weeks after laser surgery. Note the symmetric gingival contours and the emergence profiles of the laminate veneers.

Purpose of the procedure	Crown lengthening
The gingival margin around the maxillary central and lateral incisors is recontoured prior to placement of porcelain laminate veneers.	

Wavelength and settings

Diode laser, 810 nm, set to 0.8 W, continuous wave, with a 400 μm fiber.

Alternate wavelengths that may be used

Any laser can be used to perform this procedure.

Recontouring of the Gingival Margin for Crown Lengthening: Case 2

Crown lengthening in an adult female patient.

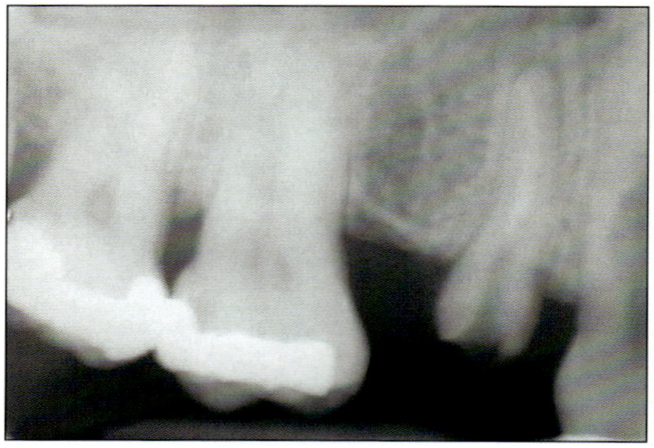

Fig 6-7a A preoperative radiograph reveals a shadow of excess soft tissue around the tooth preparation.

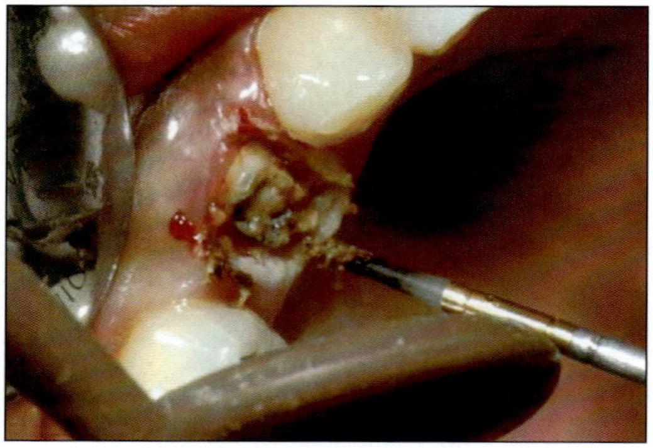

Fig 6-7b The laser retracts gingiva around the preparation.

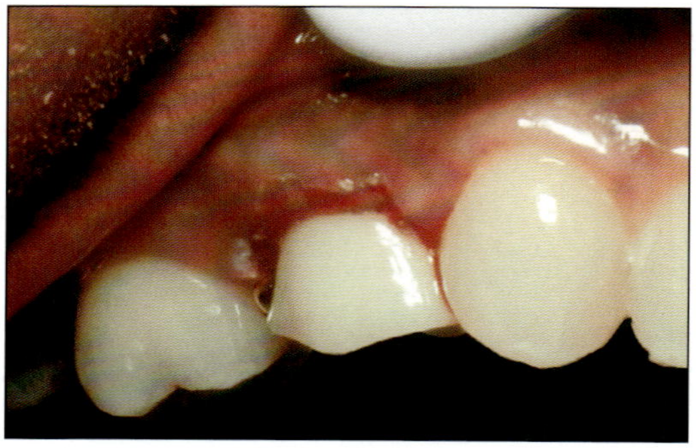

Fig 6-7c Postoperative view immediately following laser crown lengthening. The existing crown was recemented in place.

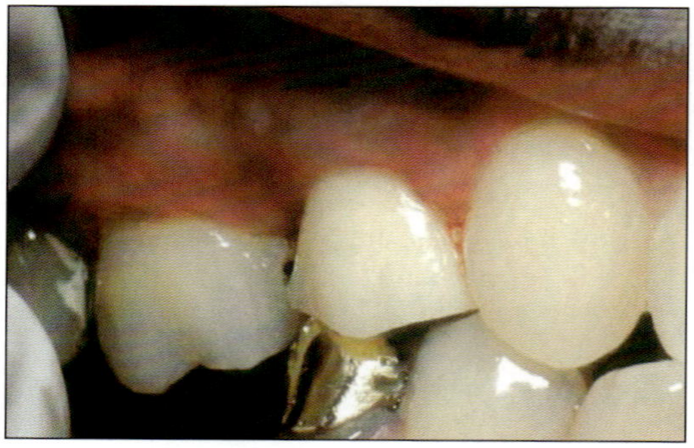

Fig 6-7d Two-week postoperative view following laser crown lengthening. The soft tissue looks healthy and shows no sign of recession.

Purpose of the procedure	Crown lengthening
Following removal of excess soft tissue around the preparation, the crown can be recemented.	

Wavelength and settings

Nd:YAG laser set to 3 W, continuous wave, with a 250 μm sapphire tip.

Alternate wavelengths that may be used

Any laser can be used to perform this procedure.

Recontouring of the Gingival Margin for Crown Lengthening: Case 3

Crown lengthening in an adult female patient.

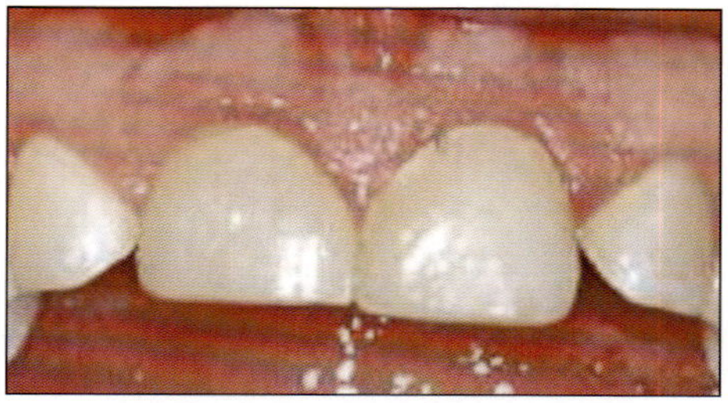

Fig 6-8a Preoperative view of short clinical crowns.

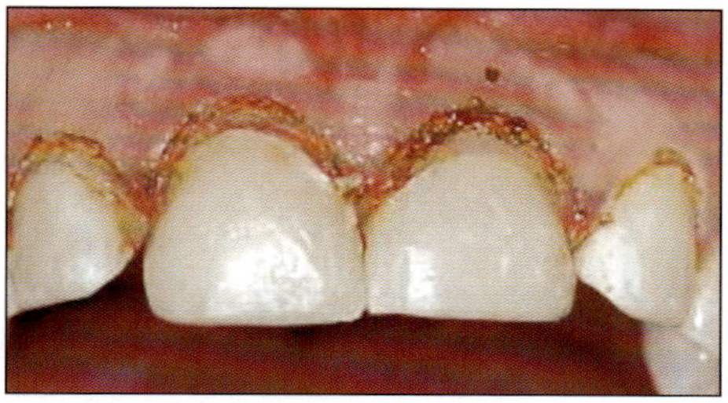

Fig 6-8b Immediate postoperative view showing completed laser crown lengthening.

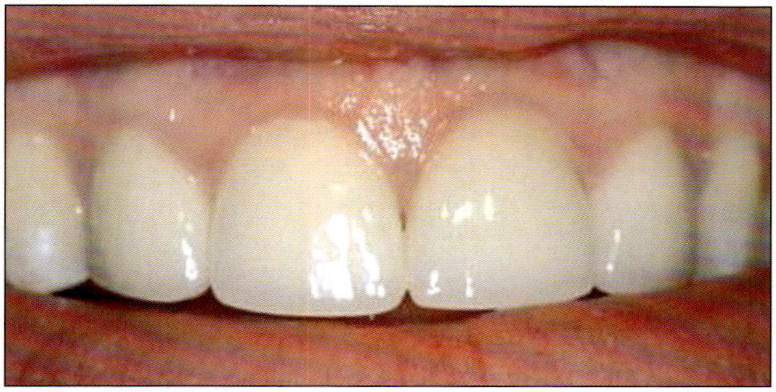

Fig 6-8c Four-week postoperative view with the definitive restorations in place.

Purpose of the procedure	Crown lengthening
The soft tissue is ablated to lengthen the clinical crowns of the maxillary incisors.	

Wavelength and settings

Nd:YAG laser set to 100 mJ, 20 Hz, with a 320 μm fiber.

Alternate wavelengths that may be used

Any laser can be used to perform this procedure.

Recontouring of the Gingival Margin for Crown Lengthening: Case 4

Crown lengthening in an adult male patient.

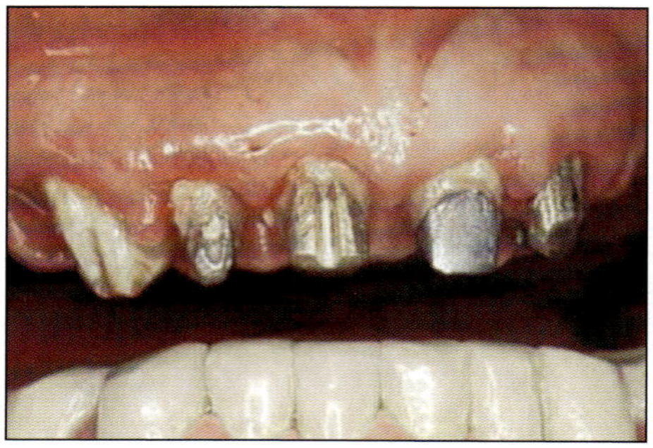

Fig 6-9a Preoperative view revealing excess soft tissue around the tooth preparations.

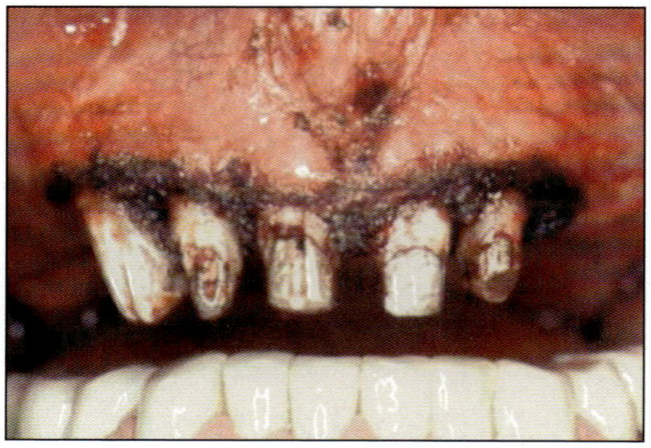

Fig 6-9b Postoperative view immediately following laser crown lengthening.

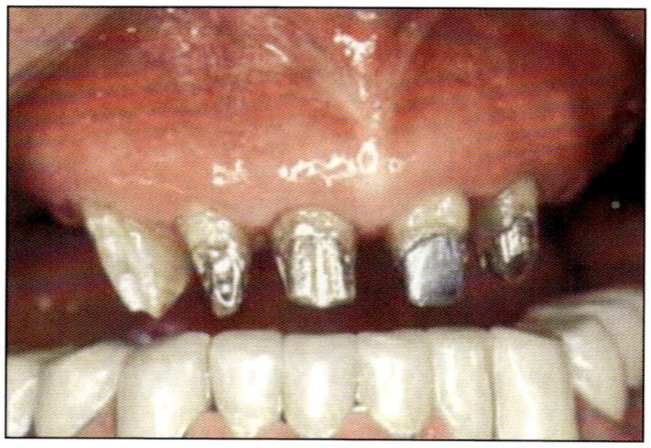

Fig 6-9c One-month postoperative view showing excellent soft tissue tone and improved crown length around the tooth preparations prior to restoration. (Case courtesy of Dr Stuart Coleton, White Plains, NY.)

Purpose of the procedure

Crown lengthening

Excess gingiva is removed to lengthen the clinical crowns prior to restoration.

Wavelength and settings

CO_2 laser, 10,600 nm, set to 6 W, continuous wave.

Clinical tip

During the laser procedure, a periosteal elevator was placed between the gingiva and teeth so the laser energy would not inadvertently interact with the dentin.

Recontouring of the Gingival Margin for Crown Lengthening: Case 5

Crown lengthening in a 30-year-old female patient.

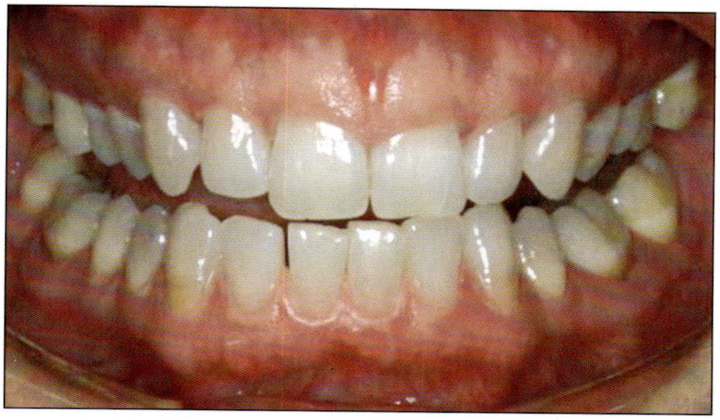

Fig 6-10a Preoperative view of thick gingiva covering the necks of the teeth with an uneven contour.

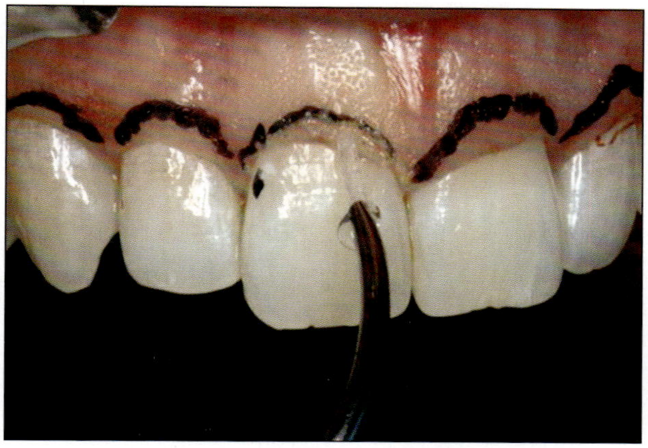

Fig 6-10b The laser ablates the excess soft tissue. The gingiva is marked in pen to outline the desired gingival contour.

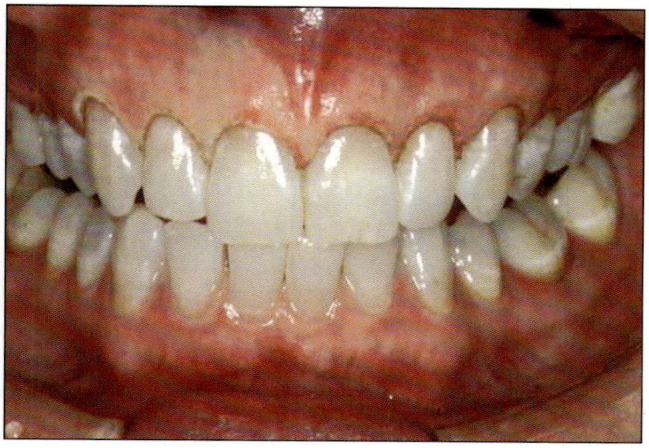

Fig 6-10c Postoperative view immediately following laser crown lengthening.

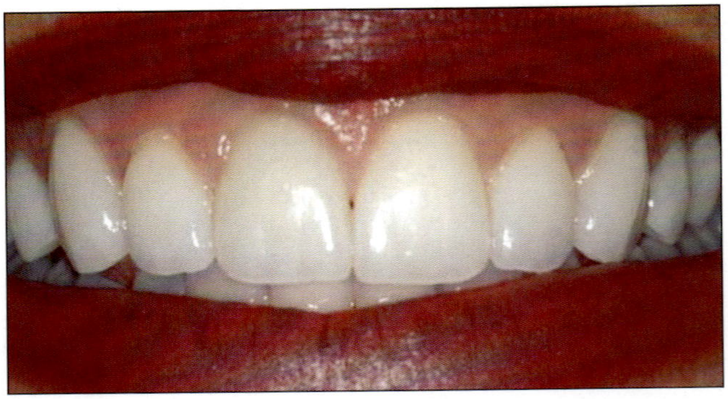

Fig 6-10d The 3-month postoperative view shows the porcelain veneer restorations that were placed once tooth whitening was accomplished.

Purpose of the procedure	Crown lengthening

Excess tissue covering the necks of the anterior teeth is removed to lengthen the clinical crowns.

Wavelength and settings

Diode laser, 810 nm, set to 1 W, continuous wave, with a 400 μm fiber.

Alternate wavelengths that may be used

Any laser can be used to perform this procedure.

Clinical tip

Outlining the new gingival margin with an indelible pencil allows the clinician to refine the contour before removing any gingival tissue. This step is particularly useful when the clinician is first learning how to perform laser crown lengthening.

Edentulous Site Preparation

Edentulous sites often need to be reshaped to provide esthetic emergence profiles for restorations. Both the soft tissue and the alveolar crest can be contoured with laser instruments. Any laser can be used to reshape soft tissue, but only Er lasers can be used to recontour the underlying osseous structure.

Edentulous Site Preparation: Case 1

Preparation of an edentulous site for a fixed partial denture in the esthetic zone in an adult female patient.

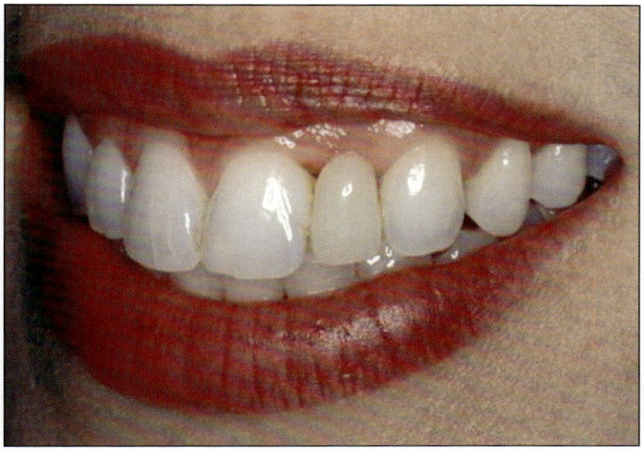

Fig 6-11a Preoperative view showing a fixed partial denture in the maxillary left anterior dentition. The pontic sits at the maxillary left lateral incisor site and is buccal to rather than emerging from the soft tissue. Without an emergence profile, the pontic is unesthetic and disharmonious with the rest of the dentition.

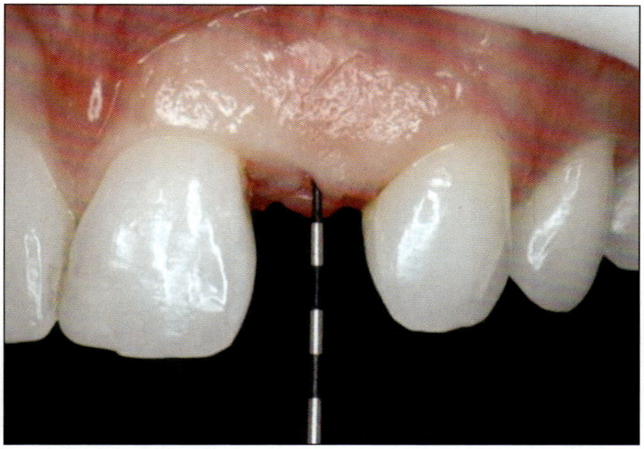

Fig 6-11b Measurement of available soft tissue for removal. The fixed partial denture has been removed to reveal dense, bulky soft tissue with a flat rather than concave shape.

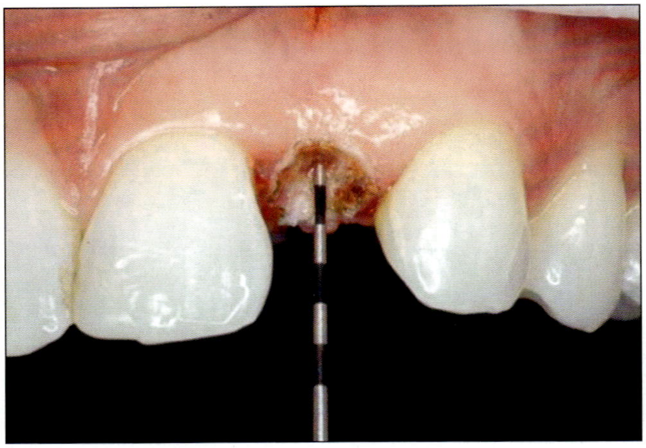

Fig 6-11c Intraoperative view of soft tissue contouring. The laser removes excess soft tissue to shape a physiologic and esthetic site for the restorative pontic.

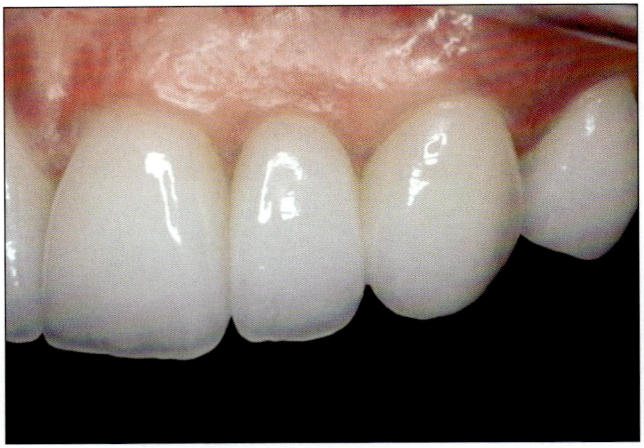

Fig 6-11d One-year postoperative view of the definitive fixed partial denture. The recontoured pontic site provides a natural-looking emergence profile and a more realistic-looking and esthetic restoration. (Case courtesy of Dr David Hornbrook, La Mesa, CA.)

Purpose of the procedure	Site preparation
Once the edentulous site is prepared, an esthetic pontic can be placed.	

Wavelength and settings

Diode laser, 810 nm, set to 1 W, continuous wave, with a 400 μm fiber.

Alternate wavelengths that may be used

Any laser can be used to perform this procedure.

Clinical tip

The edentulous site must be accurately measured with a periodontal probe. The apex and buccolingual position of the pontic must be aligned with those of adjacent teeth. The edentulous site must be recontoured with a concave shape to fit the convex form of the pontic. If an insufficient amount of tissue is removed, the pontic will appear shorter than adjacent teeth. However, if too much tissue is removed, the pontic will appear to be too long. Periodontal consideration requires a minimum of 1 mm of soft tissue to cover the osseous crest.

Edentulous Site Preparation: Case 2

Preparation of an edentulous site for a fixed partial denture in an adult male patient.

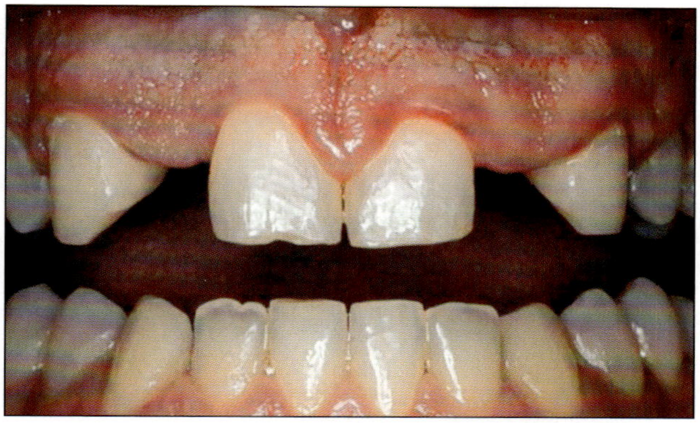

Fig 6-12a Preoperative view of the maxillary anterior dentition. The edentulous gaps in the maxillary lateral incisor sites will be restored with two fixed partial dentures.

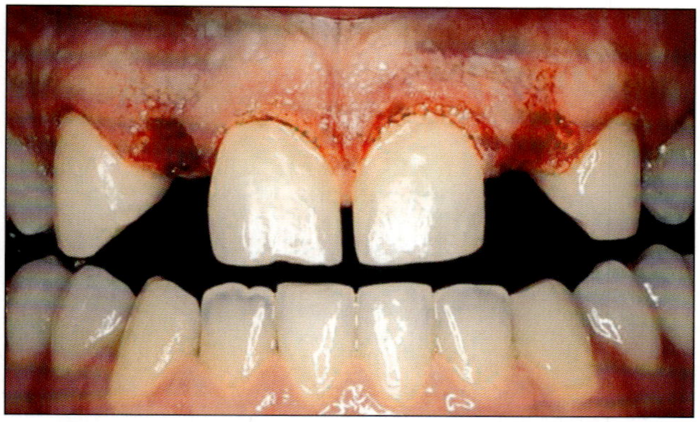

Fig 6-12b Postoperative view immediately following laser surgery. The edentulous sites have been recontoured to a concave shape.

Purpose of the procedure

Site preparation

Esthetic pontics can be placed after edentulous sites are prepared.

Wavelength and settings

Diode laser, 810 nm, set to 0.8 W, continuous wave, with a 400 µm fiber.

Alternate wavelengths that may be used

Any laser can be used to perform this procedure.

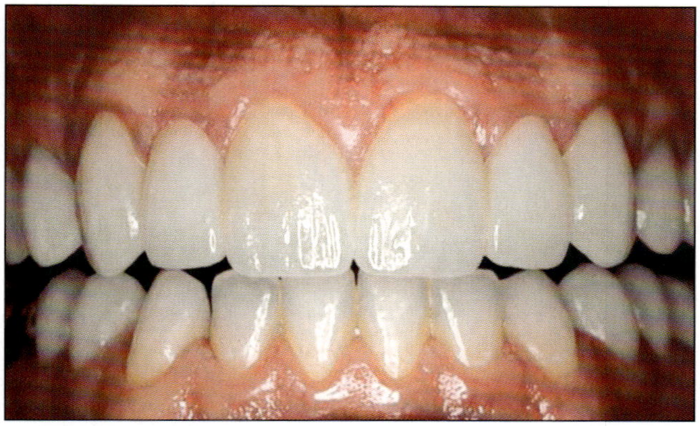

Fig 6-12c Six-month postoperative view with the definitive restorations. Note the natural appearance of the emergence profile of the pontics.

Edentulous Site Preparation: Case 3

Preparation of an edentulous site for a fixed partial denture in an adult male patient.

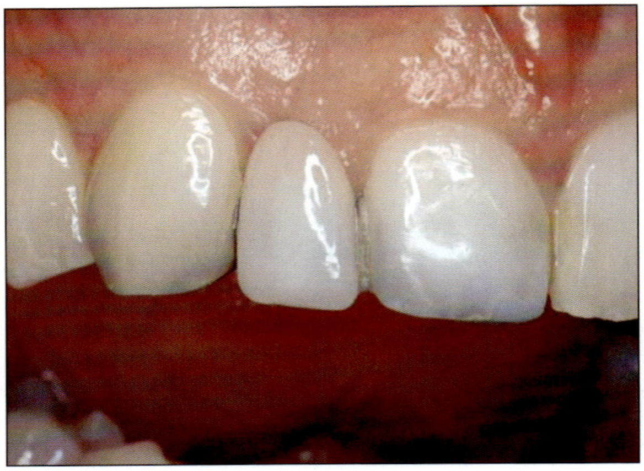

Fig 6-13a Preoperative view of a resin-bonded fixed partial denture. Note the unesthetic pontic in the maxillary right lateral incisor site.

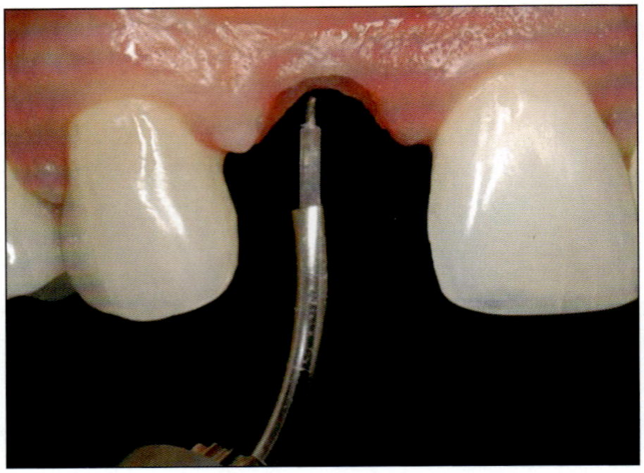

Fig 6-13b Intraoperative view of laser surgery to prepare the pontic site. Both hard and soft tissue were removed in this procedure.

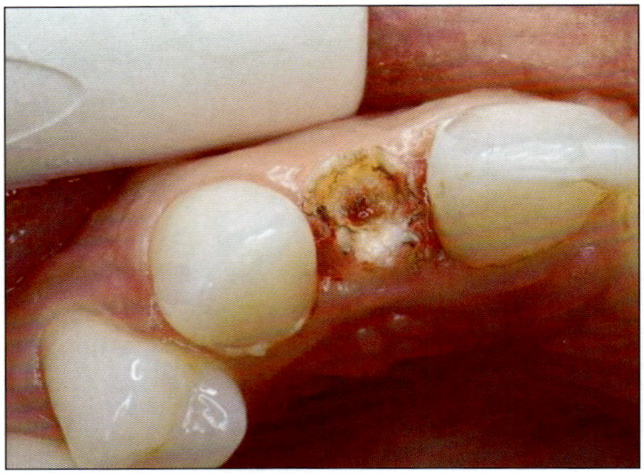

Fig 6-13c Immediate postoperative view of the new contour of the edentulous site.

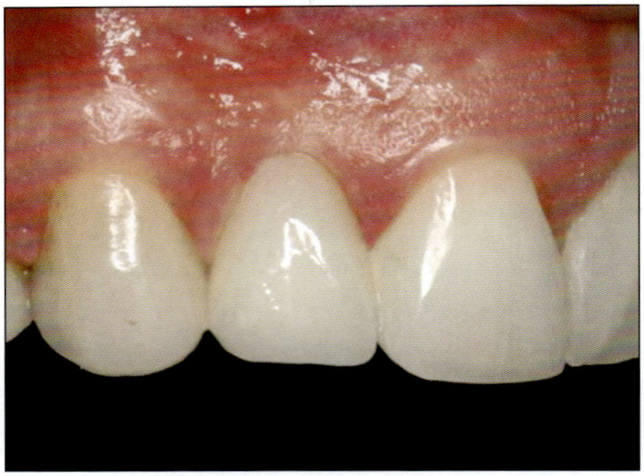

Fig 6-13d One-year postoperative view with the definitive prosthesis in place. (Case courtesy of Dr David Hornbrook, La Mesa, CA.)

Purpose of the procedure

Site preparation

A fixed partial denture with a pontic in the maxillary right lateral incisor site can be placed once the soft tissue is contoured to fit the pontic.

Wavelength and settings

Er:YAG laser, 2940 nm, set to 50 mJ, 30 Hz, with water spray, and a 400 µm tip. Since this procedure was performed as one continuous surgery, the water spray was used for both hard and soft tissue ablation, and the laser maintained light contact with the target tissues.

Alternate wavelengths that may be used

Only an Er laser can be used from start to finish because this procedure requires both hard and soft tissue removal. If an Er laser is not available, an alternate method can be used. A soft tissue laser or scalpel blade can be used to reflect a soft tissue flap. Osseous tissue can be removed using traditional instruments (eg, rongeur, bone file, or round bur in a high-speed handpiece with water spray). After the soft tissue flap has been sutured in place and sufficient healing has occurred, it may need to be reshaped with a soft tissue laser.

Clinical tip

The Er family of lasers will ablate soft tissue more efficiently and with better hemostasis when the water spray is turned off. When edentulous site preparation is performed, the laser must be properly positioned over the crest of the alveolar ridge so that the proper anatomic shape can be produced.

Osseous Recontouring for Crown Lengthening

When crown lengthening is planned in a clinical site with inadequate biologic width, the treatment plan must include bone removal. Contouring the osseous tissue to conform to the natural anatomy of the periodontium may require open-flap surgery. However, a closed-flap procedure may be employed when treatment involves removal of only a small amount of bone and the surgical site provides adequate visibility and access. The potential problems associated with closed-flap procedures include creating an undercut on the osseous crest; an uneven surface can compromise both esthetic and functional treatment objectives. Some practitioners use only closed-flap procedures for osseous recontouring. The authors, however, do not advocate procedures that disregard conventional periodontal protocols and are not supported by peer-reviewed research.

Osseous Recontouring for Crown Lengthening: Case 1

Osseous crown lengthening in an adult male patient.

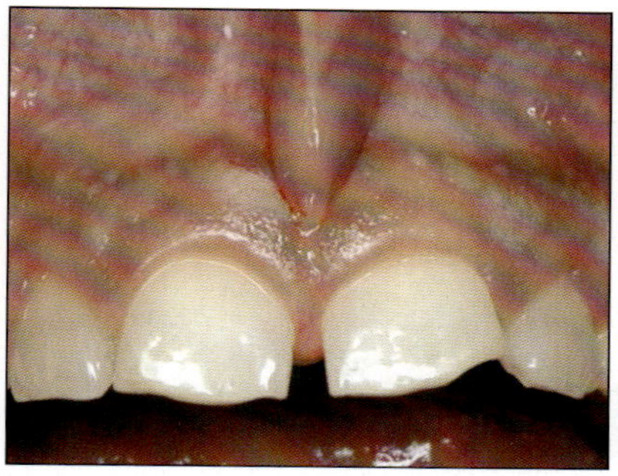

Fig 6-14a Preoperative view of a patient who wants to change the esthetics of his smile. Note the short gingivoincisal length of the anterior teeth.

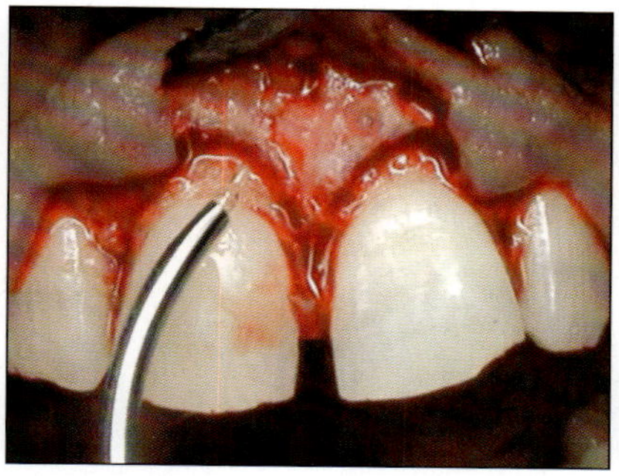

Fig 6-14b An Er:YAG laser removes osseous structure to lengthen the clinical crowns. Conventional instruments were used to reflect the soft tissue flap.

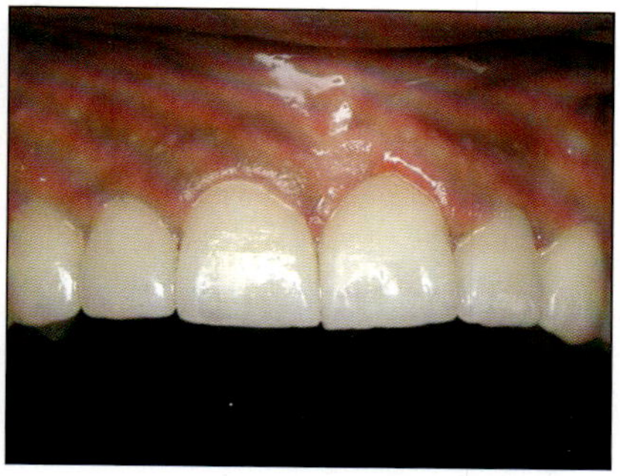

Fig 6-14c Four-month postoperative view with the definitive restorations in place. (Case courtesy of Dr Enrique Trevino, Juarez, Chihuahua, Mexico.)

Purpose of the procedure	Crown lengthening
The clinical crowns are lengthened via a combination of soft and hard tissue procedures.	

Wavelength and settings

Er:YAG laser, 2940 nm, set to 50 mJ, 30 Hz, with a 400 μm tip.

Alternate wavelengths that may be used

Since osseous tissue was recontoured, only an Er laser can be used to accomplish this procedure from start to finish.

Clinical tip

This procedure may be performed using a number of different instruments. The soft tissue flap can be reflected with any laser or a conventional scalpel. Once the soft tissue flap is reflected, the osseous tissue can be recontoured with an Er laser or conventional instruments (eg, rongeur, round bur in a high-speed handpiece, bone chisels, etc).

Osseous Recontouring for Crown Lengthening: Case 2

Crown lengthening in an adult male patient.

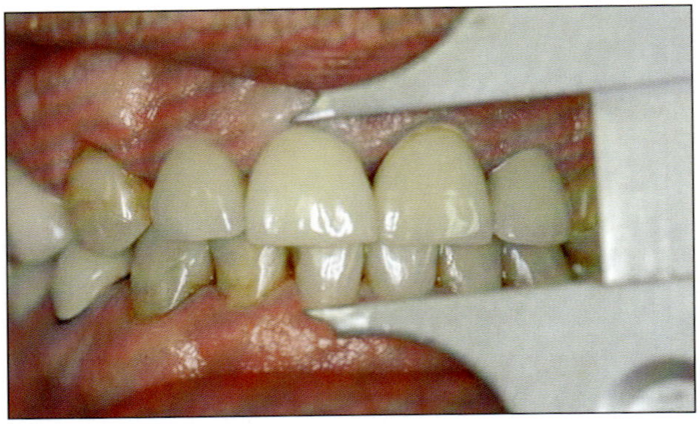

Fig 6-15a Measurement of preoperative tooth length.

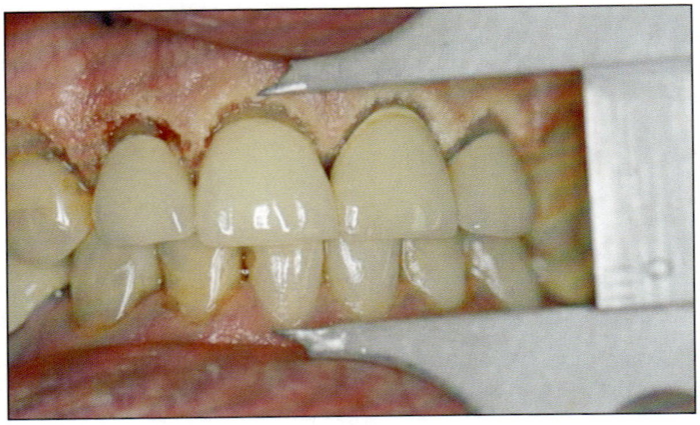

Fig 6-15b Immediate postoperative measurement of new incisal length following a closed-flap crown lengthening procedure. The Er:YAG laser was used to remove both soft and hard tissue.

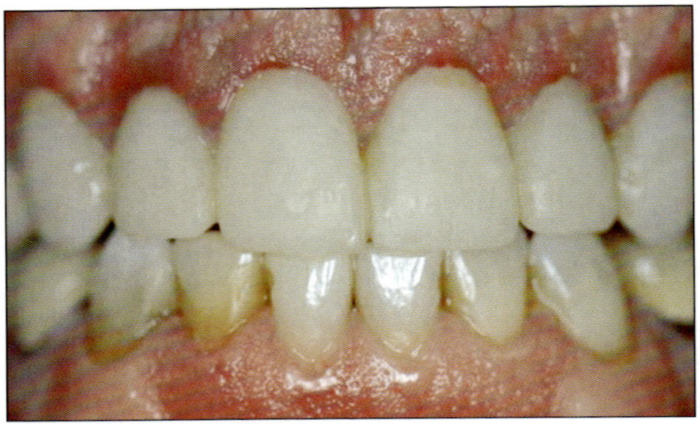

Fig 6-15c Provisional restorations in place.

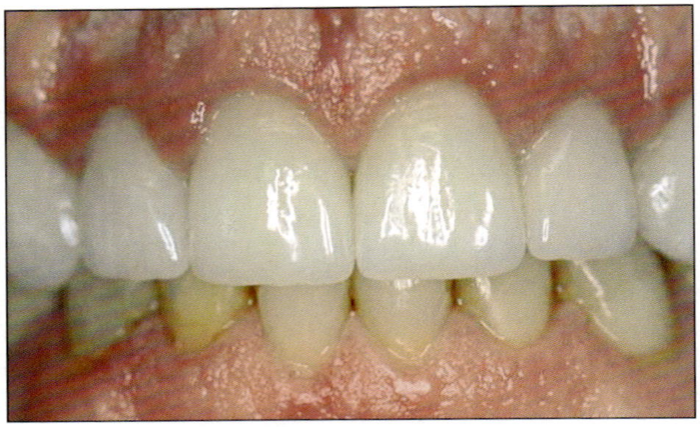

Fig 6-15d Two-month postoperative view with the definitive porcelain laminate veneers in place surrounded by healthy periodontal tissue. The anterior dentition now has a softer, more tapered shape. (Case courtesy of Dr F. Jay Ohmes, Dardenne Prairie, MO.)

Purpose of the procedure	Crown lengthening
The clinical crowns are lengthened via a combination of soft and hard tissue procedures.	

Wavelength and settings
Er:YAG laser, 2940 nm, set to 50 mJ, 30 Hz, with a 400 μm tip with water spray.
Alternate wavelengths that may be used
A closed-flap procedure cannot be accomplished without an Er laser. If an Er laser is not available, a soft tissue flap must be reflected conventionally or with a laser and the osseous tissue removed with conventional instruments.

Osseous Recontouring for Crown Lengthening: Case 3

Crown lengthening in an adult female patient.

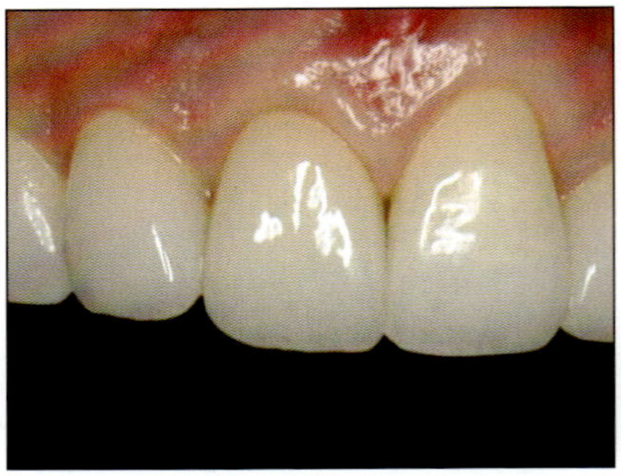

Fig 6-16a The preoperative view shows an uneven gingival contour over the veneers on the maxillary central incisors.

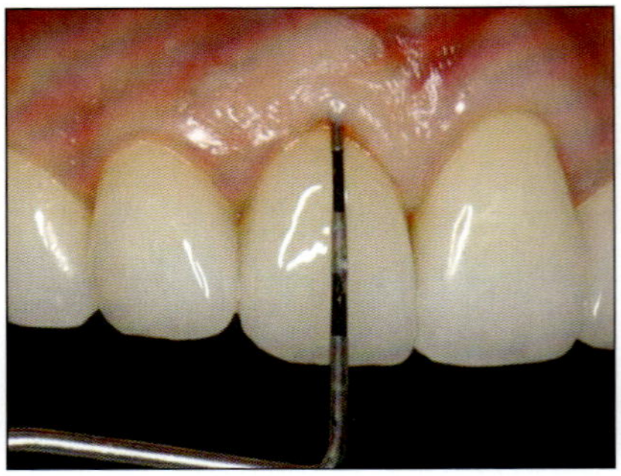

Fig 6-16b Initial measurement of biologic width. Periodontal probing indicates that soft tissue removal would violate the biologic width.

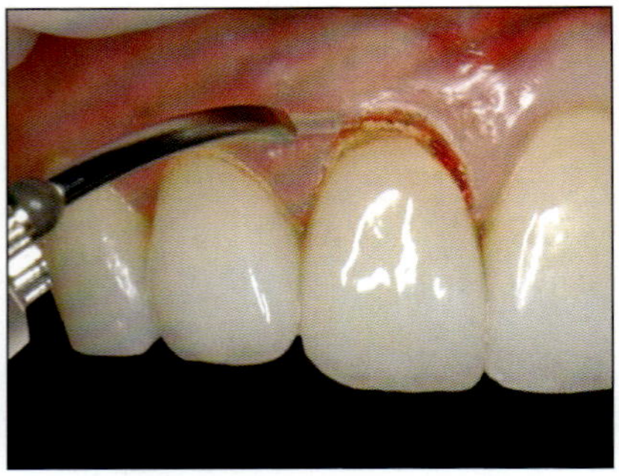

Fig 6-16c The Er:YAG laser is used without water spray to first carefully ablate the soft tissue.

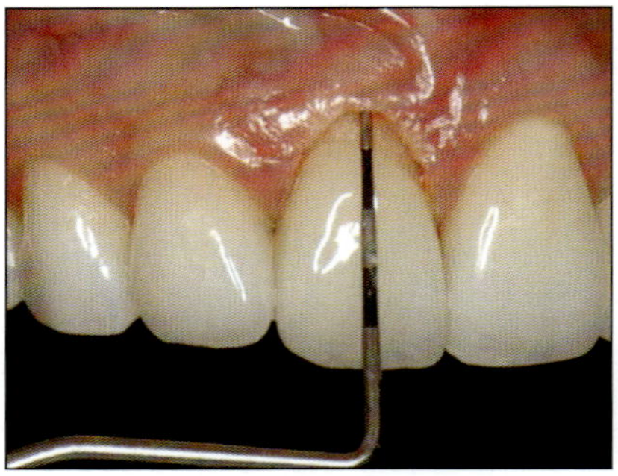

Fig 6-16d Second measurement of biologic width. Probing of the area immediately following soft tissue surgery indicates that the biologic width has been violated.

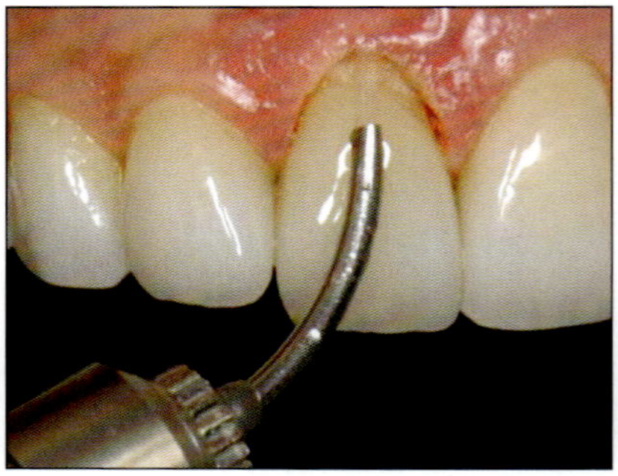

Fig 6-16e Intraoperative view of bone removal. The osseous tissue is recontoured via a closed-flap procedure, which will reestablish an adequate biologic width.

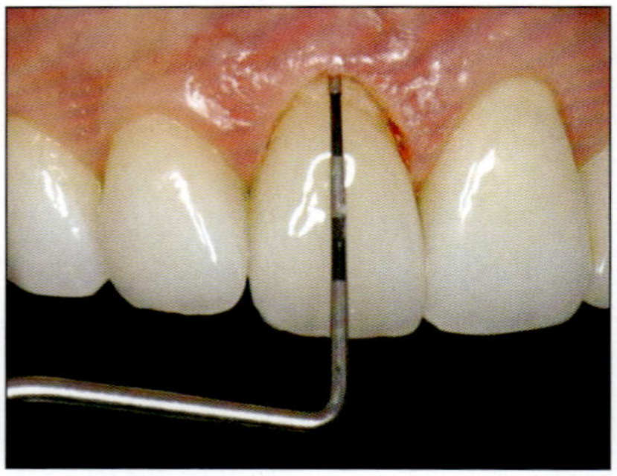

Fig 6-16f Immediate postoperative view of final probing to confirm stable biologic width.

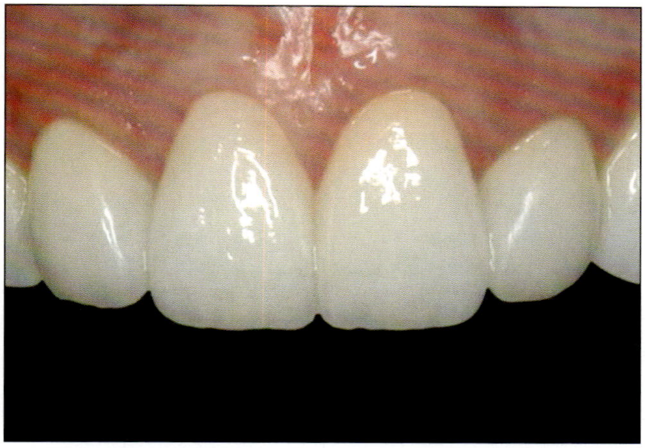

Fig 6-16g Six-month postoperative view of the maxillary anterior dentition. The desired esthetic result was achieved without any physiologic compromises. (Case courtesy of Dr David Hornbrook, La Mesa, CA.)

Purpose of the procedure	Crown lengthening

The esthetics of the anterior dentition is improved by using hard and soft tissue procedures to lengthen previously restored maxillary central incisors.

Wavelength and settings

Er:YAG laser, 2940 nm; settings for soft tissue contouring: 50 Hz, 30 mJ, with a 400 μm tip with no water spray; settings for osseous contouring: 30 Hz, 50 mJ, with a 400 μm tip with water spray.

Clinical tip

In this case, the Er laser was first used without water spray to efficiently ablate the soft tissue. The water spray was subsequently turned on and the energy was increased to proceed with recontouring of the osseous structure.

References

1. Walsh LJ. The current status of laser applications in dentistry. Aust Dent J 2003;48:146–155.
2. Nanami T, Shiba H, Ikeuchi S, Nagai T, Asanami S, Shibata T. Clinical applications and basic studies of lasers in dentistry and oral surgery. Keio J Med 1993;42:199–201.
3. Janda P, Sroka R, Mundweil B, Betz CS, Baumgartner R, Leunig A. Comparison of thermal tissue effects induced by contact application of fiber guided laser systems. Lasers Surg Med 2003;33:93–101.
4. Rowson JE. The contact diode laser—A useful instrument for excising oral lesions [abstract]. Br J Oral Maxillofac Surg 1995; 33:123.
5. White JM, Goodis HE, Rose CL. Use of the pulsed Nd:YAG laser for intraoral soft tissue surgery. Lasers Surg Med 1991;11:455–461.
6. Baraldi CE, Puricelli E, Kulkes S, Martins GL. Er:YAG laser in oral soft tissue surgery [abstract 59]. J Oral Laser Appl 2001;1:24.
7. Wilder-Smith P, Arrastia AM, Liaw LH, Berns M. Incision properties and thermal effects of three CO_2 lasers in soft tissue. Oral Surg Oral Med Oral Pathol Oral Radiol Endod 1995;79:685–691.
8. Gargiulo AW, Wentz FM, Orban B. The dimensions of the dentogingival junction in humans. J Periodontol 1961;32:261–267.
9. Kois JC. New paradigms for anterior tooth preparation: Rationale and technique. Contemp Esthet Dent 1996;2:1–8.
10. Newcomb GM. The relationship between the location of subgingival crown margins and gingival inflammation. J Periodontol 1974;45:151–154.
11. Schalter R. The Er,Cr:YSGG laser in various restorative treatments. J Acad Laser Dent 2005;13:26–29.
12. Parker S. The use of lasers in fixed prosthodontics. Dent Clin North Am 2004;48:971–978.

7

LASER APPLICATIONS IN REMOVABLE PROSTHODONTICS

Long-term success of a removable prosthesis is dependent on the support provided by hard and soft tissues. A comprehensive prosthodontic treatment plan may need to incorporate surgery to maximize this support. Surgery of healthy tissues may include removal of a torus, reduction of a hard or soft tissue tuberosity, removal of hyperplastic or redundant soft tissue, contouring of irregular ridge anatomy, and vestibuloplasty. Surgery may also be indicated to treat irritated or inflamed tissues underneath or adjacent to a denture base, such as removal of an epulis or management of generalized denture stomatitis. Dental lasers can be successfully used for all of these procedures because laser energy reduces bacteria at the surgical site, coagulates blood vessels, minimizes scar formation, reduces swelling and postoperative pain, and facilitates the overall treatment of prosthodontic patients. All dental wavelengths can perform soft tissue surgeries, but the erbium (Er) family of lasers is the only group of lasers indicated for treatment of osseous tissue.

Treatment of Inflamed Soft Tissues: Case 1

Irritated epulis fissurata in a 54-year-old female patient.

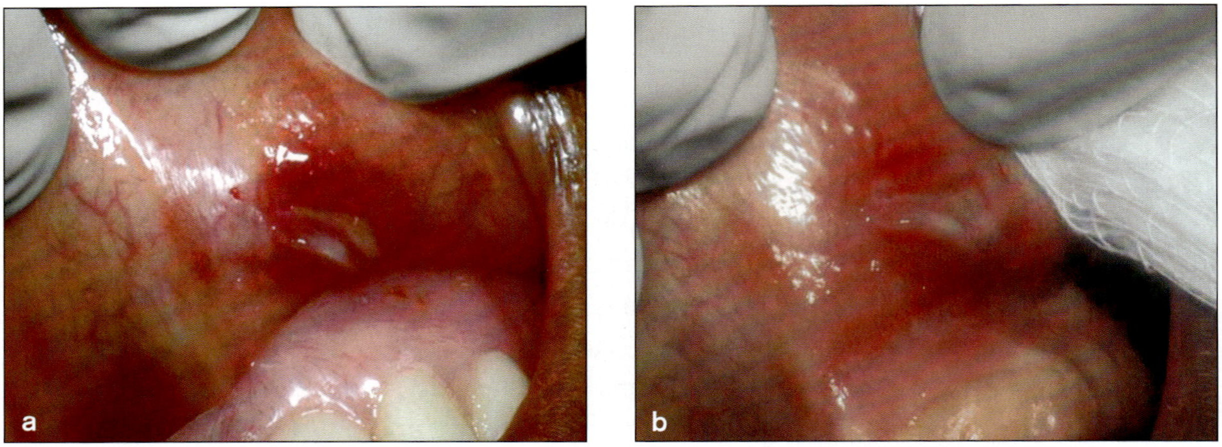

Figs 7-1a and 7-1b Irritated epulis fissurata with the denture in place *(a)* and with the denture removed *(b)*.

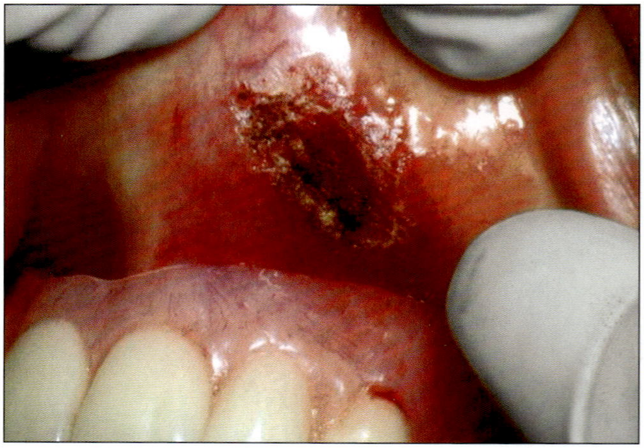

Fig 7-1c Immediate postoperative view of the affected area.

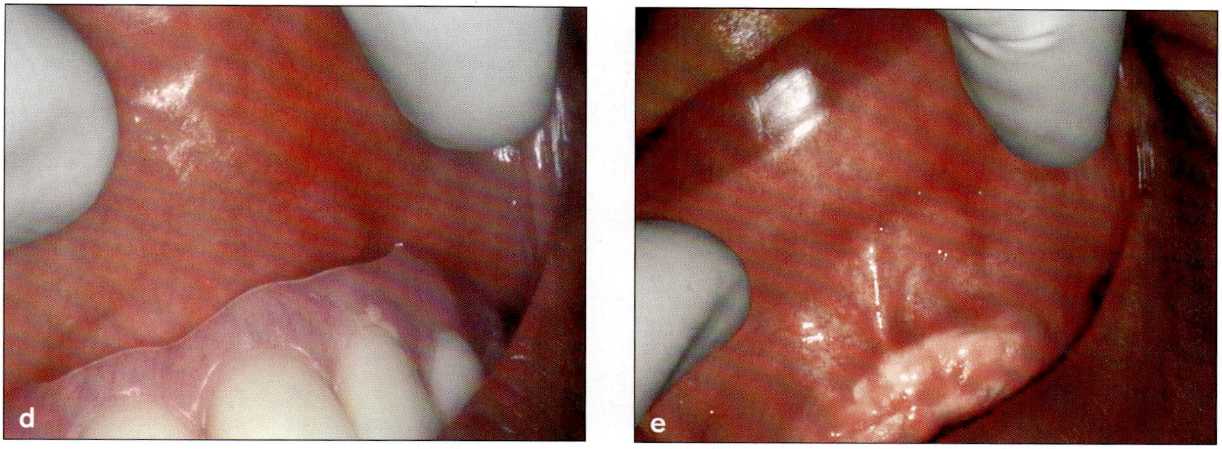

Figs 7-1d and 7-1e Ten-day postoperative views with the denture in place *(d)* and with the denture removed *(e)*.

Purpose of the procedure	Treatment of epulis fissurata
The inflamed epulis fissurata is treated with laser ablation to promote healing.	

Wavelength and settings

CO_2 laser set to 4 W, continuous wave, with an 800 μm ceramic tip.

Alternate wavelengths that may be used

Any laser can be used to perform this procedure.

Clinical tip

Laser ablation of an epulis allows the mucosa to heal with no tissue shrinkage, whereas more conventional methods (eg, using a scalpel) may result in tissue shrinkage during healing. In a patient with a buccal vestibule of inadequate depth, tissue shrinkage may adversely affect denture fit. As with any lesion treatment, the denture base must also be adjusted to prevent recurrent irritation in the area.

Treatment of Inflamed Soft Tissues: Case 2

Chronic denture stomatitis in a 76-year-old female patient.

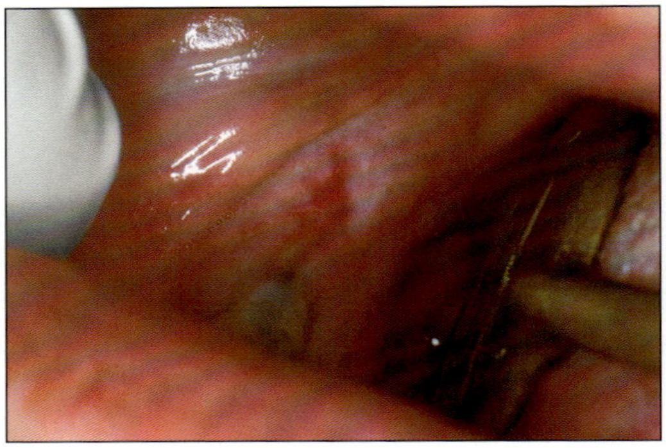

Fig 7-2a Denture sore on the right mandibular ridge.

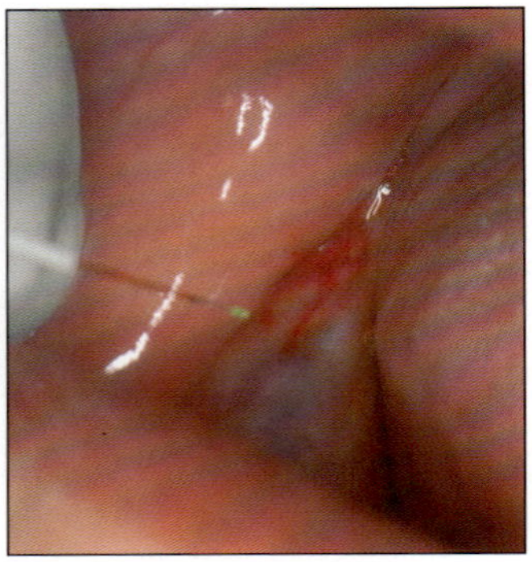

Fig 7-2b A laser fiber-optic tip is used to treat the area.

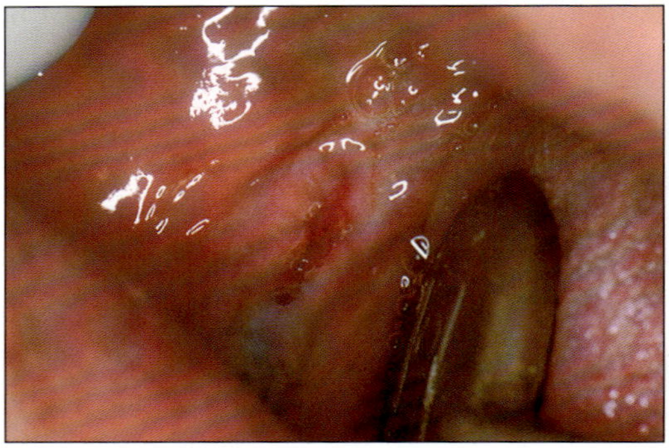

Fig 7-2c Postoperative view of soft tissue area immediately following laser treatment.

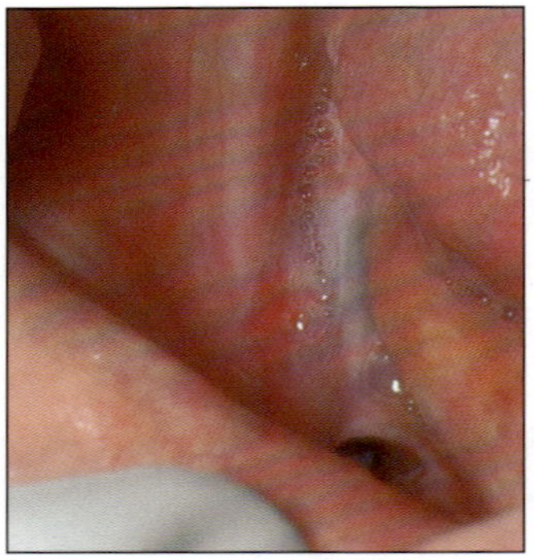

Fig 7-2d One-week postoperative view showing complete healing.

Purpose of the procedure	Treatment of denture sore
Laser ablation on the denture sore results in healing of chronic denture stomatitis.	

Wavelength and settings

Nd:YAG laser set to 1.75 W, 87 mJ, 20 Hz, with a 320 μm fiber.

Alternate wavelengths that may be used

Any laser can be used to perform this procedure.

Soft Tissue Denture Base Modification: Case 1

Contouring of the maxillary denture base in a 50-year-old male patient.

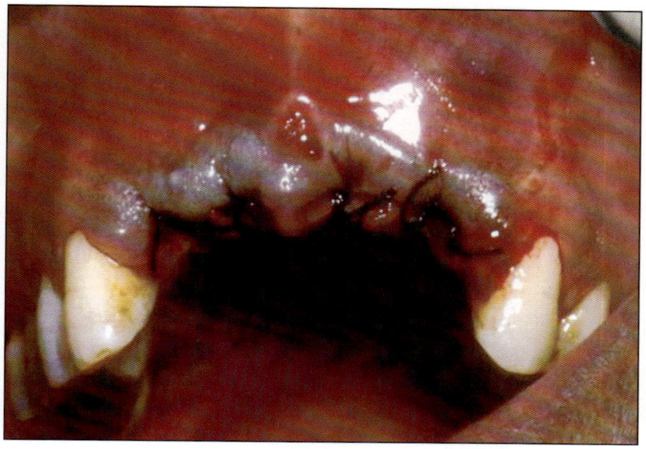

Fig 7-3a Preoperative view showing a partially edentulous maxilla immediately following extraction of the anterior dentition.

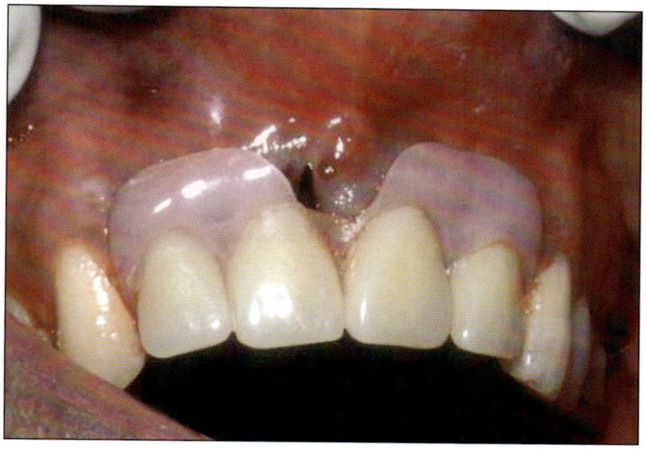

Fig 7-3b Immediate placement of a removable partial prosthesis. Due to the excessive granulomatous tissue at the extraction sites, the denture binds and will not seat properly. Note the blanched tissue gingival to the prosthetic central incisors.

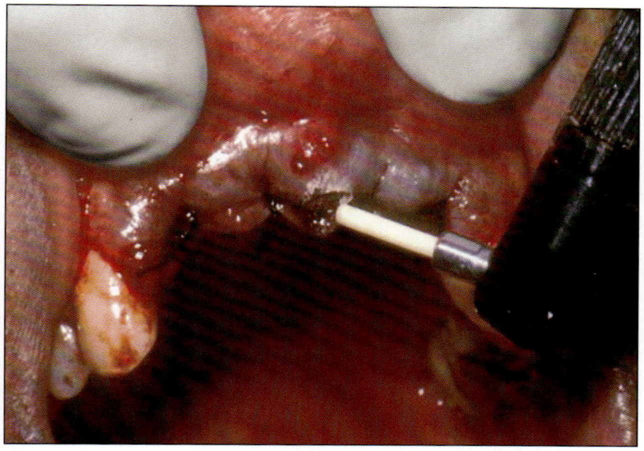

Fig 7-3c Laser removal of the granulomatous tissue. Recontouring the soft tissue will create a better support base for the prosthesis.

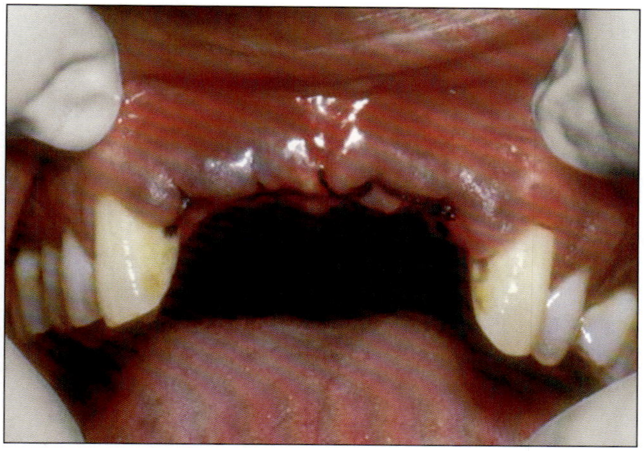

Fig 7-3d Immediate postoperative view showing the recontoured soft tissue of the anterior maxilla.

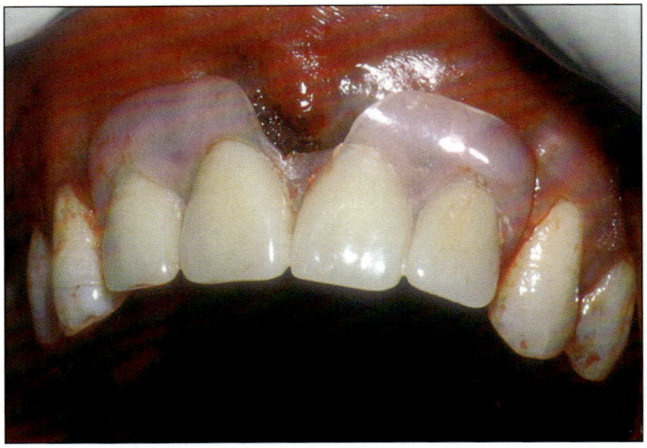

Fig 7-3e The denture is fully reseated on the alveolar ridge, and the gingival tissue is no longer blanched.

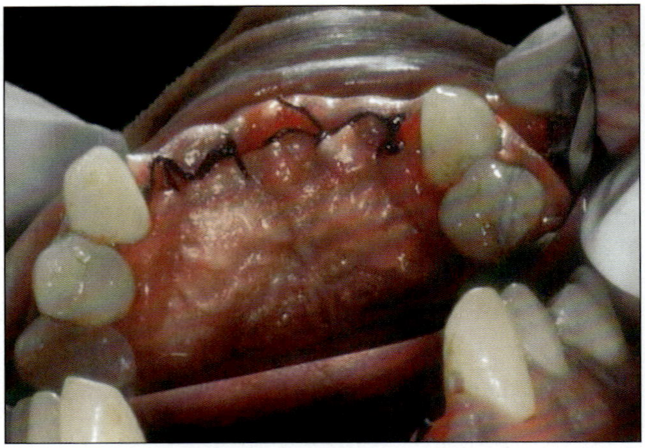

Fig 7-3f Soft tissue healing 1 week following tooth extraction and soft tissue recontouring.

Purpose of the procedure	Soft tissue recontouring
The removable partial denture is fully seated on the alveolar ridge once the granulomatous tissue is removed and the soft tissue has been recontoured.	

Wavelength and settings

CO_2 laser set to 3 W, continuous wave, with an 800 μm ceramic tip.

Alternate wavelengths that may be used

Although any dental laser will work, a wavelength with superior hemostatic ability (ie, CO_2, diode, or Nd:YAG) will ensure that blood clots formed in the coagulated extraction sockets will not be displaced and cause new bleeding.

Soft Tissue Denture Base Modification: Case 2

Contouring of the mandibular denture base in a 74-year-old male patient.

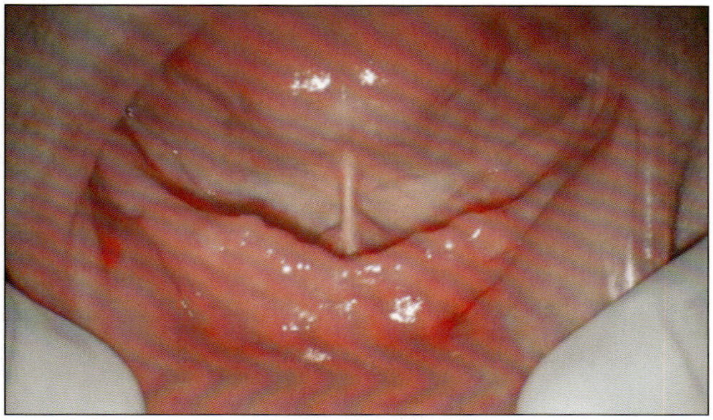

Fig 7-4a Chronically inflamed hyperplastic tissue on the mandibular ridge.

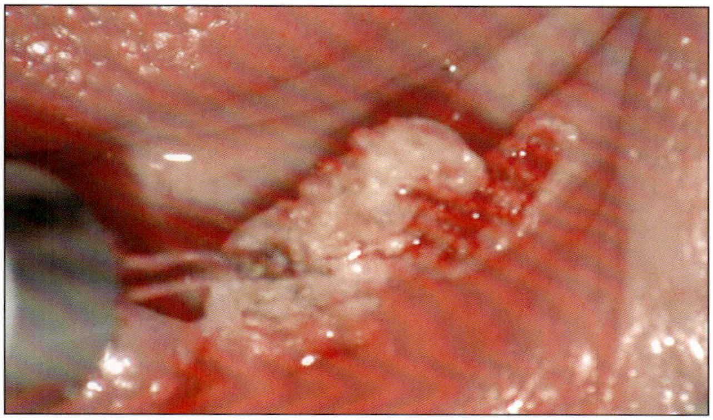

Fig 7-4b Soft tissue laser ablation.

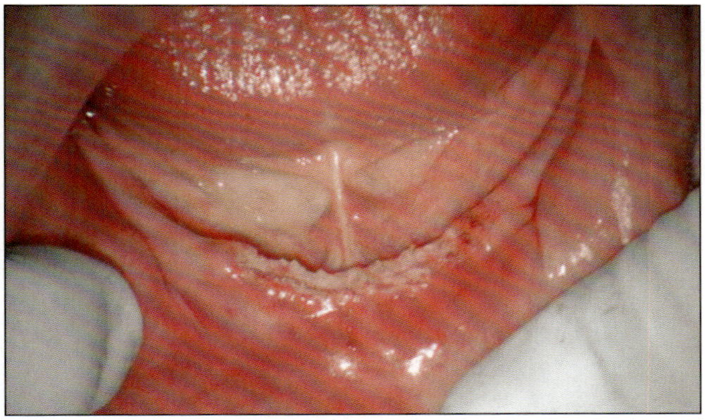

Fig 7-4c Immediate postoperative view of the soft tissue denture base.

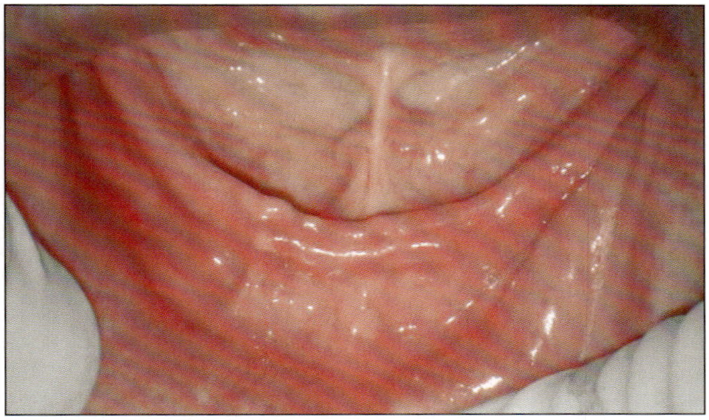

Fig 7-4d The 1-month postoperative view shows complete healing. (Case courtesy of Dr Glen van As, North Vancouver, BC, Canada.)

Purpose of the procedure

Soft tissue recontouring

Laser instrumentation is used to remove chronically inflamed hyperplastic tissue from the mandibular arch.

Wavelength and settings

Er:YAG laser set to 1.5 W, 30 mJ, 50 Hz, with no water spray.

Alternate wavelengths that may be used

Any laser can be used to perform this procedure.

Soft Tissue Denture Base Modification: Case 3

Vestibuloplasty in a 73-year-old male patient.

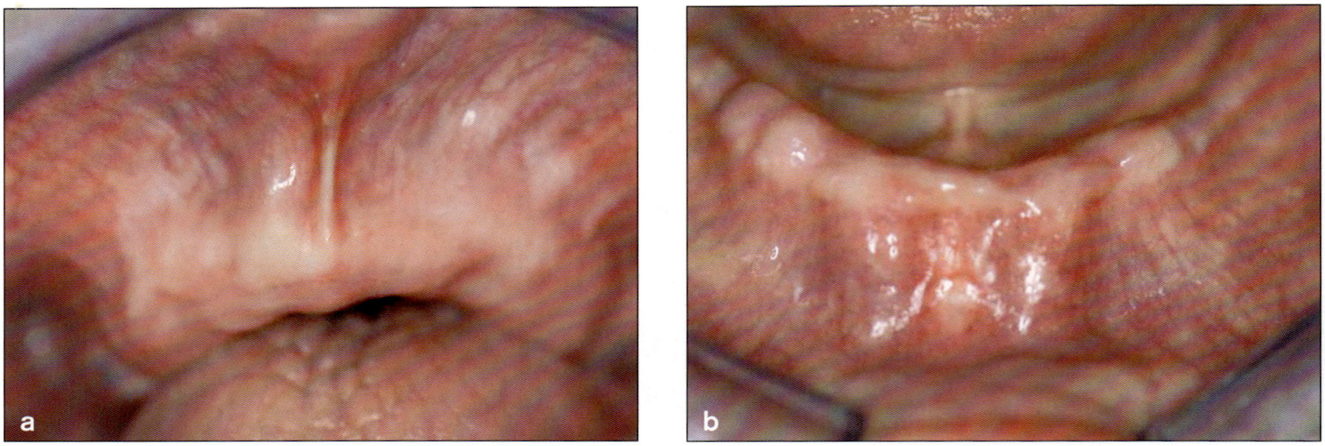

Figs 7-5a and 7-5b Preoperative views of a maxilla *(a)* with both a buccal vestibule of inadequate depth and an anterior frenum attached to the crest of the alveolar ridge, and a mandible *(b)* with a buccal vestibule of inadequate depth.

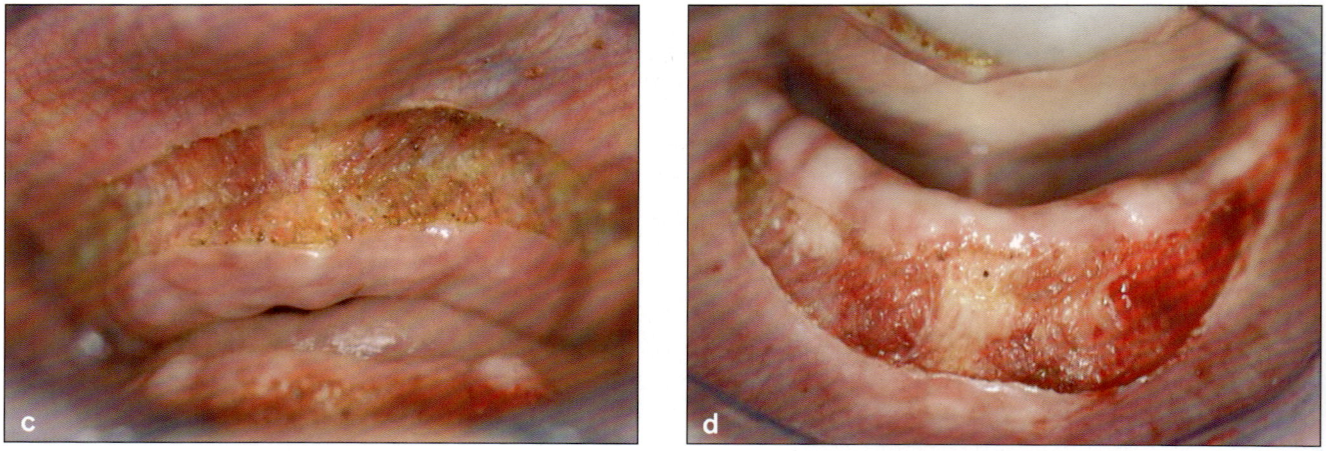

Figs 7-5c and 7-5d Immediate postoperative views of the maxilla *(c)* following the frenectomy and vestibuloplasty and the mandible *(d)* following vestibuloplasty.

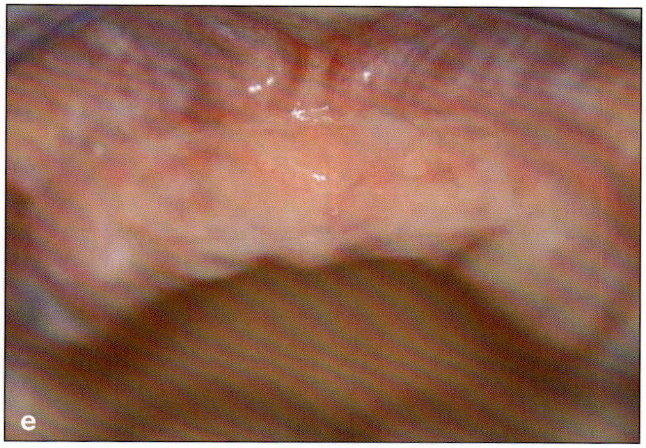

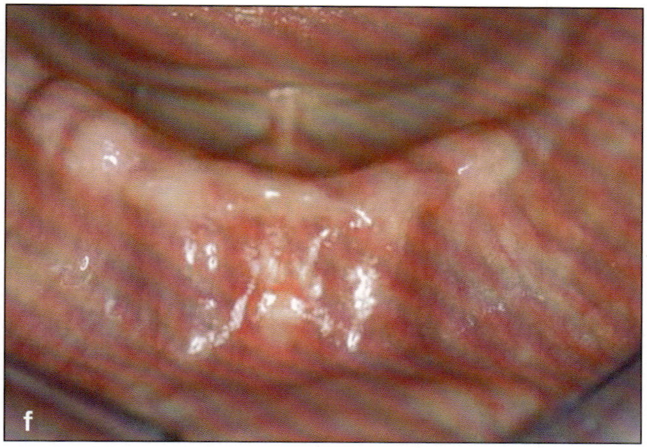

Figs 7-5e and 7-5f Three-month postoperative views of the maxilla *(e)* and mandible *(f)*. (Case courtesy of Dr F. Jay Ohmes, Dardenne Prairie, MO.)

Purpose of the procedure	Vestibuloplasty

The vestibuloplasty increases the amount of keratinized tissue available to support a new removable prosthesis by increasing the depth of the buccal vestibule.

Wavelength and settings

Diode laser, 810 nm, set to 1 W, continuous wave, with a 400 μm fiber.

Alternate wavelengths that may be used

Any laser can be used to perform this procedure.

Clinical tip

The laser incision is made at the junction of keratinized and nonkeratinized tissue. The surface of the nonkeratinized tissue is gently ablated, which allows for a new band of keratinized tissue to form as it heals. This procedure is much simpler than conventional techniques, such as palatal grafts.

Soft Tissue Denture Base Modification: Case 4

Tuberosity reduction in the posterior maxilla in a 65-year-old female patient.

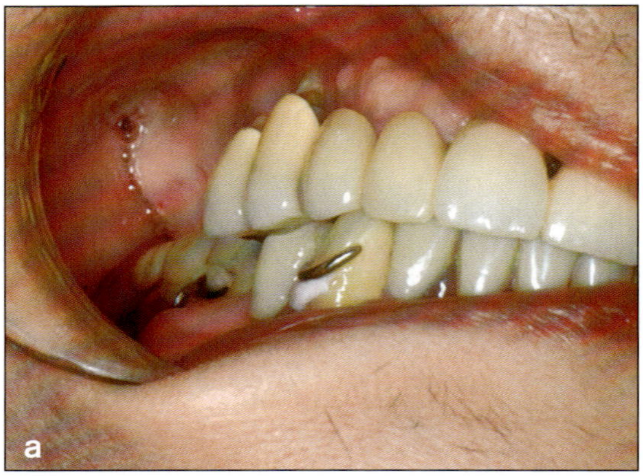

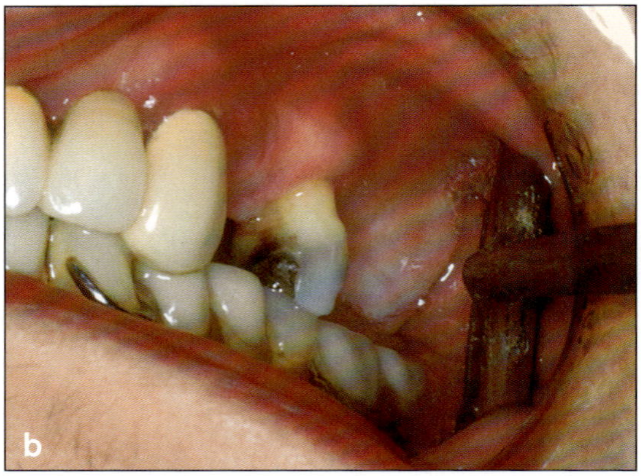

Figs 7-6a and 7-6b Preoperative views of a posterior maxillary tuberosity on the right *(a)* and left *(b)* sides. Because the tuberosities are in occlusion with the mandibular dentition, there is insufficient interocclusal space for a new removable prosthesis.

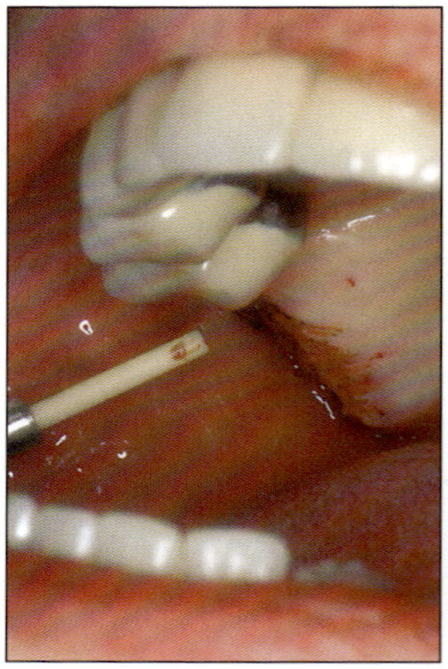

Fig 7-6c Tuberosity reduction in the posterior right maxilla.

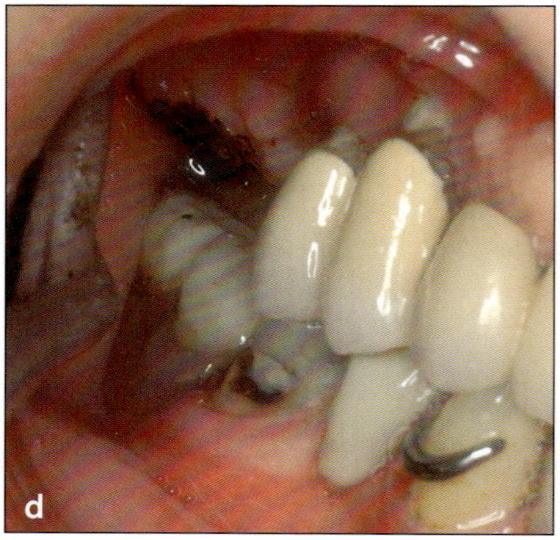

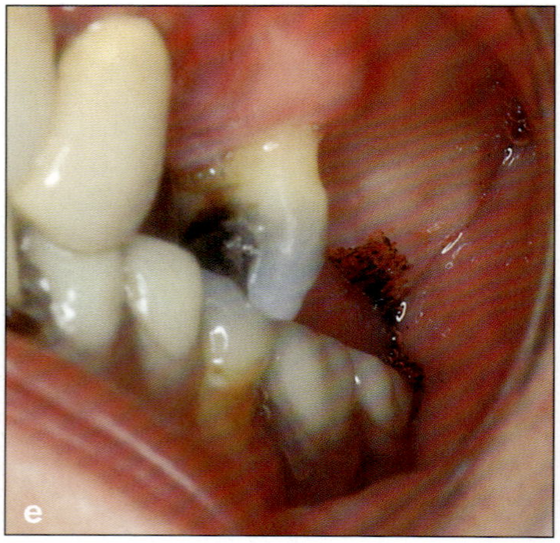

Figs 7-6d and 7-6e Immediate postoperative views of the right *(d)* and left *(e)* sides of the posterior maxilla following laser ablation. This soft tissue surgery is in preparation for a complete maxillary denture.

Purpose of the procedure

Tuberosity reduction

A bilateral soft tissue tuberosity reduction provides room for the placement of an immediate complete maxillary denture.

Wavelength and settings

CO_2 laser set to 4 W, continuous wave, with an 800 μm ceramic tip.

Alternate wavelengths that may be used

Any laser can be used to reduce soft tissue tuberosities. For hard tissue tuberosity reduction, the Er family of lasers is necessary to ablate bone.

Alternate procedure

Tuberosity reductions can also be performed using a combination of a scalpel and a laser. A conventional Y incision is made over the crest of the tuberosity with either the laser or scalpel. Once reflected, the tissue may be ablated with the laser until a sufficient amount is removed.

Clinical tip

Diagnosis is critical for this type of procedure. The clinician must determine whether the tuberosity involves a pneumatized maxillary sinus or hyperplastic tissue. In the case of a pneumatized sinus, a sinus elevation would be an ideal treatment. Preoperative periapical radiographs of the maxillary posterior quadrants or a preoperative panoramic radiograph help to determine the most appropriate treatment plan.

Torus Reduction: Case 1

Removal of a mandibular torus in a 68-year-old female patient.

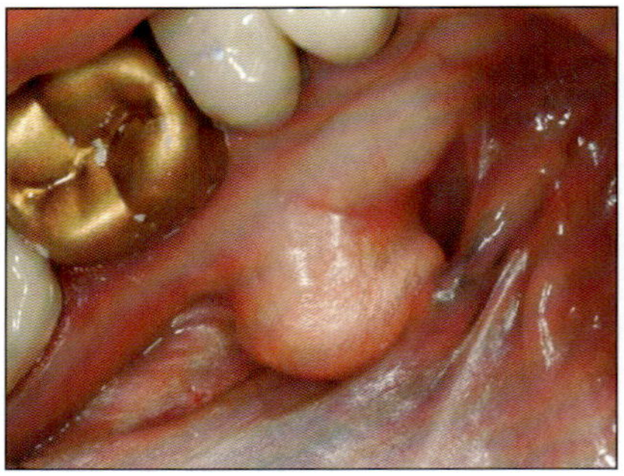

Fig 7-7a Large torus on the lingual aspect of the left mandible.

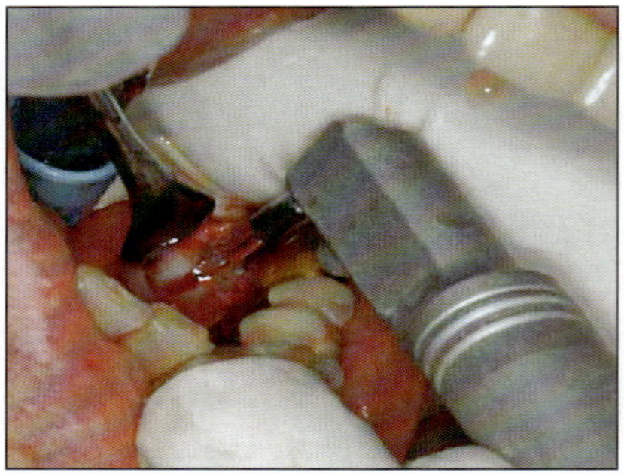

Fig 7-7b An Er laser cuts the osseous protuberance.

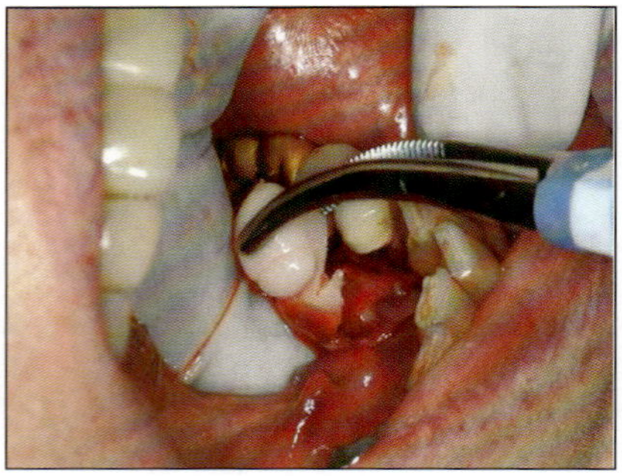

Fig 7-7c Torus removal with a hemostat.

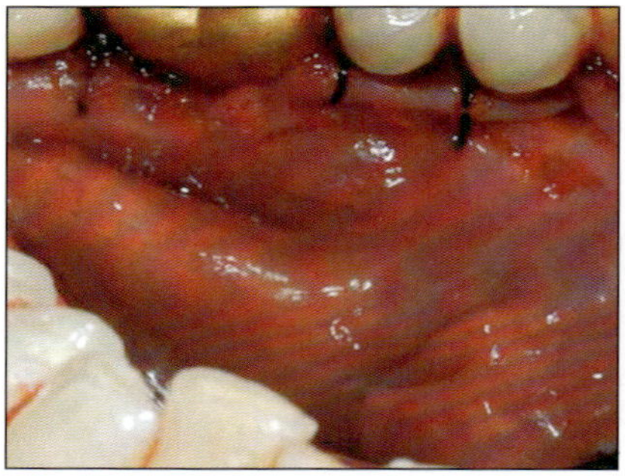

Fig 7-7d Immediate postoperative view.

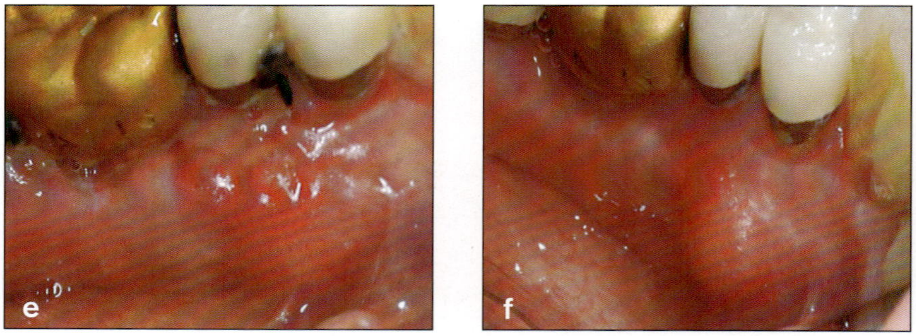

Figs 7-7e and 7-7f Postoperative views 24 hours *(e)* and 2 weeks *(f)* following surgery.

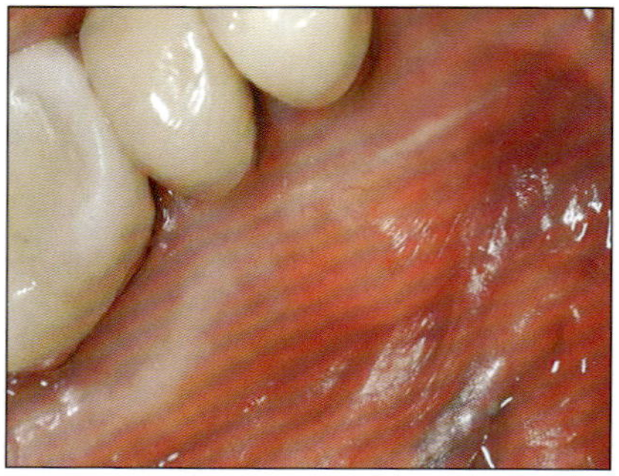

Fig 7-7g At 3 months, the surgical site has completely healed. (Case courtesy of Dr Glenda Payas, Tulsa, OK.)

Purpose of the procedure

Reduction of a mandibular torus

Removal of a torus allows the clinician to recontour the osseous tissue on the lingual aspect of the mandible.

Wavelength and settings

Er:YAG laser set to 500 mJ, 12 Hz, with an 800 μm sapphire tip with water spray. CO_2 laser set to 3 W, continuous wave, defocused.

Alternate wavelengths that may be used

Reflection of the soft tissue flap and hemostasis can be accomplished using any wavelength. However, the osseous reduction can only be performed with Er family lasers.

Alternate procedures

There are many different methods to treat this case. The soft tissue flap may be reflected with either a laser (any wavelength) or a scalpel. The osseous reduction may be performed only with an Er family laser (Er:YAG or Er,Cr:YSGG). If an Er laser is unavailable, a rongeur, bone file, or large round bur in a high-speed handpiece with copious water spray would be acceptable. For hemostasis, any laser would be acceptable, including a CO_2 laser, or a diode or Nd:YAG laser, either of which is absorbed by the pigmented hemoglobin.

Clinical tip

This procedure was performed using a scalpel and two different laser wavelengths. The scalpel was used to reflect a soft tissue flap to gain access to the torus. An Er laser was used to section the torus for removal and to smooth the bone. A CO_2 laser was used to obtain hemostasis at the surgical site.

Torus Reduction: Case 2

Removal of a mandibular torus in an adult patient.

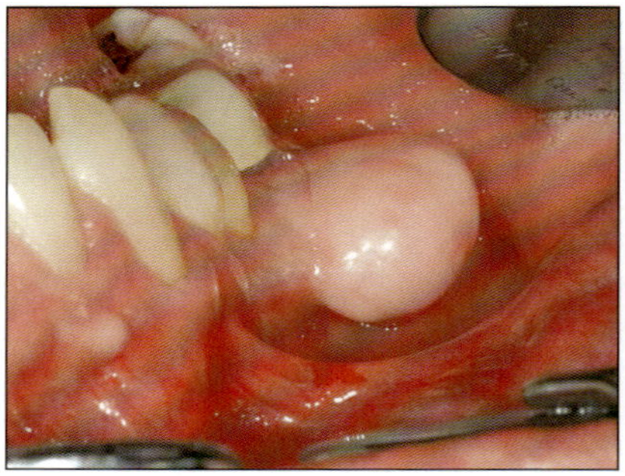

Fig 7-8a Torus on the facial aspect of the mandible.

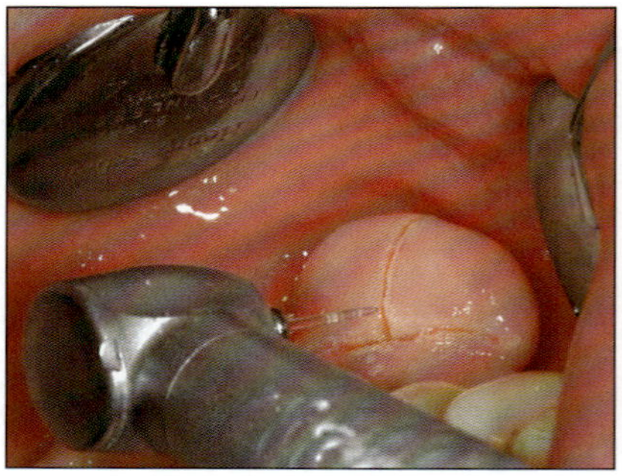

Fig 7-8b A laser incision is made prior to reflection of a soft tissue flap.

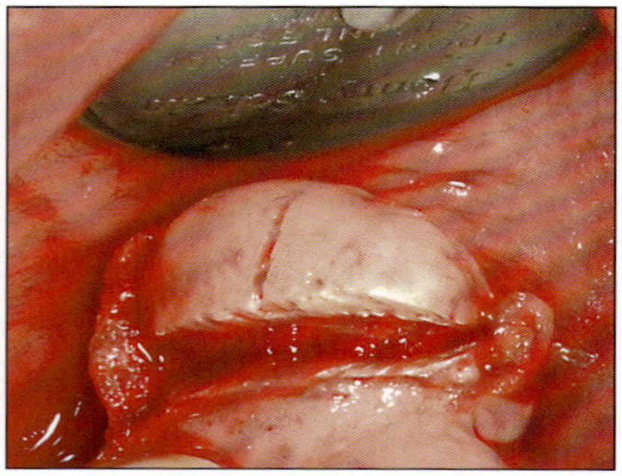

Fig 7-8c Exposed osseous protruberence sectioned by laser energy.

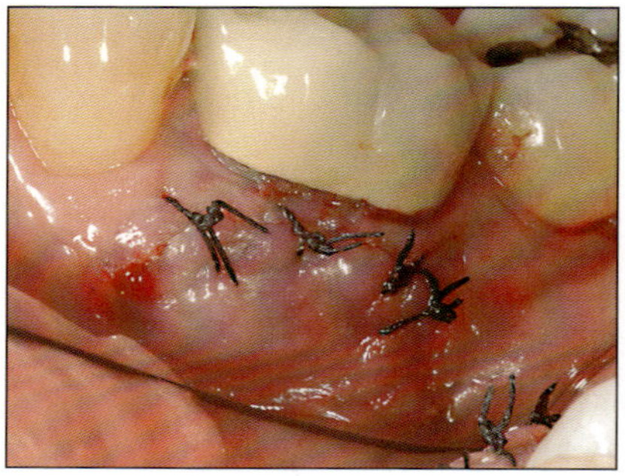

Fig 7-8d Immediate postoperative view following the removal of the torus, the contouring of the osseous tissue, and the suturing of the soft tissue in place.

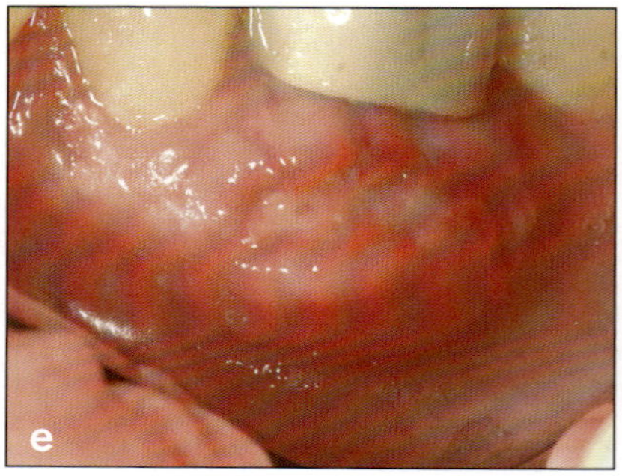

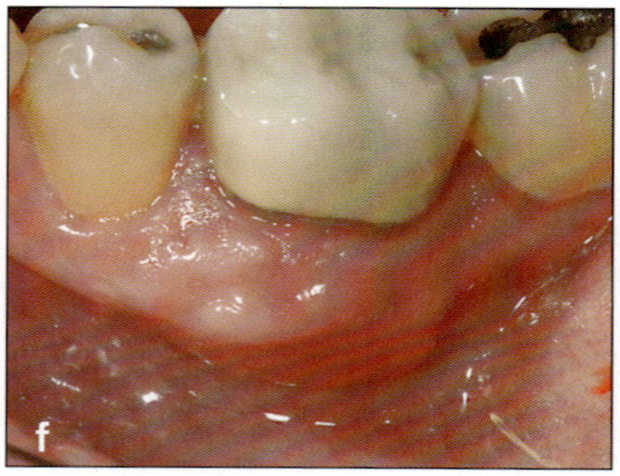

Figs 7-8e and 7-8f Postoperative views showing the surgical site following suture removal at 8 days *(e)* and with evident redundant soft tissue at 1 month *(f)*.

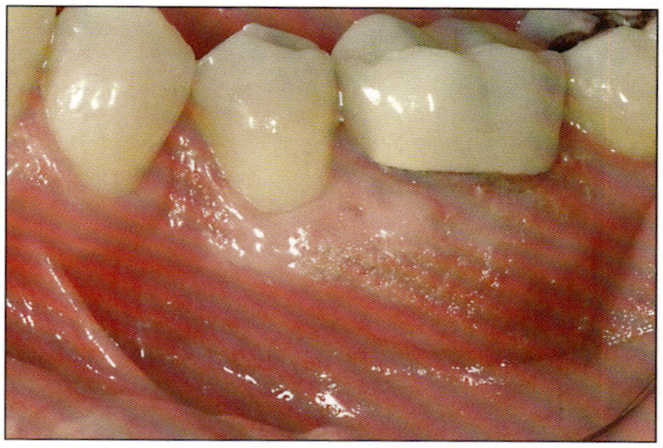

Fig 7-8g Immediate postoperative view following soft tissue contouring with the laser.

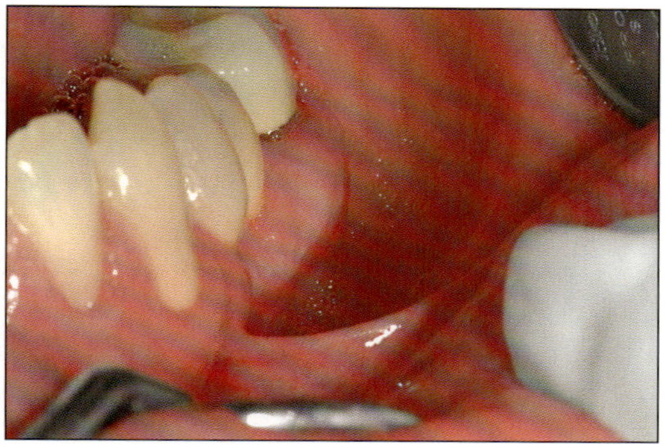

Fig 7-8h Two months following the removal of the torus, the surgical site has completely healed. (Case courtesy of Dr Arthur Scott, Metairie, LA.)

Purpose of the procedure

Reduction of a mandibular torus

Removal of the torus allows the clinician to recontour the osseous tissue on the facial aspect of the mandible.

Wavelength and settings

Er,Cr:YSGG laser; settings for soft tissue ablation: 1.5 W, 75 mJ, 20 Hz, with a 400 µm sapphire tip and 7% water spray; settings for osseous tissue ablation: 3.5 W, 175 mJ, 20 Hz, with a 600 µm sapphire tip and 40% water spray.

Alternate wavelengths that may be used

Reflection of the soft tissue flap and hemostasis can be accomplished using any wavelength. However, the osseous reduction can only be performed with the Er family of lasers.

Alternate procedures

As with the previous case, there are many different techniques to perform this surgical procedure. Lasers or scalpels can be used to reflect the soft tissue flap. The Er:YAG or Er,Cr:YSGG laser can be used to remove the bone. If an Er laser is not available, conventional techniques would be necessary for the osseous surgery. Postoperative recontouring of the soft tissue can be performed with any soft tissue laser.

Suggested Reading

Baraldi CE, Puricelli E, Kulkes S, Martins GL. Er:YAG laser in oral soft tissue surgery [abstract 59]. J Oral Laser Appl 2001;1:24.

Convissar RA, Gharemani EH. Laser treatment as an adjunct to removable prosthetic care. Gen Dent 1995;43:336–341.

Hopkins R. Textbook of Preprosthetic Oral Surgery. London: Wolfe Medical, 1987.

Ishikawa I, Aoki A, Takasaki AA. Potential applications of Erbium:YAG laser in periodontics. J Periodont Res 2004;39:275–285.

Kesler G. Clinical applications of lasers during removable prosthetic reconstruction. Dent Clin North Am 2004;48:963–969.

Pick RM, Pecaro BC. Use of the CO_2 laser in soft tissue dental surgery. Lasers Surg Med 1987; 7:207–213.

Rowson JE. The contact diode laser—A useful instrument for excising oral lesions [abstract]. Br J Oral Maxillofac Surg 1995;33:123.

White JM, Goodis HE, Rose CL. Use of the pulsed Nd:YAG laser for intraoral soft tissue surgery. Lasers Surg Med 1991;11:455–461.

8

ESTHETIC LASER DENTISTRY

Some procedures in cosmetic dentistry do not involve treatment of disease or pathology, and, in many cases, there is no need for restoration. This chapter deals with esthetic treatment plans that do not require dental restoration and have the primary objective of enhancing the patient's smile. Shaping of the gingival contour and overall osseous architecture for esthetic symmetry (eg, recontouring gingival margins to reduce a "gummy" smile) may be achieved with lasers. Laser instruments can be used to remove gingival hyperpigmentation, which is a part of cosmetic treatment plans in many cultures. In addition, tooth discoloration can be treated by laser-activated tooth whitening. Dental lasers are ideal for use in esthetic treatment plans because all dental laser wavelengths may be used for soft tissue surgery. However, recontouring or removal of bone or tooth structure can only be performed by lasers from the erbium (Er) family.

Good periodontal health demands a stable dentogingival complex. Clinicians must maintain a viable biologic width when manipulating hard or soft tissues for a desired esthetic outcome. No matter which laser wavelength is used to accomplish the treatment plan, a successful outcome must be based on sound biologic principles. Violation of the biologic width, whether by scalpel, rotary instrument, or laser, will compromise the success of the treatment plan.

Esthetic Crown Lengthening

Clinical tip

In all cases of crown lengthening, a complete periodontal and radiographic examination must be performed, including pocket depth measurement (Fig 8-1), before planning treatment. The clinical cases presented in this section followed the established protocol of measuring the biologic width preoperatively and confirming it postoperatively. Once the biologic width is determined, various methods may be used to guide tissue removal during treatment. An indelible marker can outline the desired gingival contour (Figs 8-2 and 8-3), and lasers can mark the tissue contours as well. In Fig 8-4, a CO_2 laser ablates a few layers of tissue, while the diode laser used in Fig 8-5 ablates an outline of dots through the soft tissue.

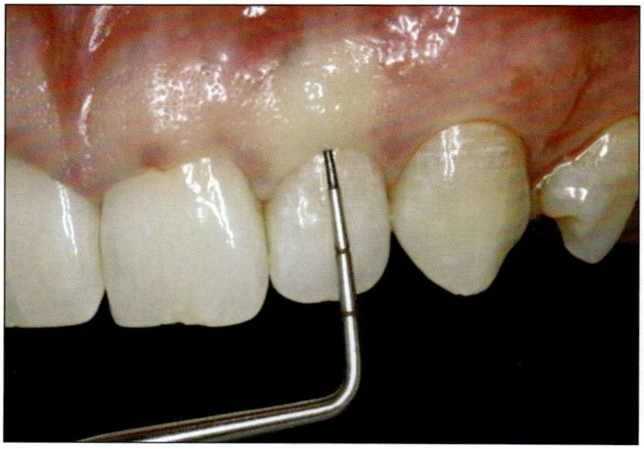

Fig 8-1 Measurement of periodontal probling to determine biologic width.

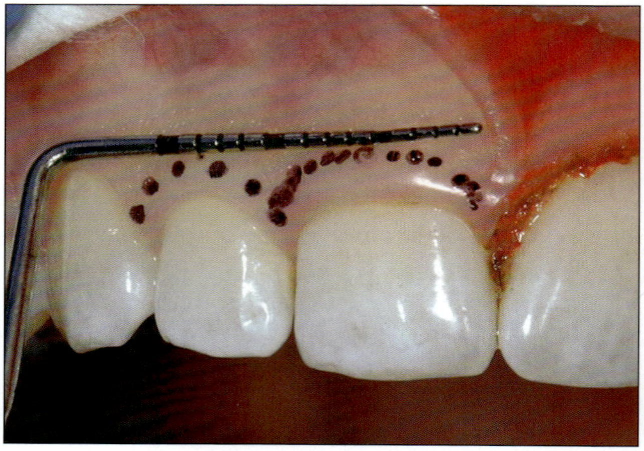

Fig 8-2 Gingival contour outlined by dots made with an indelible marker.

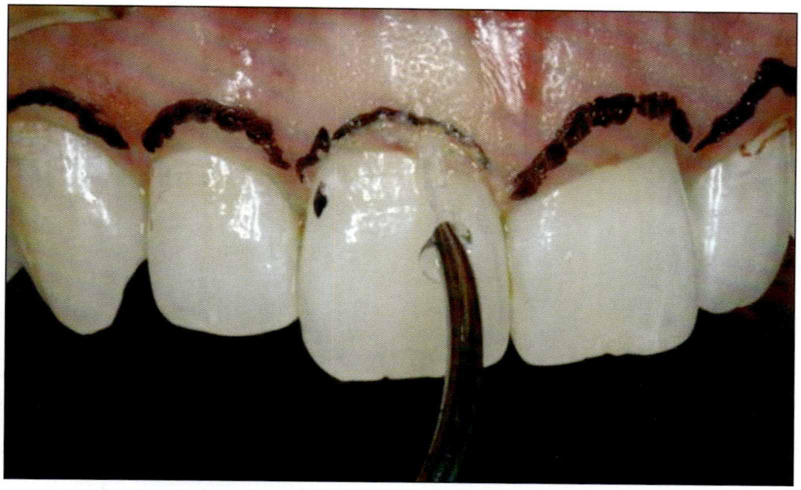

Fig 8-3 A line of indelible ink outlines the new gingival contour. (Figs 8-1 to 8-3 courtesy of Dr David Hornbrook, La Mesa, CA.)

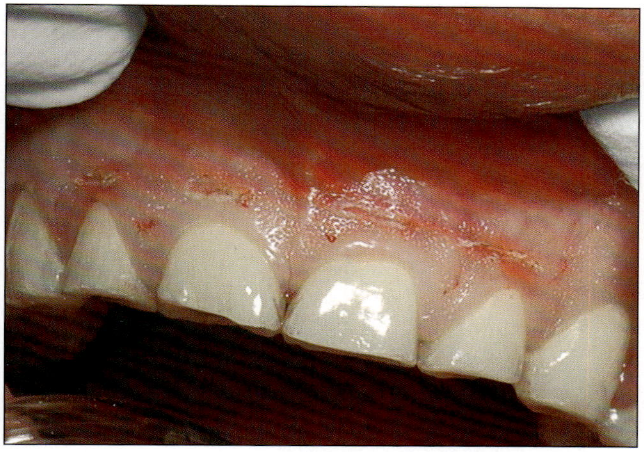

Fig 8-4 A CO_2 laser lightly marks the apices of the new gingival contour.

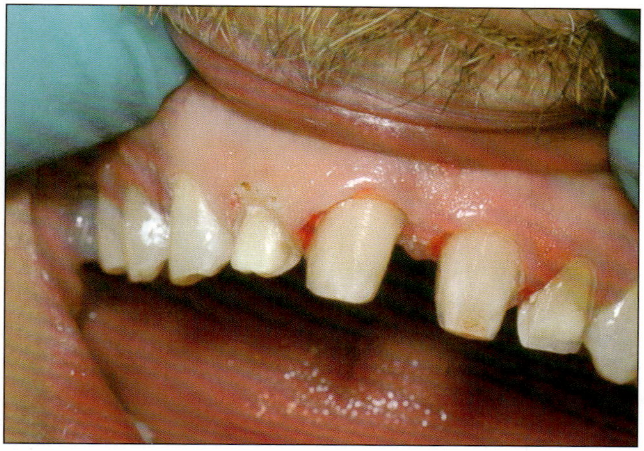

Fig 8-5 A diode laser is used to outline the desired tissue contour in dots of ablated tissue.

Esthetic Crown Lengthening: Case 1

Crown lengthening in a 26-year-old female patient.

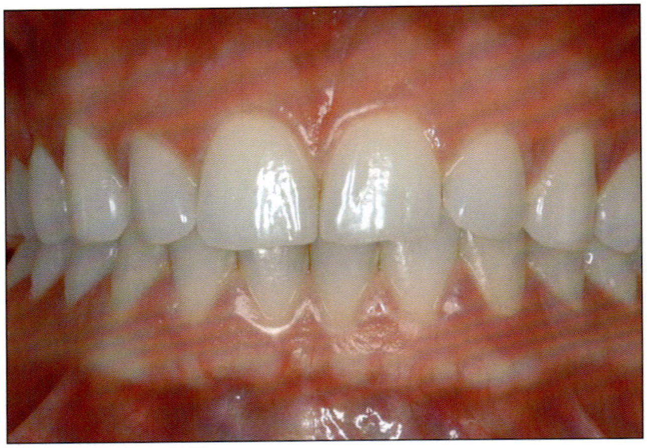

Fig 8-6a Preoperative view showing short clinical crowns with square shapes.

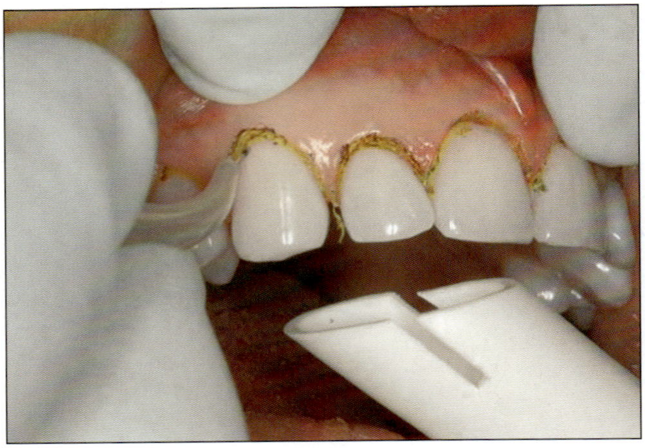

Fig 8-6b Resculpting of the gingival contours during laser ablation.

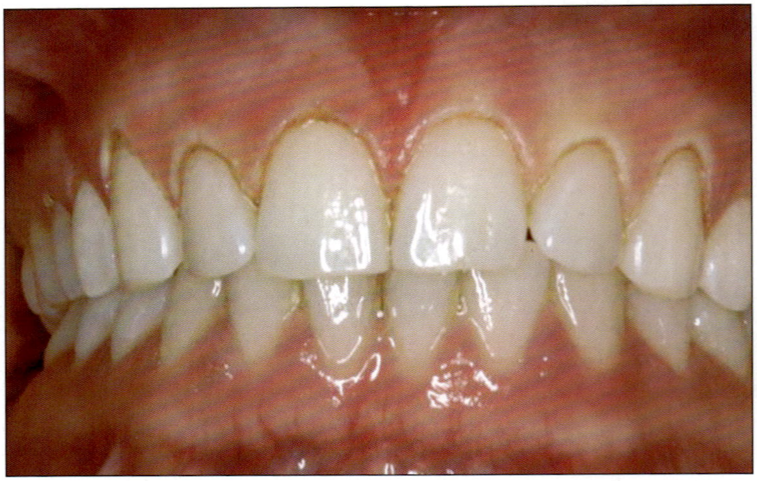

Fig 8-6c Postoperative view immediately following the procedure. The new gingival contour gives the appearance of longer anterior teeth.

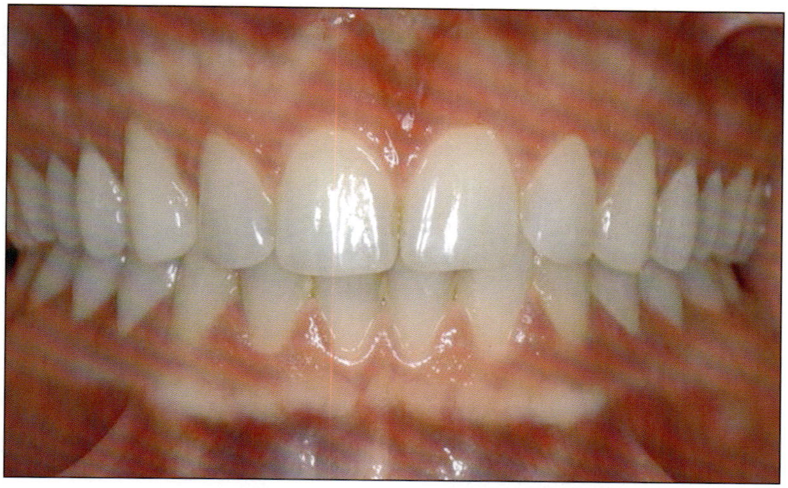

Fig 8-6d Two-week postoperative view of the completed treatment. The gingival tissue is completely healed and shows no evidence of the recent surgical procedure. The beautiful gingival contours add to an esthetically pleasing smile. (Case courtesy of Dr Timothy Adams, Las Vegas, NV.)

Purpose of the procedure	Crown lengthening
The longer and more rectangular clinical crowns reduce the amount of gingiva that the patient reveals when smiling.	

Wavelength and settings

Diode laser, 810 nm, set to 0.8 W, continuous wave, with a 400 μm fiber.

Alternate wavelengths that may be used

While any dental laser wavelength can be used to accomplish the same procedure, extra care must be taken when using CO_2 and Er lasers because their wavelengths can ablate the enamel tissue if too much power is used during exposure. When using an Er family or CO_2 laser, the clinician should carefully direct the laser energy away from the tooth structure or place an instrument (eg, periosteal elevator) between the tooth and the gingiva to act as a shield.

Esthetic Crown Lengthening: Case 2

Crown lengthening in a 22-year-old female patient.

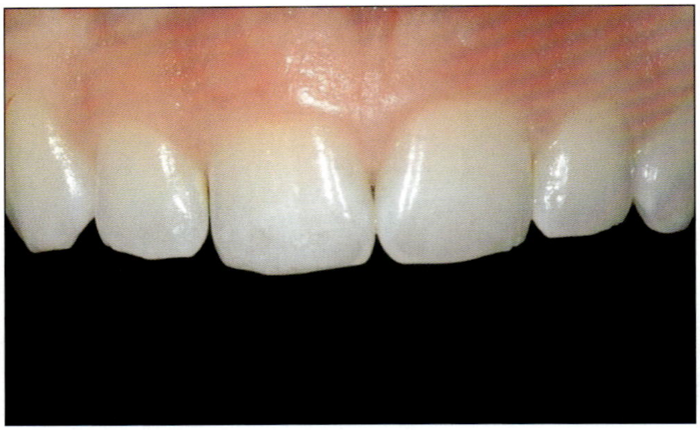

Fig 8-7a Short clinical crowns and overabundance of gingiva are evident in the initial clinical situation.

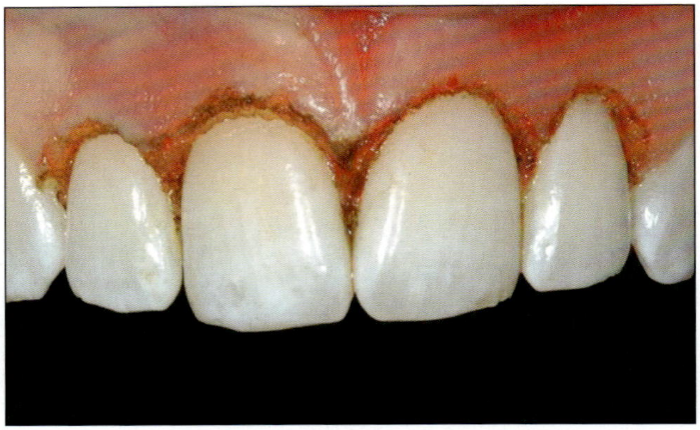

Fig 8-7b Intraoperative view of the progressing tissue ablation.

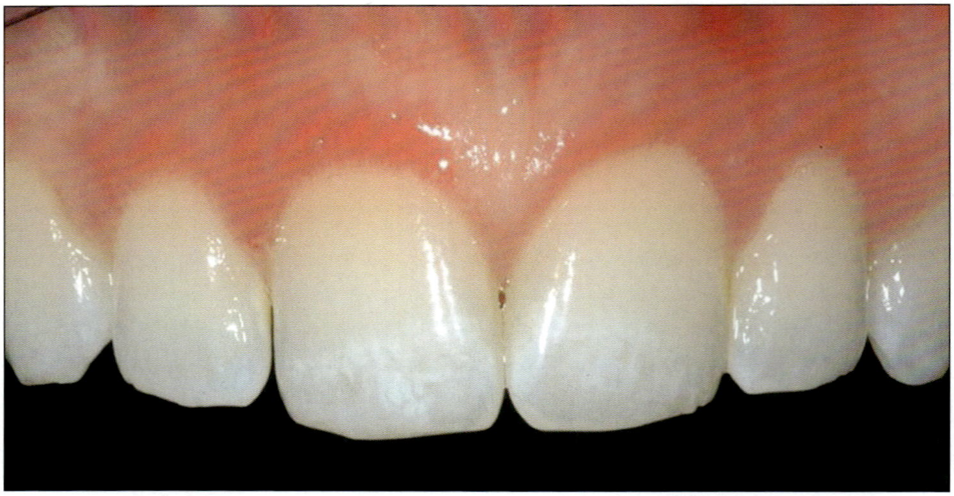

Fig 8-7c Definitive gingival contour 1 month postoperative. Repositioning the gingiva has dramatically lengthened the clinical crowns. (Case courtesy of Dr David Hornbrook, La Mesa, CA.)

Purpose of the procedure	Crown lengthening

By increasing the clinical crown length of the anterior dentition, the clinician reduces the amount of gingiva that the patient reveals when smiling.

Wavelength and settings

Er laser set to 2 W, 40 mJ, 50 Hz, with a 400 μm tip.

Alternate wavelengths that may be used

While any dental laser wavelength can be used to accomplish the same procedure, extra care must be taken when using CO_2 and Er lasers because their wavelengths can ablate the enamel tissue if too much power is used during exposure. When using an Er family or CO_2 laser, the clinician should carefully direct the laser energy away from the tooth structure or place an instrument (eg, periosteal elevator) between the tooth and the gingiva to act as a shield.

Esthetic Crown Lengthening: Case 3

Crown lengthening in a 30-year-old male patient.

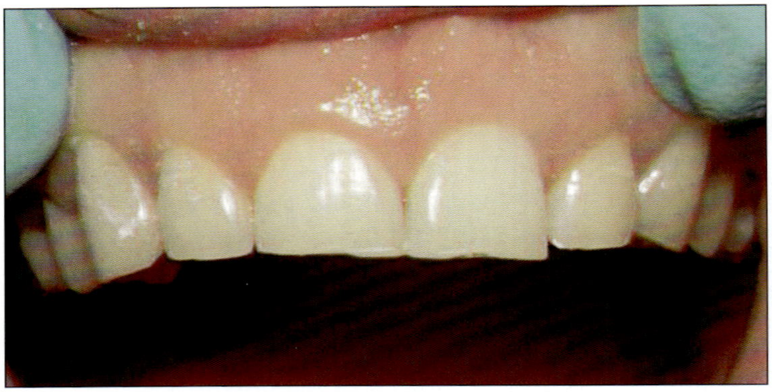

Fig 8-8a The preoperative view shows thick gingival tissue covering the necks of the teeth and creating an uneven contour.

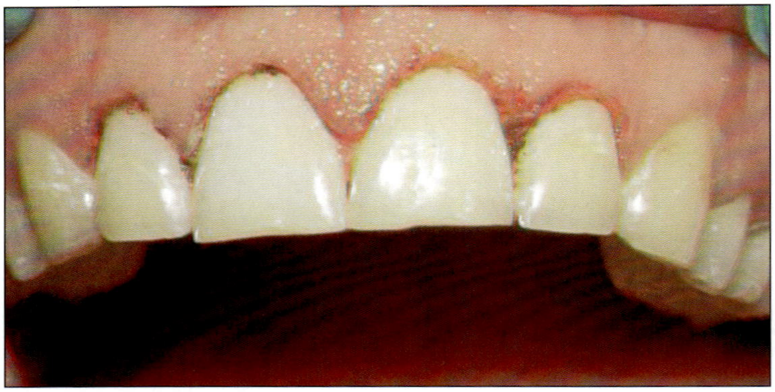

Fig 8-8b Postoperative view immediately following the tissue recontouring. The beveling and thinning of the gingival margin creates good physiologic contours.

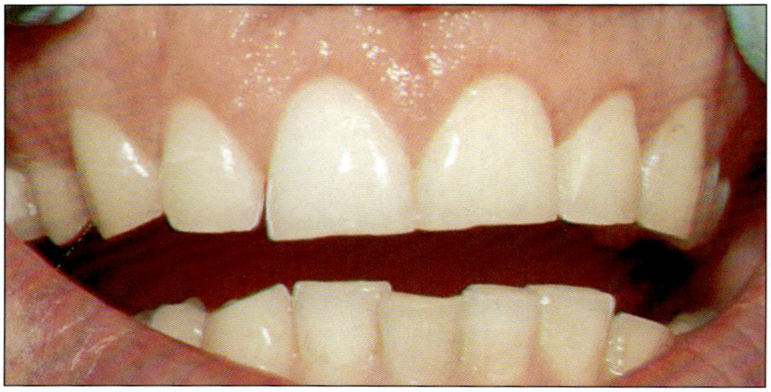

Fig 8-8c Four-month postoperative view showing an esthetic gingival contour with no tissue regrowth.

Purpose of the procedure	Crown lengthening

Once the excessive tissue covering the necks of the anterior teeth is removed, the sizes of the clinical crowns can be balanced by creating an even marginal contour.

Wavelength and settings

Diode laser, 810 nm, set to 1 W, continuous wave, with a 400 μm fiber.

Alternate wavelengths that may be used

While any dental laser wavelength can be used to accomplish the same procedure, extra care must be taken when using CO_2 and Er lasers because their wavelengths can ablate the enamel tissue if too much power is used during exposure. When using an Er family or CO_2 laser, the clinician should carefully direct the laser energy away from the tooth structure or place an instrument (eg, periosteal elevator) between the tooth and the gingiva to act as a shield.

Clinical tip

The initial ablation for tissue removal often leaves a thick, blunt gingival edge. The clinician must shape and bevel the edge to create a more esthetic gingival margin with a natural contour and to minimize tissue regrowth. Crown lengthening in case 1 was performed with a diode laser at 0.8 W, continuous wave, while the same diode laser was used in case 3 with a setting at 1 W, continuous wave. As previously discussed in chapter 2, clinicians must be aware of the quality of the soft tissue (eg, thickness and degree of melanin pigment) and adjust the variable properties of the laser instrument accordingly.

Hyperpigmentation Removal

Laser energy may be used to remove gingival hyperpigmentation and lighten tissue pigment. In many cultures, lighter-colored gingiva is considered more esthetic. Because melanin, the primary pigment chromophore in gingiva, readily absorbs diode and neodymium-doped yttrium aluminum garnet (Nd:YAG) wavelengths, these lasers are ideal for pigment removal. However, some studies favor the Er family or CO_2 wavelengths, which easily ablate soft tissue because of the high water content of the gingiva.[1–3] The three cases presented in this section deal specifically with melanin hyperpigmentation. The same technique is also applicable to amalgam tattoos and other soft tissue discolorations of similar etiology.

Clinical tip

Dentists must discuss the patient's desires and expectations prior to performing the procedure in order to ensure success. In certain cases, some repigmentation may occur after several months, but, generally, patients are pleased with the results of the procedure.

Hyperpigmentation Removal: Case 1

Gingival depigmentation in a 28-year-old female patient.

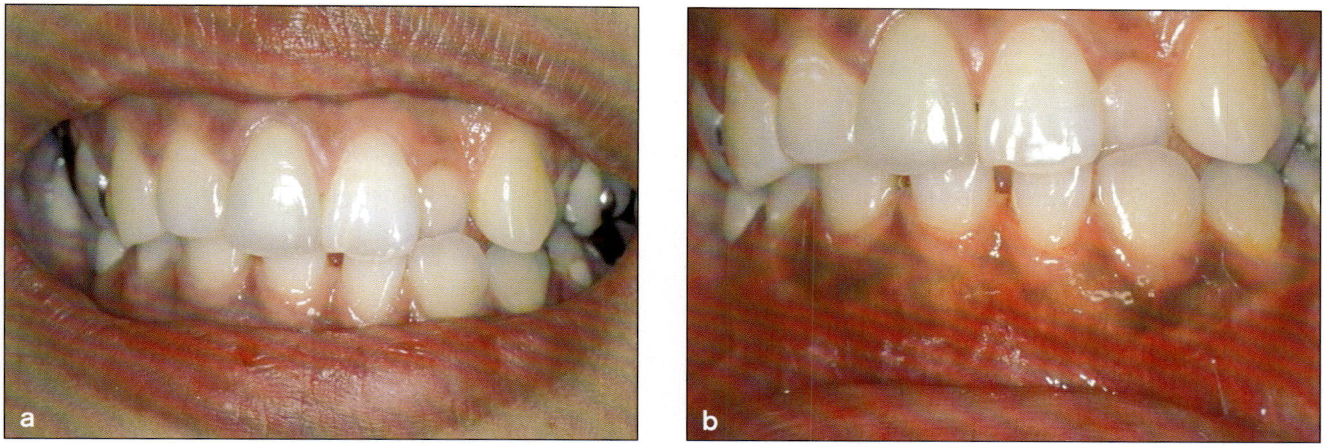

Figs 8-9a and 8-9b Preoperative views of the dark, melanotic gingiva in the maxillary *(a)* and mandibular *(b)* arches.

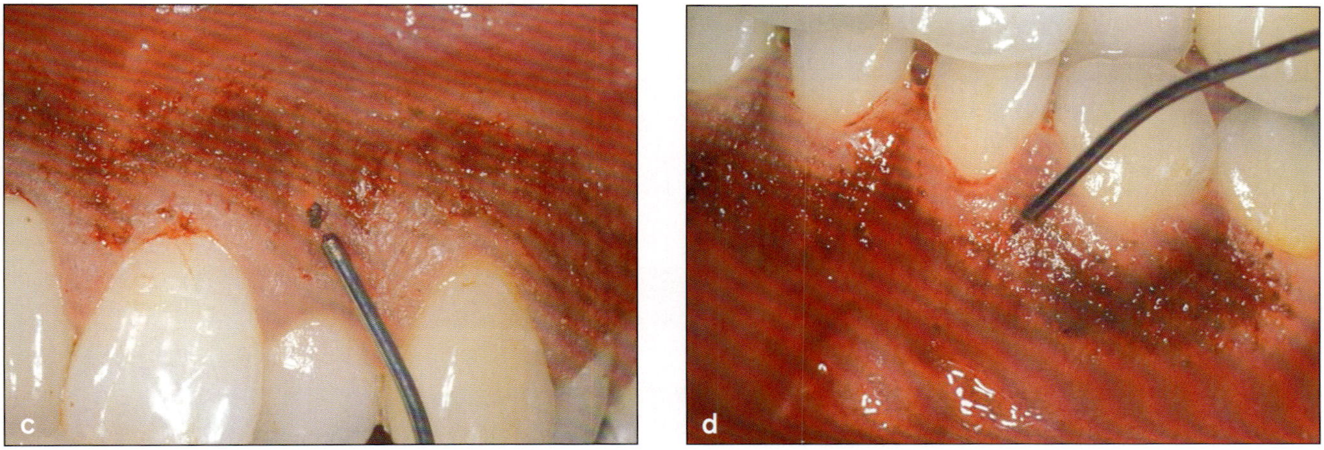

Figs 8-9c and 8-9d Intraoperative views of laser depigmentation in the maxillary *(c)* and mandibular *(d)* arches.

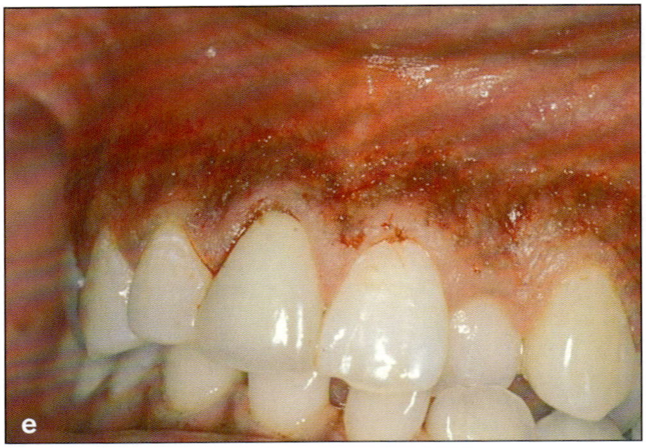

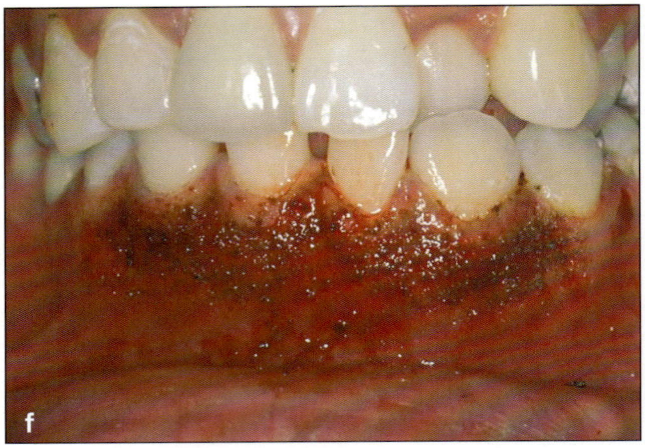

Figs 8-9e and 8-9f Postoperative views of the maxillary *(e)* and mandibular *(f)* arches immediately following the procedure.

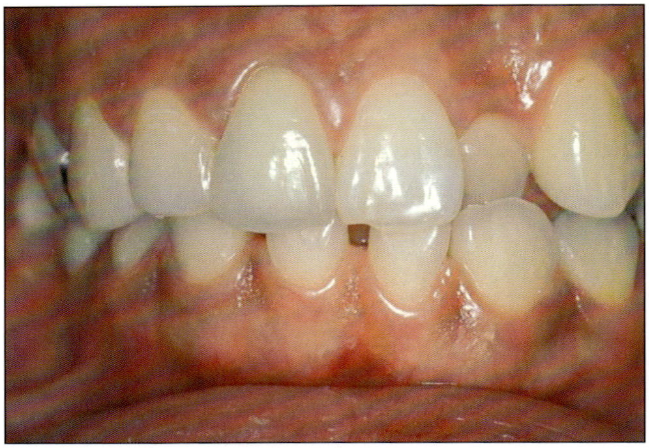

Fig 8-9g One-week postoperative view showing complete healing and dramatic depigmentation.

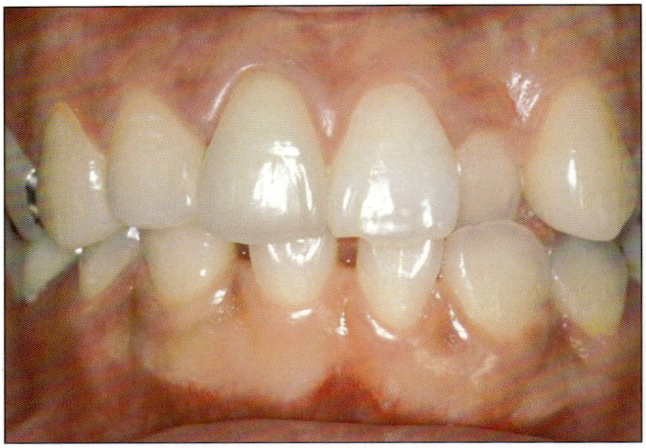

Fig 8-9h After 3 months, no repigmentation had occurred. (Case courtesy of Dr Hiroshi Umemoto, Kawasaki, Japan.)

Purpose of the procedure	Removal of gingival hyperpigmentation

Wavelength and settings
Nd:YAG laser set to 80 mJ, 20 Hz, with a 320 µm fiber.
Alternate wavelengths that may be used
Any laser can be used to perform this procedure.

Hyperpigmentation Removal: Case 2

Gingival depigmentation in a 26-year-old female patient.

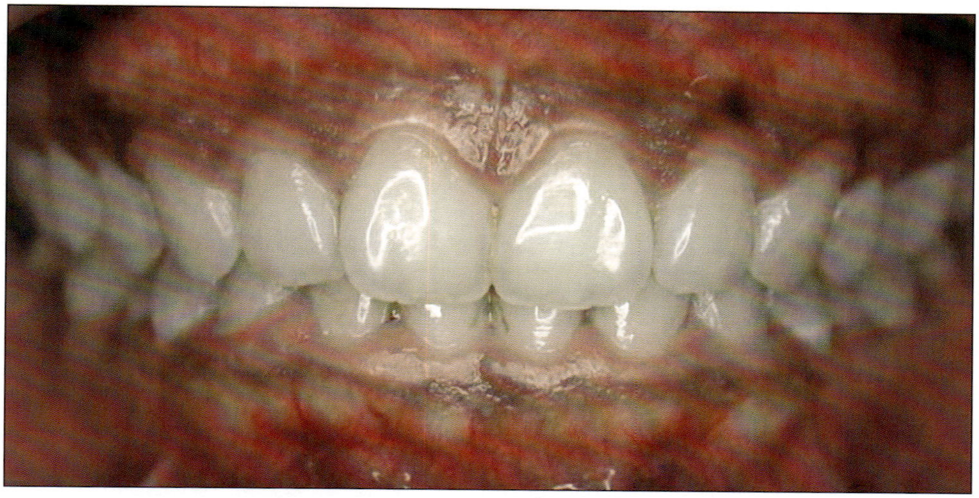

Fig 8-10a Preoperative view of hyperpigmented gingiva.

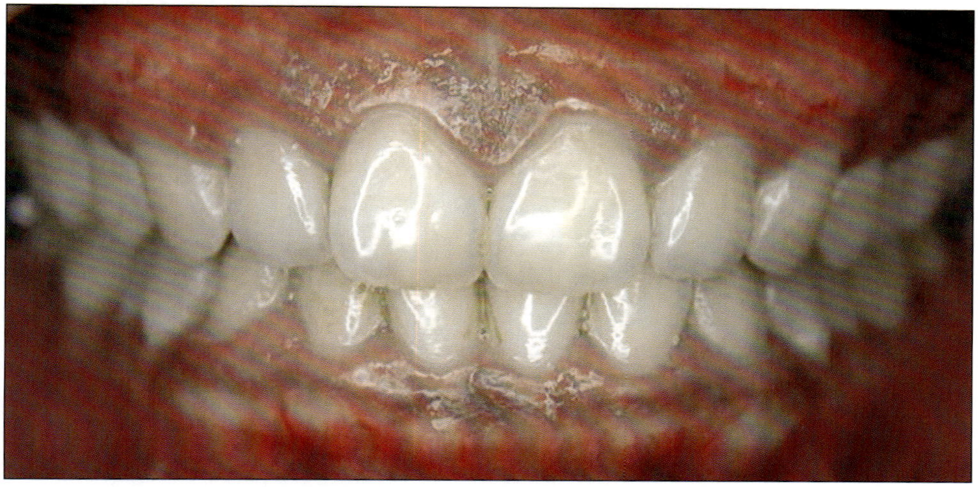

Fig 8-10b Six-day postoperative view.

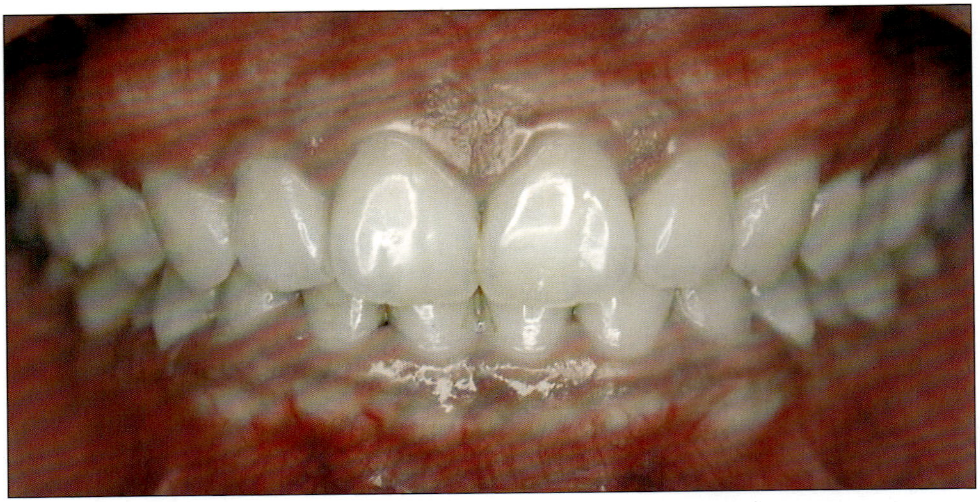

Fig 8-10c Six-month postoperative view. (Case courtesy of Dr Kenneth Luk, Hong Kong, China.)

Purpose of the procedure	Removal of gingival hyperpigmentation

Wavelength and settings

Diode laser, 810 nm; settings at average power: 9.9 W, with a 600 μm fiber, and copious water irrigation; settings at peak power: 30 W, 20,000 Hz.

Alternate wavelengths that may be used

Any laser can be used to perform this procedure.

Clinical tip

In this case, a digitally pulsed diode instrument was used, which allows for repetition rates up to 20,000 pulses per second (Hz). Most diode lasers only provide between 10 and 50 pulses per second. Although a high-power setting was used, the continuous water flow ensured that minimal thermal damage would occur.

Hyperpigmentation Removal: Case 3

Gingival depigmentation in a 23-year-old female patient.

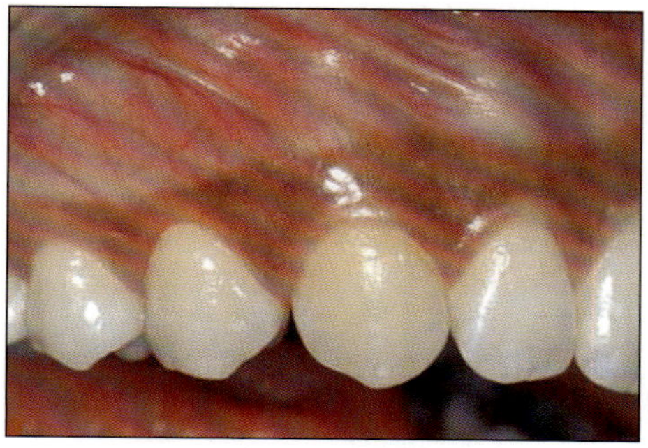

Fig 8-11a Preoperative view showing a dark band of melanotic gingiva in the maxilla.

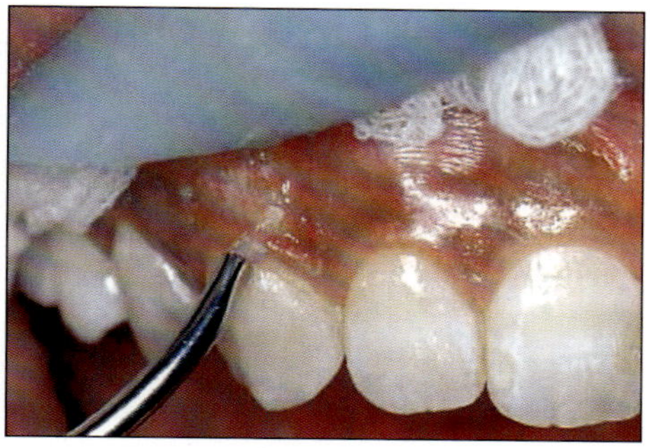

Fig 8-11b Intraoperative view at beginning of the laser procedure.

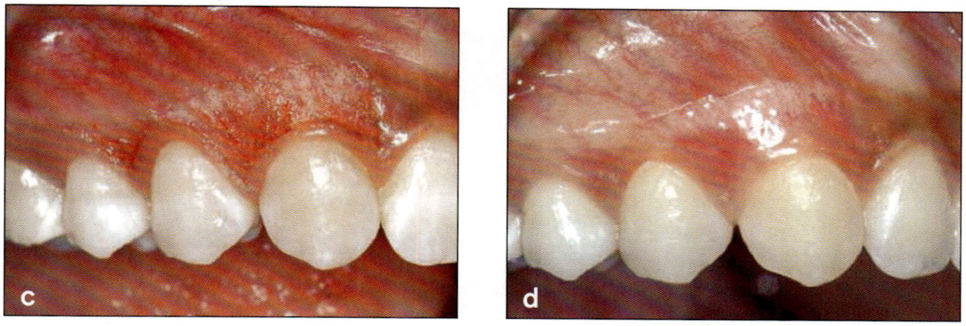

Figs 8-11c and 8-11d Immediate *(c)* and 1-month *(d)* postoperative views. (Case courtesy of Dr Akira Aoki, Tokyo, Japan.)

Purpose of the procedure	Removal of gingival hyperpigmentation

Wavelength and settings

Er:YAG laser; average settings: 1.5 W, 30 mJ, 50 Hz, with a 600 μm tip and no water spray.

Alternate wavelengths that may be used

Any laser can be used to perform this procedure.

Laser-Activated Tooth Whitening

Most of the proprietary whitening agents that are available to the dental practitioner contain hydrogen peroxide or carbamide peroxide. Some agents, which are activated by heat, light, or a combination of both, can be used with specific lasers for rapid tooth whitening. Certain dental lasers can be used with bleaching products containing the specific chromophore that will absorb the laser's wavelength. Studies have documented the laser's ability to achieve lighter tooth shades and have recommended laser exposure times to minimize the rise of pulpal temperatures.[4–6] The longevity of whitening procedures varies because of patients' postoperative habits (eg, diet), but most patients are satisfied with the results.

Clinical tip

To ensure the effectiveness of the whitening with lasers, many practitioners suggest that patients follow an in-office laser-activated tooth whitening with an at-home beaching regimen.

Laser-Activated Tooth Whitening: Case 1

Tooth whitening in a 35-year-old female patient.

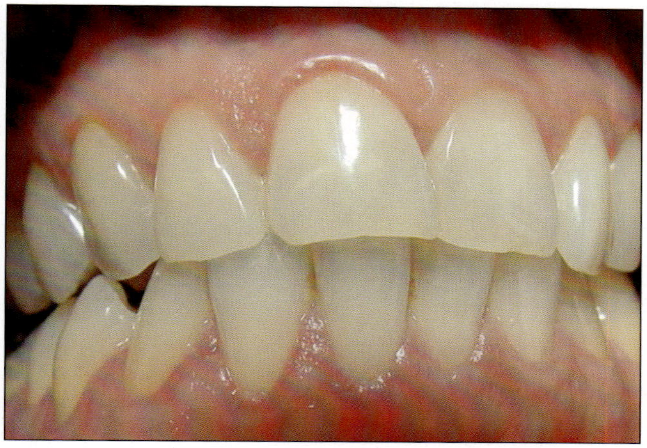

Fig 8-12a Preoperative view of discolored dentition prior to whitening.

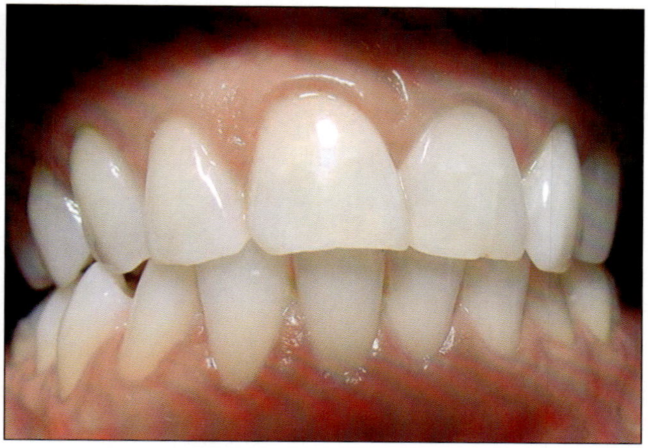

Fig 8-12b Postoperative view of dentition following whitening procedure. (Case courtesy of DEKA Lasers, Florence, Italy.)

Purpose of the procedure	Whitening of discolored teeth

Wavelength, settings, and frequency

KTP laser, 532 nm, set to 0.6 W, continuous wave, with a 0.7 mm spot size and a frequency of 30 seconds per tooth in sequence, then repeat.

Alternate wavelengths that may be used

The wavelength used is determined by the chromophore of the bleaching material. Only a laser wavelength that is absorbed by the chromophore in the bleaching material can be used for optimal results.

Laser-Activated Tooth Whitening: Case 2

Tooth whitening in a 27-year-old male patient.

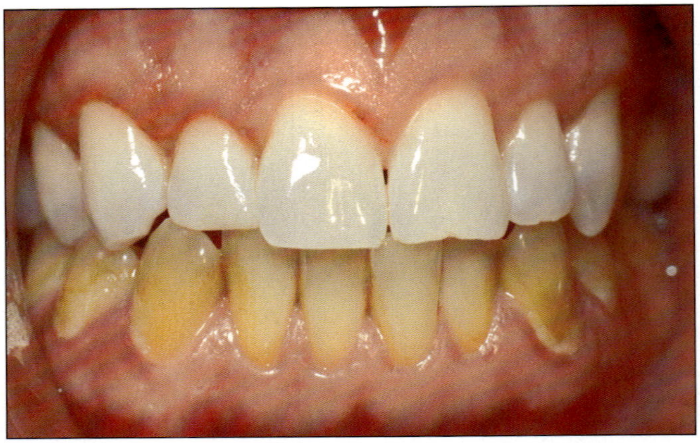

Fig 8-13 Postoperative view immediately following the whitening of the maxillary teeth. The dramatic whitening of the maxillary teeth is evident when juxtaposed to the mandibular teeth.

Purpose of the procedure	Whitening of discolored teeth

Wavelength and settings

CO_2 laser set to 1 W, continuous wave.

Alternate wavelengths that may be used

The wavelength used is determined by the chromophore of the bleaching material.

References

1. White JM, Goodis HE, Rose CL. Use of the pulsed Nd:YAG laser for intraoral soft tissue surgery. Lasers Surg Med 1991;11:455–461.
2. Dickinson MR, Charlton A, King TA, Freemont AJ, Bramley R. Studies of Er:YAG laser interactions with soft tissue. Lasers Med Sci 1991;6:125–131.
3. Pick RM, Pecaro BC. Use of the CO_2 laser in soft tissue dental surgery. Lasers Surg Med 1987;7:207–213.
4. Baik JW, Rueggeberg FA, Liewehr FR. Effect of light-enhanced bleaching on in vitro surface and intrapulpal temperature rise. J Esthet Restorative Dent 2001;13:370–378.
5. Eldeniz AU, Usumez A, Usumez S, Ozturk N. Pulpal temperature rise during light-activated bleaching. J Biomed Mater Res B Appl Biomater 2005;72:254–259.
6. Sulieman M, Addy M, Rees JS. Surface and intra-pulpal temperature rises during tooth bleaching: An in vitro study. Br Dent J 2005; 199:37–40.

Suggested Reading

Adams TC, Pang PK. Lasers in aesthetic dentistry. Dent Clin North Am 2004;48:833–860.

Atsawasuwan P, Greethong K, Nimmanon V. Treatment of gingival hyperpigmentation for esthetic purposes by Nd:YAG laser: Report of 4 cases. J Periodontol 2000;71:315–321.

Esen E, Haytac MC, Oz IA, Erdogan O, Karsli ED. Gingival melanin pigmentation and its treatment with the CO_2 laser. Oral Surg Oral Med Oral Pathol Oral Radiol Endod 2004;98: 522–527.

Garber DA. Dentist-monitored bleaching: A discussion of combination and laser bleaching. J Am Dent Assoc 1997;128(suppl):26S–30S.

Ingber JS, Rose LF, Coslet JG. The "biologic width"—A concept in periodontics and restorative dentistry. Alpha Omegan 1977;70(3): 62–65.

Manni JG. Dental Applications of Advanced Lasers. Burlington, MA: JGM Associates, 2005.

Myers TD. The future of lasers in dentistry. Dent Clin North Am 2000;44:971–980.

Reyto R. Laser tooth whitening. Dent Clin North Am 1998;42:755–762.

Sun G. The role of lasers in cosmetic dentistry. Dent Clin North Am 2000;44:831–850.

Tal H, Oegiesser D, Tal M. Gingival depigmentation by erbium:YAG laser: Clinical observations and patient responses. J Periodontol 2003;74: 1660–1667.

Yousuf A, Hossain M, Nakamura Y, Yamada Y, Kinoshita J, Matsumoto K. Removal of gingival melanin pigmentation with the semiconductor diode laser: A case report. J Clin Laser Med Surg 2000;18:263–266.

9

ENDODONTIC LASER THERAPY

Dental lasers can be used in virtually every phase of endodontic therapy, from opening access to the root canal to the final step of obturation.[1] A primary goal of endodontic therapy is to eliminate microbial pathogens from the root canal system. Any laser wavelength can be used to significantly decrease bacteria in root canal systems, which is extremely beneficial for long-term endodontic success.[2–7] However, only the erbium (Er) family of wavelengths has the capability to clean and shape the dentin walls during canal preparation for obturation.[8,9] When an Er laser is used to prepare the dentin, the smear layer is eliminated (Fig 9-1).[10] Compared to conventional instrumentation, the use of Er wavelengths in the root canal improves disinfection of the dentinal tubules and adhesion of the endodontic sealers to the root canal walls. Though most laser tips are end cutting, manufacturers are developing side-firing tips for endodontic treatment (Figs 9-2 to 9-4).

Lasers also may be used during endodontic surgery for making a soft tissue incision, ablating diseased periapical tissue, amputating the root, and preparing the root for a retrograde restoration. Each step is enhanced by the laser's hemostatic and bactericidal properties.[11]

In addition, dental lasers can be used adjunctively in performing pulp capping. Unlike pediatric pulpotomies (see chapter 11), pulp capping in permanent teeth is traditionally performed on small areas of exposed vital tissue to form a dentinal bridge over the exposed area, thereby maintaining pulpal vitality. Studies using neodymium-doped yttrium aluminum garnet

(Nd:YAG), carbon dioxide (CO_2), and Er family lasers set at low-power parameters report success and improved prognosis over results obtained with conventional chemical methods.[12–15]

Well-documented studies also demonstrate reduction in hypersensitivity after laser exposure of the dentinal surface. Three techniques have been proposed to reduce hypersensitivity: the use of very low output from a visible red or an invisible near infrared laser may produce an anti-inflammatory effect; the use of moderate levels of Nd:YAG or CO_2 laser energy modifies the dentin structures by fusing or narrowing the tubules; and the use of moderate levels of Er laser energy evaporates the intracellular fluid and seals the ends of the odontoblastic processes. Varying degrees of success have been reported for each procedure.[16–20]

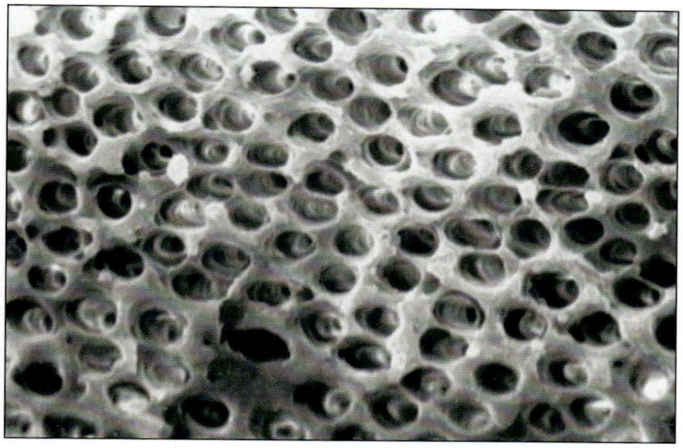

Fig 9-1 Root canal walls at 1200× magnification after exposure to Er:YAG energy. The dentinal tubules are completely patent, and the removal of the smear layer from the canal walls assures superior bactericidal disinfection of the root canal system. (Courtesy of Dr Adam Stabholz, Jerusalem, Israel.)

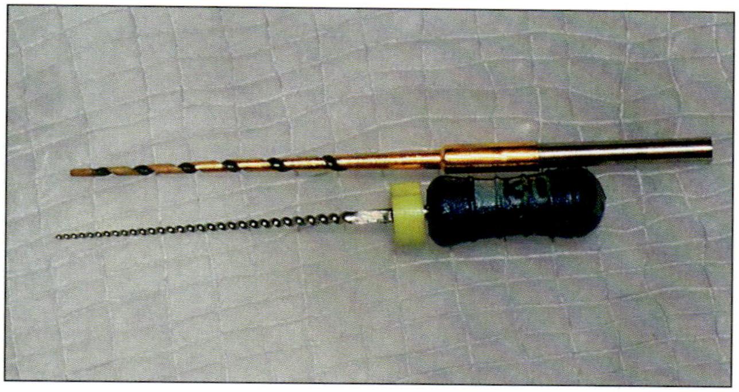

Fig 9-2 Side-by-side comparison of endodontic instruments: a side-firing laser tip and a no. 30 file.

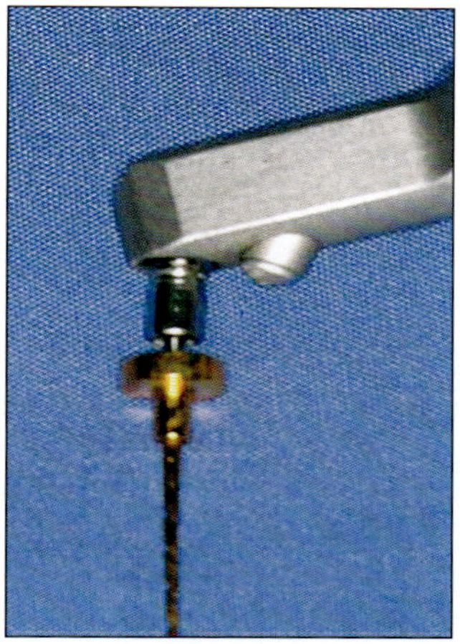

Fig 9-3 Side-firing endodontic tip in an Er:YAG handpiece. As with conventional endodontic instruments, a rubber stop can be placed on the laser tip to correspond to the working length of the canal. (Courtesy of Dr Adam Stabholz, Jerusalem, Israel.)

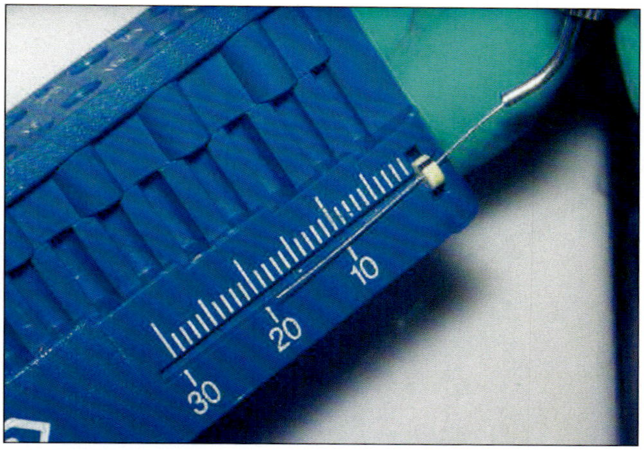

Fig 9-4 Setting the working length of an end-cutting endodontic laser tip.

Pulp Capping: Case 1

Direct pulp capping in a primary mandibular left second molar.

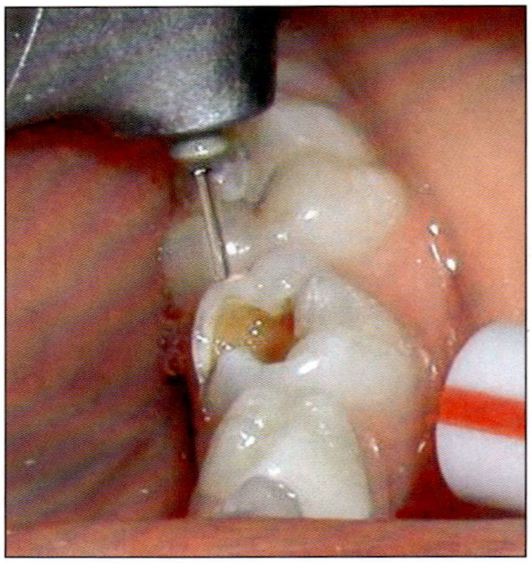

Fig 9-5a Caries removal in a primary mandibular left second molar. A pinpoint carious exposure occurred during laser excavation.

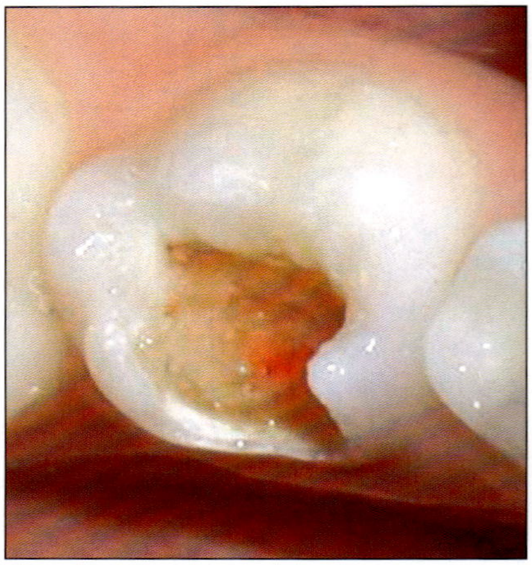

Fig 9-5b Pink pinpoint exposure. A pulp-capping procedure was performed using laser energy.

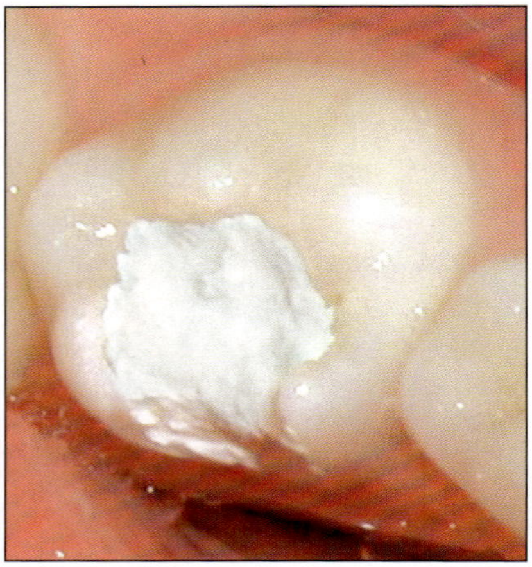

Fig 9-5c Postoperative view of a provisional restoration of zinc oxide and eugenol material. The definitive restoration will involve a stainless steel crown. (Case courtesy of Dr Fred Margolis, Buffalo Grove, IL.)

Purpose of the procedure	Direct pulp capping

Performing a direct pulp cap on a pinpoint exposure in a primary molar maintains the vitality of the tooth.

Wavelength and settings

Er,Cr:YSGG laser set to 1.5 W and 25 Hz.

Alternate wavelengths that may be used

Any laser can be used to perform this procedure. Please note that as of this writing, use of any laser wavelength for pulp capping (including the Er family of lasers) has not been cleared by the Food and Drug Administration. However, studies mentioned previously along with anecdotal reports by laser users have made this procedure relatively common.

Root Canal Disinfection: Case 1

Disinfection of the root canal system in an adult male patient.

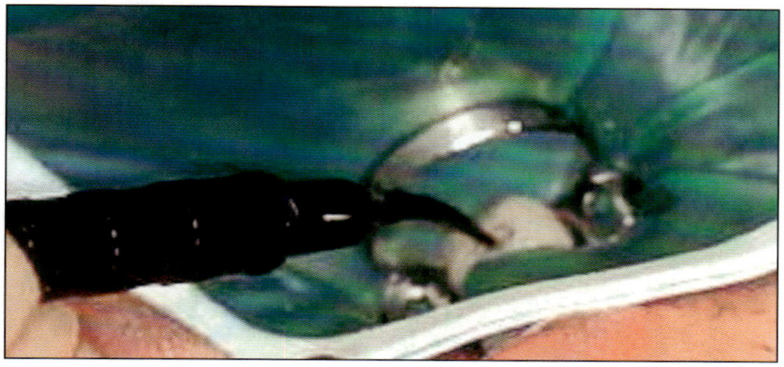

Fig 9-6 Disinfection of a root canal using an Nd:YAG laser. (Courtesy of Dr Steven Parker, Harrogate, North Yorkshire, England.)

Purpose of the procedure

Laser disinfection

When the root canal system is disinfected, the long-term stability of a tooth is increased.

Wavelength and settings

Nd:YAG laser set to 150 mJ, 10 Hz, with a 320 μm fiber, for 20 seconds of exposure per canal.

Alternate wavelengths that may be used

Any laser can be used to perform this procedure.

Clinical tip

After the working length has been measured and verified via conventional methods, the laser fiber/tip is placed between 1 and 2 mm short of the canal apex because the laser energy emanates beyond the end of the tip. The canal must be kept moist at all times to avoid charring of the dentinal walls and to enhance the bactericidal effects of the laser energy. Conventional root canal irrigants can be used.

Endodontic Treatment: Case 1

Endodontic therapy of the maxillary right central incisor in an adult male patient.

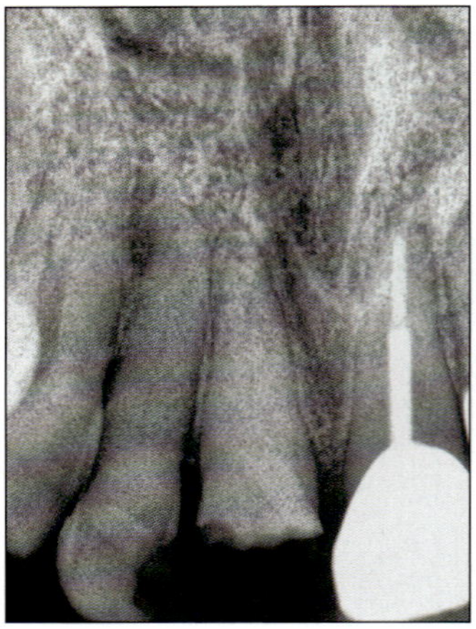

Fig 9-7a A maxillary right central incisor showing an indistinct, partially calcified root canal.

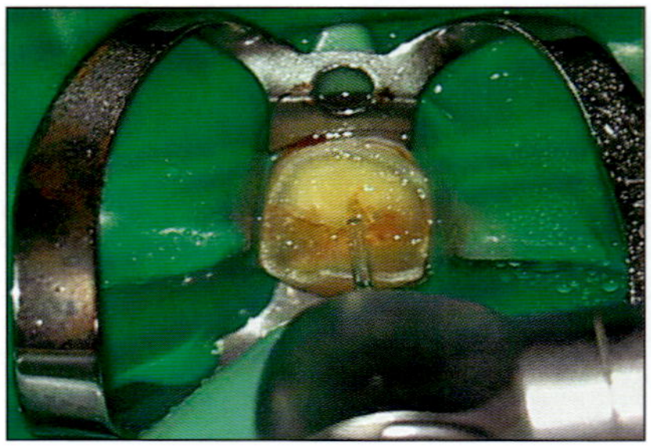

Fig 9-7b The initial root canal access is made with a laser.

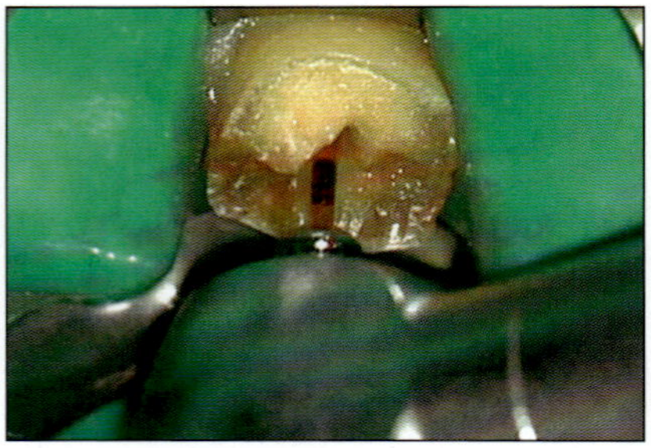

Fig 9-7c The laser is used to enlarge the opening to the root canal.

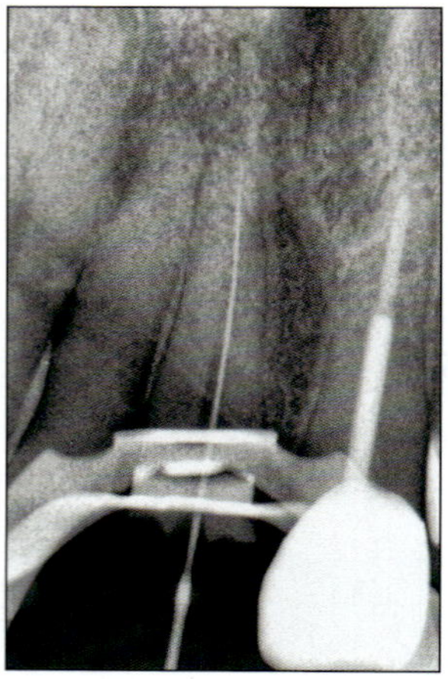

Fig 9-7d Apical patency is achieved with the laser, and the working length is verified with a no. 15 file.

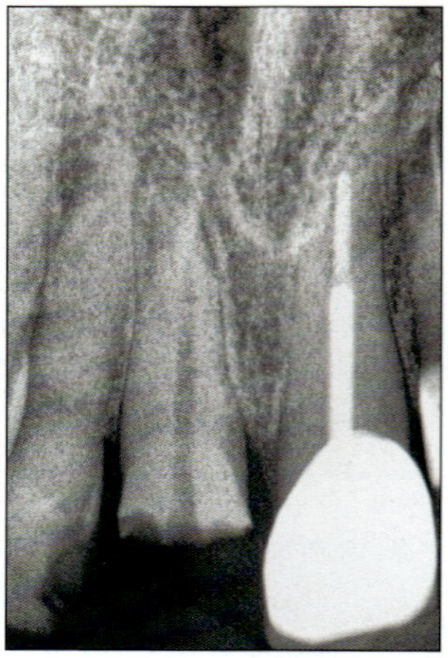

Fig 9-7e Radiograph showing completed laser instrumentation.

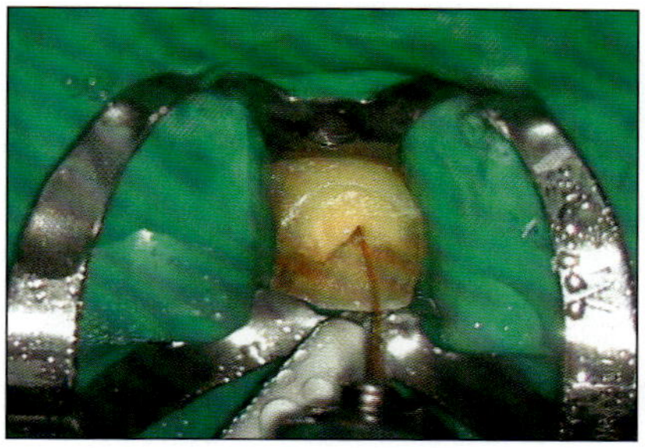

Fig 9-7f Final disinfection and debridement of the root canal.

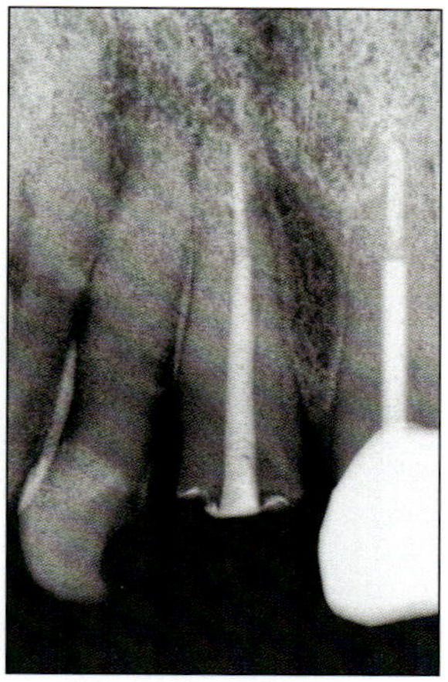

Fig 9-7g Immediate postoperative radiograph of the obturated root canal. (Case courtesy of Dr David Browdy, Lynbrook, NY.)

Purpose of the procedure	Complete endodontic therapy

The endodontic treatment includes laser instrumentation of the root canal prior to obturation.

Wavelength and settings

Er,Cr:YSGG laser; settings for initial access: 5.75 W with a G-6 tip with water spray; settings for access enlargement: 3 W with a C-6 tip with water spray; settings for canal preparation: 3 W with a Z-6 tip with water spray; settings for final disinfection and debridement: 1.5 W with a Z-2 tip with water spray.

Alternate wavelengths that may be used

Only the Er family of lasers can be used to perform this procedure.

Clinical tip

Laser instruments allow clinicians to create very conservative endodontic openings. Conventional endodontic access with rotary instruments may lead to greater loss of tooth structure and possible perforation of the root system.

Endodontic Treatment: Case 2

Endodontic retreatment of the mandibular right second molar in an adult male patient.

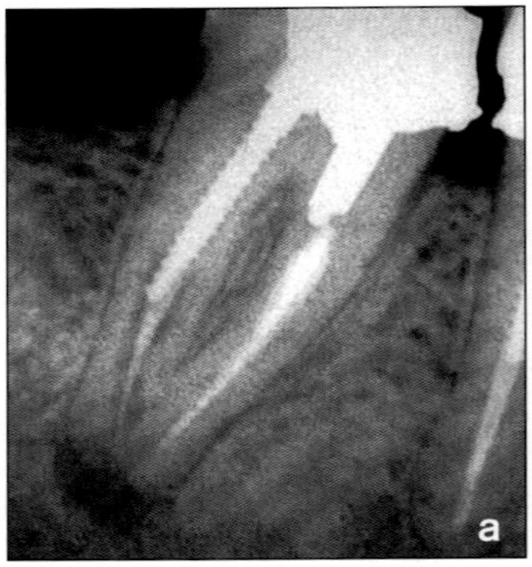

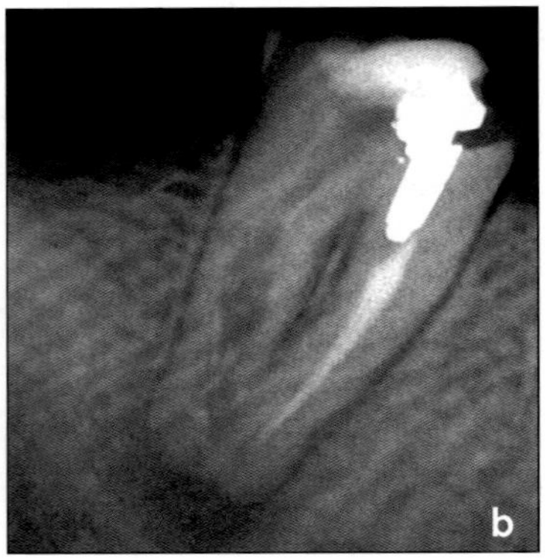

Fig 9-8a Preoperative radiograph of the mandibular right second molar. Failing endodontic treatment is evidenced by a large area of periapical radiolucency.

Fig 9-8b Intraoperative view following removal of the screw post, opened access to the root canals, and removal of gutta-percha via conventional methods.

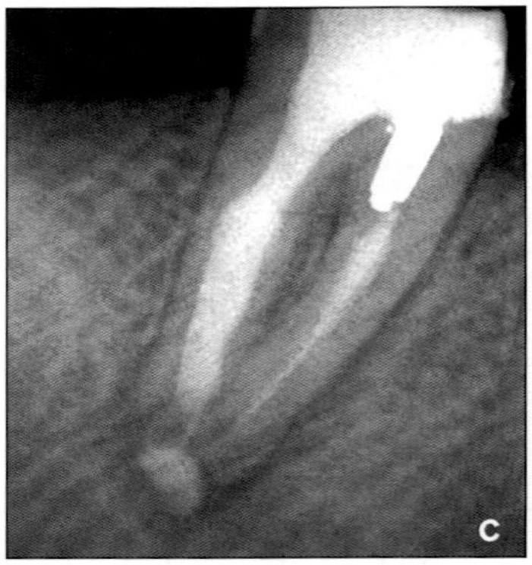

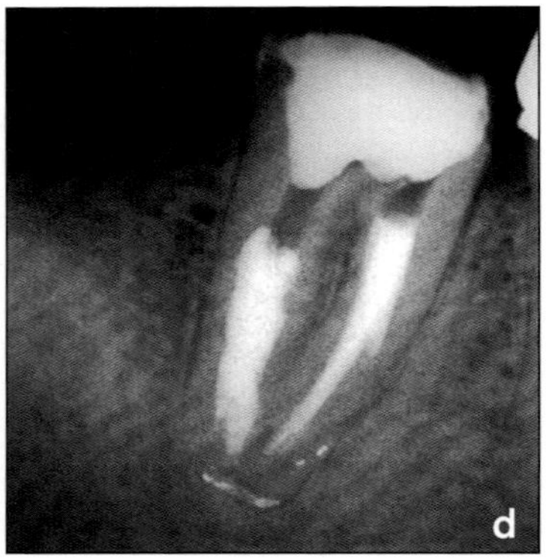

Fig 9-8c Immediate postoperative radiograph of the well-filled root canal following treatment with a side-firing laser endodontic tip.

Fig 9-8d Nine-month postoperative radiograph shows complete healing of the periapical lesion.

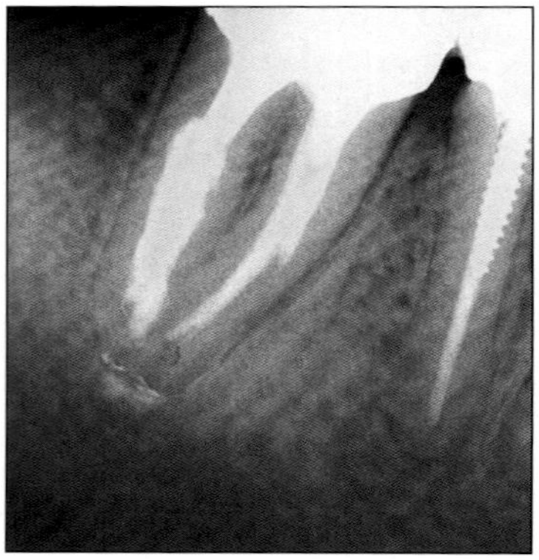

Fig 9-8e Two-year postoperative radiograph. (Case courtesy of Dr Adam Stabholz, Jerusalem, Israel.)

Purpose of the procedure

Endodontic retreatment

The periapical lesion is retreated once the failing endodontic post is removed and the canal is exposed to laser energy with a side-firing endodontic laser tip.

Wavelength and settings

Er:YAG laser set to 500 mJ and 12 Hz for 15 seconds of exposure.

Alternate wavelengths that may be used

Only the Er family of lasers can be used to perform this procedure.

Clinical tips

The entire endodontic side-firing tip (including all spirals and slits) of the laser instrument must fit completely within the canal in order to prevent unwanted laser energy from being transmitted outside the root canal (Fig 9-9). If the entire endodontic tip does not fit within the canal, either a shorter tip must be selected, or the end of the tip must be cut. To prevent charring of the canal walls and to enhance the removal of the smear layer, the canal must be kept moist with an irrigant solution, such as 17% ethylenediaminetetraacetic acid (EDTA).

After initial ablation of the canal wall, the side-firing tip of the Er family laser is rotated 90 degrees in the canal, and the root canal is exposed to laser energy for an additional 15 seconds. Rotation and ablation are repeated twice more to ensure that the entire 360-degree circumference of the root canal wall has been exposed to the laser energy.

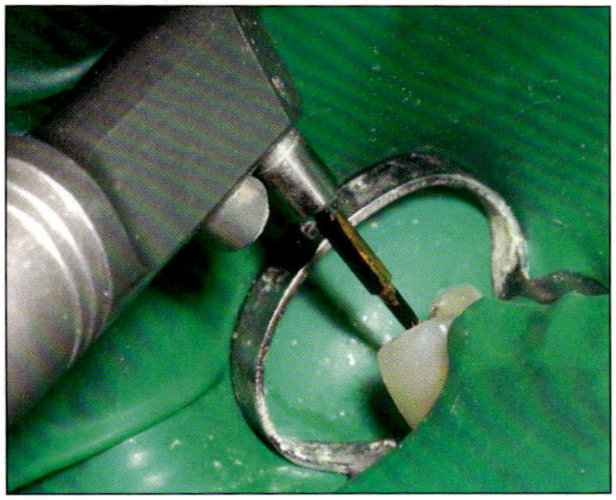

Fig 9-9 The endodontic side-firing tip entirely within a root canal.

Apicoectomy: Case 1

Apicoectomy of the maxillary left central incisor in an adult male patient.

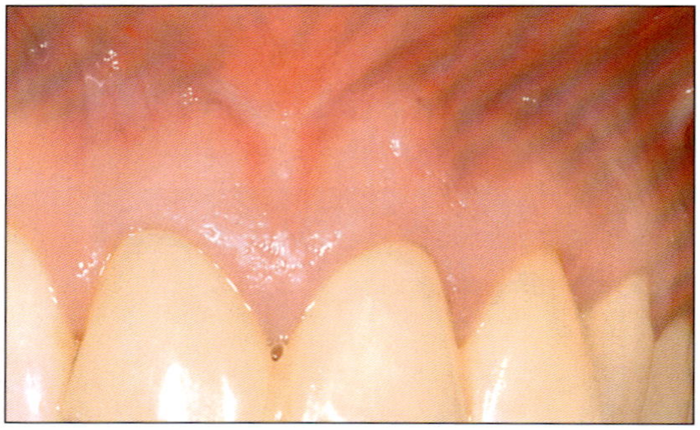

Fig 9-10a Swelling apical to the maxillary left central incisor.

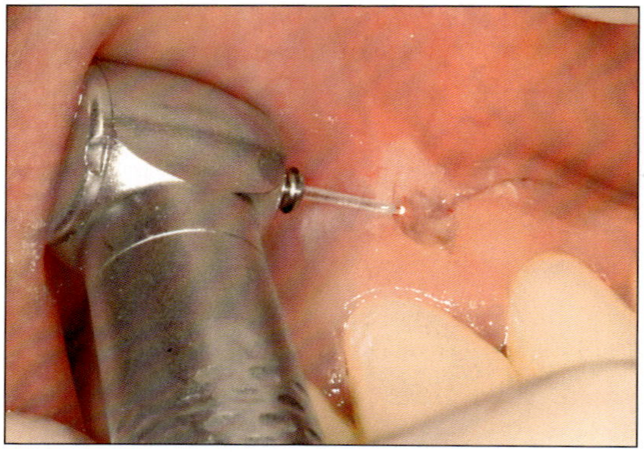

Fig 9-10b An Er,Cr:YSGG laser makes an incision.

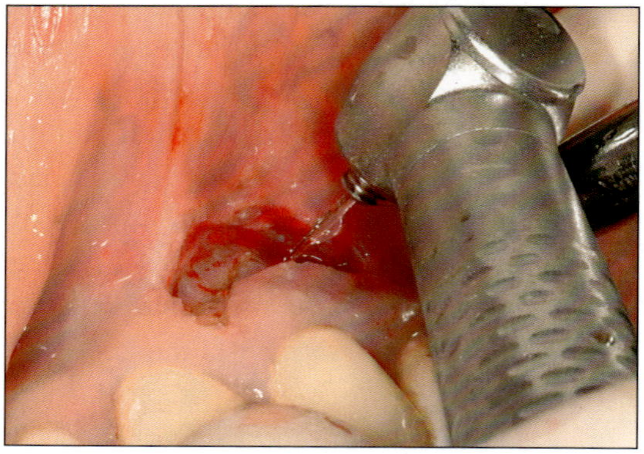

Fig 9-10c The laser removes granulomatous tissue and performs root resection.

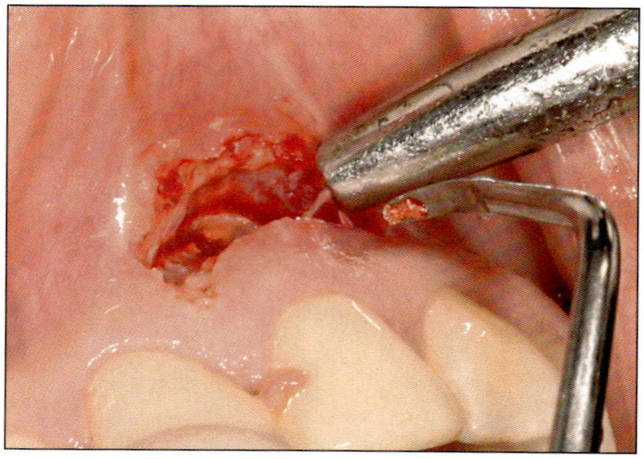

Fig 9-10d Apical gutta-percha removed with a curette.

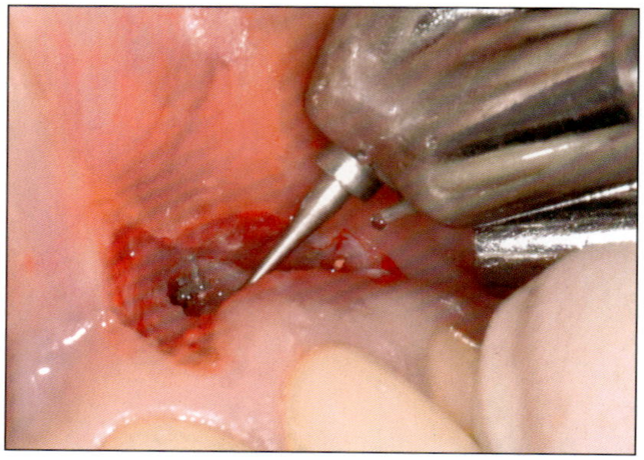

Fig 9-10e Tooth prepared with a conventional handpiece for retrograde restoration.

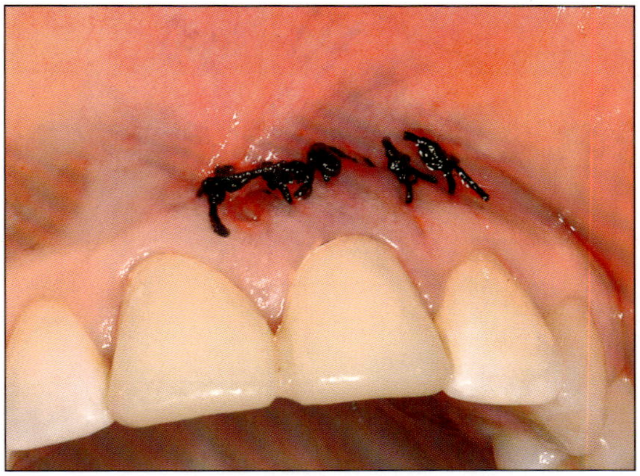

Fig 9-10f Immediate postoperative view with soft tissues sutured in place.

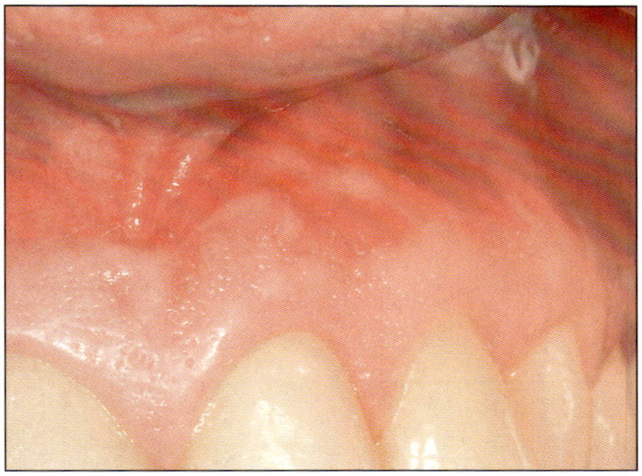

Fig 9-10g Six-month postoperative view shows complete healing. (Case courtesy of Dr Arthur Scott, Metairie, LA.)

Purpose of the procedure	Apicoectomy
A retrograde restoration is performed following a laser apicoectomy.	

Wavelength and settings

Er,Cr:YSGG laser; setting for soft tissue ablation: 1.5 W; setting for hard tissue ablation: 2.75 W.

Alternate wavelengths that may be used

Only the Er family of lasers can be used to perform this procedure.

Clinical tip

Usually 0.5 W would be sufficient to perform the soft tissue incision. However, a higher power of 1.5 W was used to make an incision through the periosteum at the same time. The laser was used to perform the root resection, but a high-speed handpiece was used to prepare for the retrograde filling since the Er,Cr:YSGG energy has difficulty ablating gutta-percha.

Apicoectomy: Case 2

Apicoectomy of the maxillary right central incisor in an adult male patient.

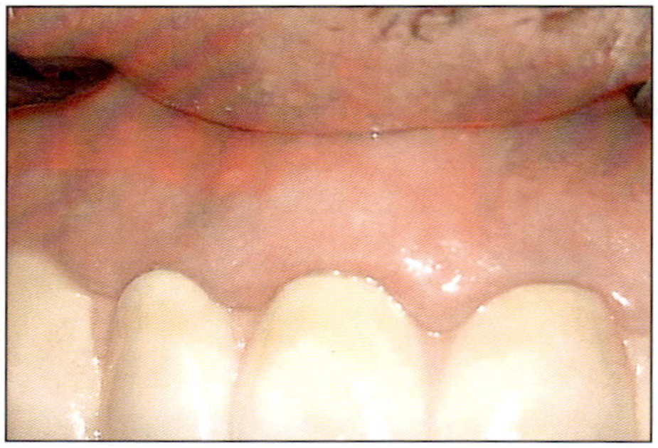

Fig 9-11a Preoperative view showing a fistulous tract between the maxillary right central and lateral incisors.

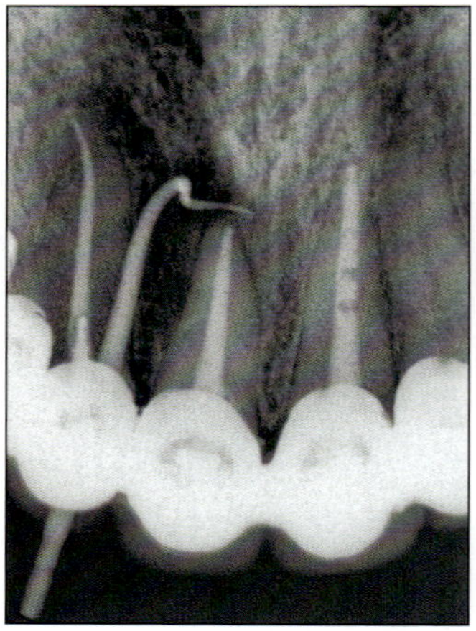

Fig 9-11b Radiographic view that traces a lesion to the apex of the maxillary right central incisor.

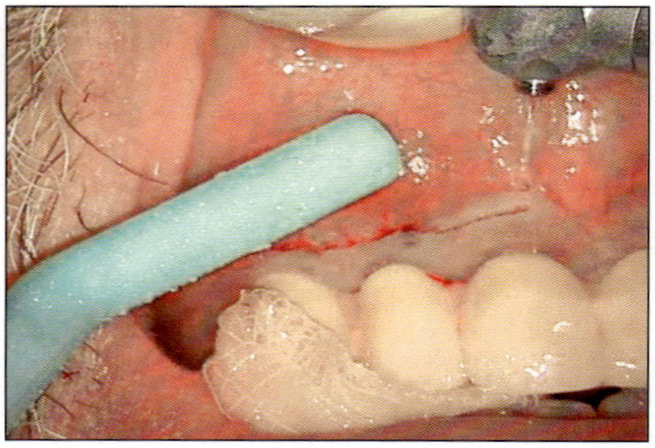

Fig 9-11c An Er,Cr:YSGG laser with a soft tissue tip makes an incision in the gingiva.

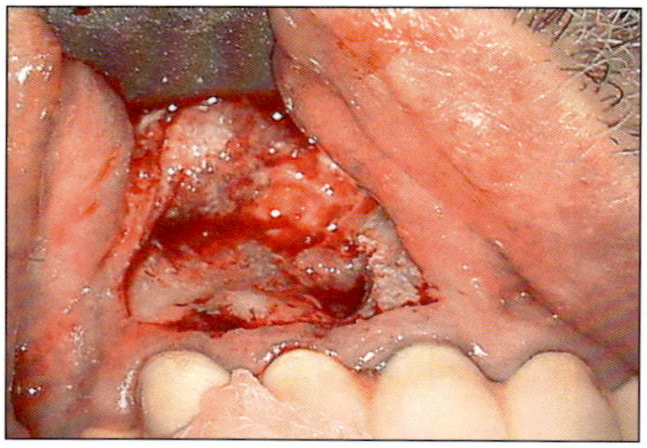

Fig 9-11d Reflection of the soft tissue reveals granulomatous tissue.

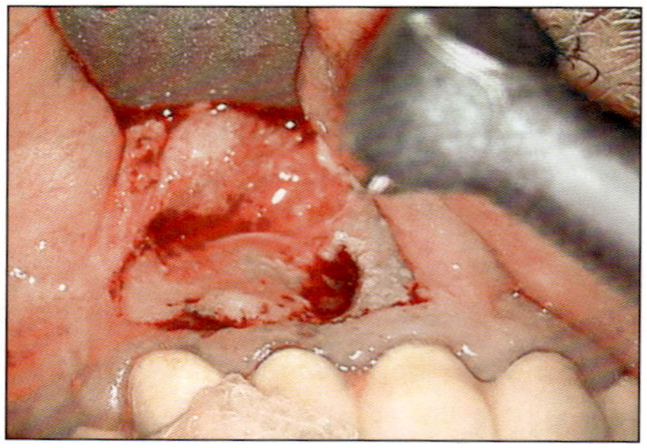

Fig 9-11e Tissue removal with the laser.

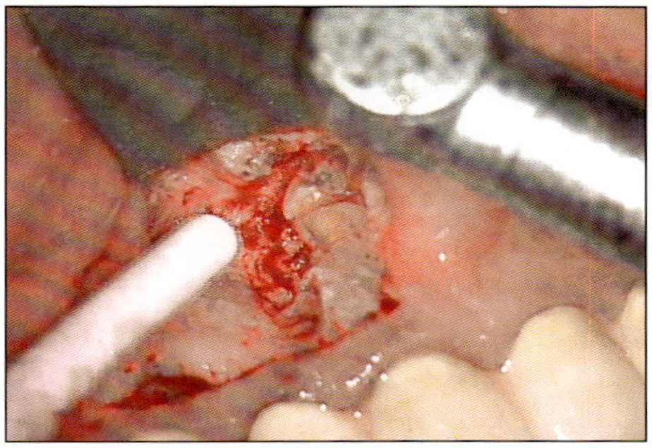

Fig 9-11f Laser root resection.

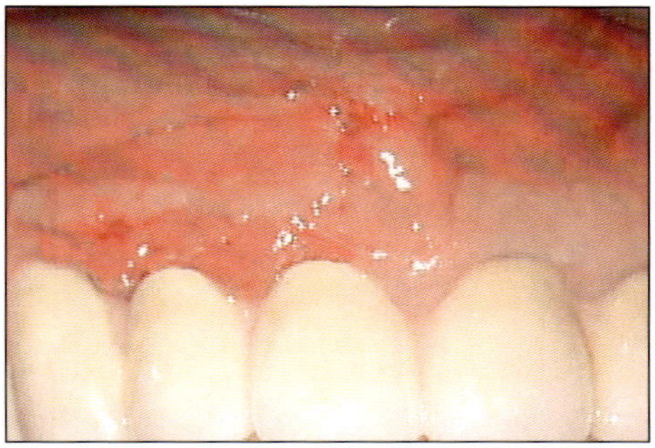

Fig 9-11g Five days after surgery, the sutures are removed. (Case courtesy of Dr David Browdy, Lynbrook, NY.)

Purpose of the procedure	Apicoectomy
The chronic apical infection is treated with a laser-assisted apicoectomy.	

Wavelength and settings

Er,Cr:YSGG laser; settings for soft tissue incision and granulomatous tissue ablation: 1.75 W with minimal water spray; settings for root resection: 4 W with water spray.

Alternate wavelengths that may be used

Only the Er family of lasers can be used to perform this procedure.

Desensitization: Case 1

Desensitization of exposed dentin in an adult male patient.

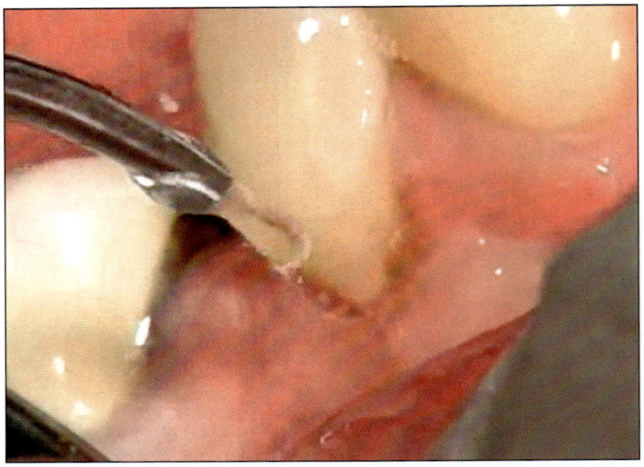

Fig 9-12 An Er:YAG laser is positioned 5 mm from the tooth surface to desensitize exposed dentin.

Purpose of the procedure	Tooth desensitization
Exposed dentin is desensitized using laser energy.	

Wavelength and settings
Er:YAG laser set to 30 mJ and 10 Hz with water spray, and with an exposure time up to 2 minutes.
Alternate wavelengths that may be used
Any laser can be used to perform this procedure.

Desensitization: Case 2

Desensitization of an exposed root surface on a maxillary first molar in an adult male patient.

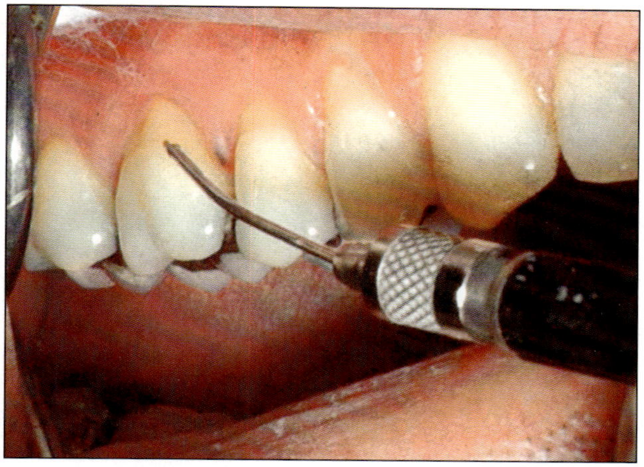

Fig 9-13 Use of an Nd:YAG laser to desensitize an exposed root surface.

Purpose of the procedure	Tooth desensitization
An exposed root surface is desensitized using laser energy.	

Wavelength and settings

Nd:YAG laser set to 10 Hz, 30 mJ, with a 320 μm fiber.

Alternate wavelengths that may be used

Any laser can be used to perform this procedure.

Clinical tip

In desensitization procedures, the clinician should start with the laser placed 10 mm from the target site and slowly bring it toward the tooth in a circling motion. If the patient begins to feel discomfort, the instrument is pulled back 1 mm, then slowly circled in again. This procedure is repeated until the laser tip is 1 mm from the tooth.

References

1. Matsumoto K. Lasers in endodontics. Dent Clin North Am 2000;44:889–906.
2. Convissar RA. The biologic rationale for the use of lasers in dentistry. Dent Clin North Am 2004;48:771–794.
3. Moritz A, Gutknecht N, Goharkhay K, Schoop U, Wernisch J, Sperr W. In vitro irradiation of infected root canals with diode laser: Results of microbiologic, infrared spectrometric, and stain penetration examination. Quintessence Int 1997;28:205–209.
4. Gutknecht N, Moritz A, Conrads G, Sievert T, Lampert F. Bactericidal effect of the Nd:YAG laser in in vitro root canals. J Clin Laser Med Surg 1996;14:77–80.
5. Yamazaki R, Goya C, Yu DG, Kimura Y, Matsumoto K. Effects of erbium, chromium: YSGG laser irradiation on root canal walls: A scanning electron microscope and thermographic study. J Endod 2001;27:9–12.
6. Dostalova T, Jelinkova H, Housova D, et al. Endodontic treatment with application of Er:YAG laser waveguide radiation disinfection. J Clin Laser Med Surg 2002;20: 135–139.
7. Le Goff A, Dautel-Morazin A, Guigand M, Vulcain JM, Bonnaure-Mallet M. An evaluation of the CO_2 laser for endodontic disinfection. J Endod 1999;25:105–108.
8. Mazeki K, Kimura Y, Yokoyama K, Matsumoto K. Preparation of root canal orifices by Er:YAG laser irradiation: In vitro and clinical observations. J Clin Laser Med Surg 2003; 21:85–91.
9. Matsuoka E, Jayawardena JA, Matsumoto K. Morphological study of the Er,Cr:YSGG laser for root canal preparation in mandibular incisors with curved root canals. Photomed Laser Surg 2005;23:480–484.
10. Biedma BM, Varela Patino P, Park SA, et al. Comparative study of root canals instrumented manually and mechanically, with and without Er:YAG laser. Photomed Laser Surg 2005;23:465–469.
11. Stabholz A, Zeltser R, Sela M, et al. The use of lasers in dentistry: Principles of operation and clinical applications. Compend Contin Educ Dent 2003;24:935–948.
12. Santucci PJ. Dycal versus Nd:YAG laser and Vitrebond for direct pulp capping in permanent teeth. J Clin Laser Med Surg 1999; 17:69–75.
13. Blanken JW. Direct pulp capping using an Er,Cr:YSGG laser. J Oral Laser Appl 2005; 5:107–114.
14. Jayawardena JA, Kato J, Moriya K, Takagi Y. Pulpal response to exposure with Er:YAG laser. Oral Surg Oral Med Oral Pathol Oral Radiol Endod 2001;91:222–229.
15. Moritz A, Schoop U, Goharkhay K, Sperr W. Advantages of a pulsed CO_2 laser in direct pulp capping: A long-term in vivo study. Lasers Surg Med 1998;22:288–293.
16. Marsilio AL, Rodrigues JR, Borges AB. Effect of the clinical application of the GaAlAs laser in the treatment of dentine hypersensitivity. J Clin Laser Med Surg 2003;21:291–296.
17. Lan WH, Liu HC. Treatment of dentin hypersensitivity by Nd:YAG laser. J Clin Laser Med Surg 1996;14:89–92.
18. Zhang C, Matsumoto K, Kimura Y, Harashima T, Takeda FH, Zhou H. Effects of CO_2 laser in treatment of cervical dentinal hypersensitivity. J Endod 1998;24:595–597.
19. Schwarz F, Arweiler N, Georg T, Reich E. Desensitizing effects of an Er:YAG laser on hypersensitive dentine. J Clin Periodontol 2002;29:211–215.
20. Watanabe H, Kataoka K, Iwami H, et al. In vitro and in vivo studies on application of erbium:YAG laser for dentin hypersensitivity. In: Ishikawa I, Frame JW, Aoki A (eds). Lasers in Dentistry: Revolution of Dental Treatment in the New Millennium. Burlington, MA: Elsevier, 2003:455–457.

10

LASER USE IN ORAL SURGERY, ORAL MEDICINE, AND ORAL PATHOLOGY

The fields of oral surgery, oral medicine, and oral pathology have greatly benefited from laser use. Whether used for excising hyperplastic tissue, ablating oral dermatopathologies, or incising pathologic tissue for a biopsy, lasers provide many advantages over conventional treatment: bloodless surgery ensures better visibility of the surgical field[1–3]; bactericidal properties minimize the possibility of infection[1–3]; minimal mechanical trauma to the surgical site reduces postoperative swelling and pain,[1–4] which may additionally lessen psychological trauma for the patient; and minimal scarring and wound contraction accelerate recovery and postoperative function.[1–3] Together, these advantages have allowed general practitioners to widen the scope of their practices to perform simple surgical procedures and biopsies that were previously referred to specialists. For example, third molar surgery is simpler and less traumatic when a soft tissue laser is used to reflect a flap, and an erbium (Er) laser is used to section partially erupted teeth for removal.[5]

The coagulative ability of lasers simplifies treatment of vascular lesions, such as venous lakes and hemangiomas and other vascular pathologies.[6] However, the most significant surgical breakthrough in using the coagulative ability of lasers for treatment of oral pathologies is the prevention of metastasis. Many carcinomas and sarcomas are thought to metastasize as a result of tumor cells being seeded via the lymphatic and circulatory systems during surgery with a scalpel. A decrease in metastasis has been reported when lasers are used to remove tumors; laser coagulation of blood vessels and lymphatic channels of up to 500 μm in diameter may play a role in preventing metastasis during laser surgery.[7–11]

Drug-induced Gingival Hyperplasia: Case 1

Removal of hyperplastic gingiva in a kidney transplant patient with high blood pressure.

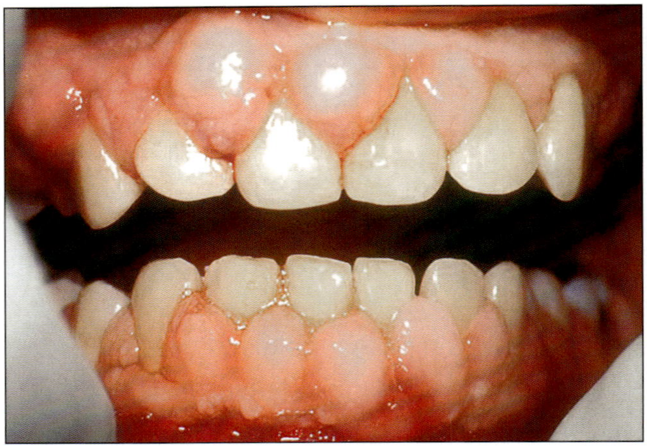

Fig 10-1a Hyperplastic gingiva secondary to cyclosporine and calcium channel blocker use. Note that the patient has immaculate hygiene.

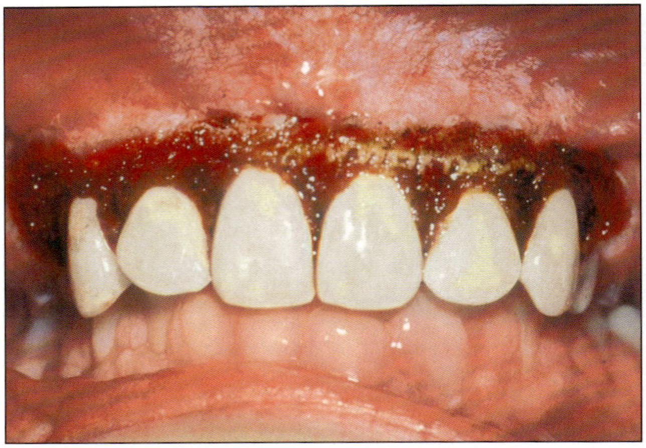

Fig 10-1b The full maxillary gingivectomy results in physiologic gingival contours with excellent hemostasis.

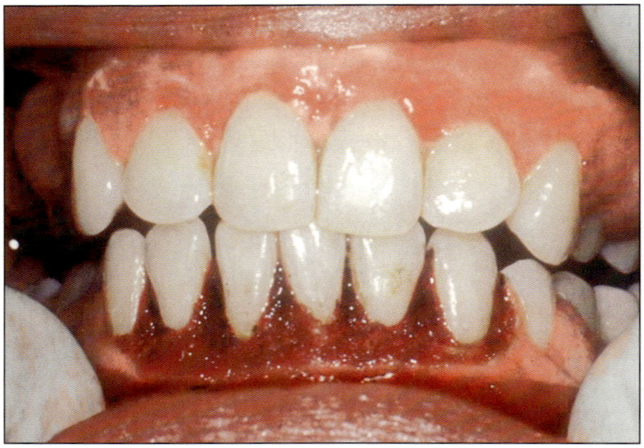

Fig 10-1c One week following the maxillary gingivectomy, the hyperplastic tissue of the mandible is likewise ablated.

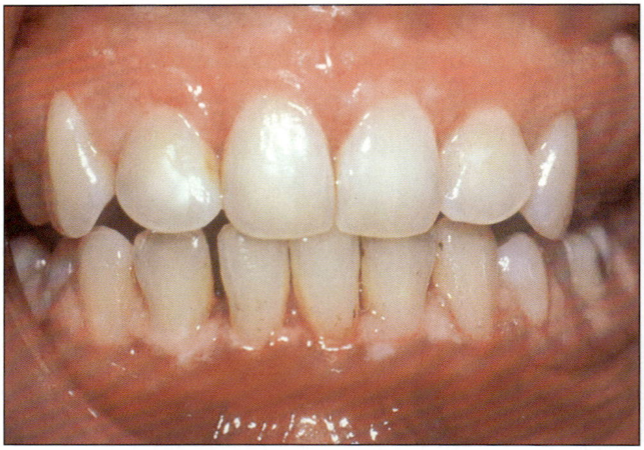

Fig 10-1d Postoperative view of the gingiva 2 weeks following the maxillary gingivectomy and 1 week after the mandibular gingivectomy.

Purpose of the procedure	Removal of drug-induced hyperplastic gingiva

Once the tissue is superficially coagulated, excessive tissue can be removed and the gingival margin refined.

Wavelength and settings

CO_2 laser; settings for initial coagulation of tissues: 3 W, continuous wave, defocused, with an 800 µm ceramic tip; settings for tissue removal: 5 W, continuous wave, with an 800 µm ceramic tip; settings for gingival contour refinement: 3 W, continuous wave, with a 250 µm metal tip.

Alternate wavelengths that may be used

Though any wavelength can be used, the CO_2 laser is ideal for this procedure. The Er family of lasers is not as efficient in providing hemostasis and may result in a bloody surgical field. Because both diode and Nd:YAG lasers must be used on high power to ablate hyperplastic tissue, there is a chance of thermal damage to subjacent and lateral tissues due to the depth of wavelength penetration, which could result in postoperative discomfort, delayed healing, and even sloughing off of tissue.

Clinical tip

There are many techniques for accomplishing this procedure. However, the ideal method would combine conventional and laser techniques. A defocused laser with excellent coagulative abilities (ie, CO_2, diode, or Nd:YAG) set to low power can superficially coagulate the gingiva. A scalpel can then be used to remove the excessive hyperplastic tissue. A large-spot-size fiber/tip can be used to further reduce the tissue before a small-spot-size fiber/tip refines the gingival contours.

Drug-induced Gingival Hyperplasia: Case 2

Removal of mandibular hyperplastic gingiva in an organ transplant patient.

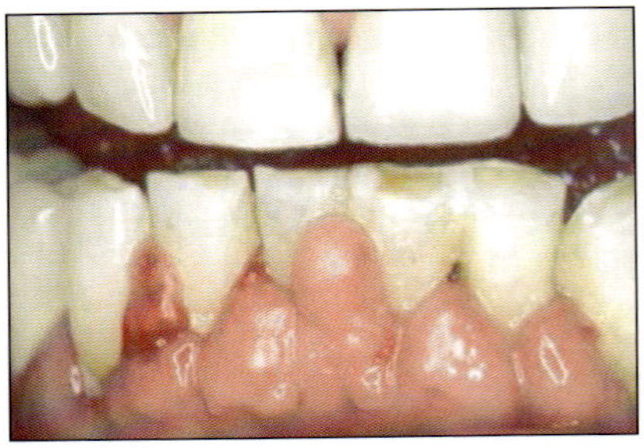

Fig 10-2a Drug-induced hyperplasia in the anterior mandibular gingiva. Poor oral hygiene has contributed to the edematous tissue quality.

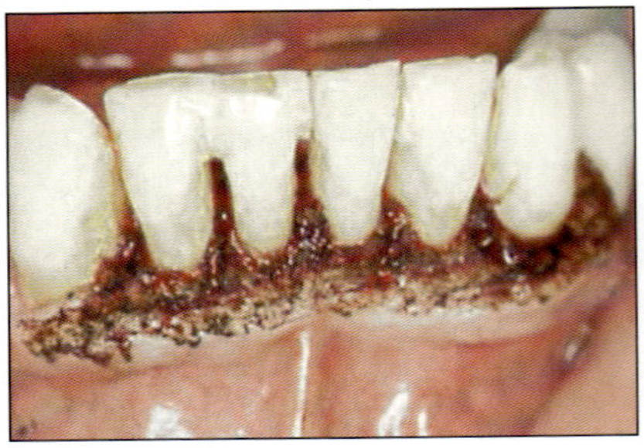

Fig 10-2b Immediate postoperative view of the mandibular gingivectomy.

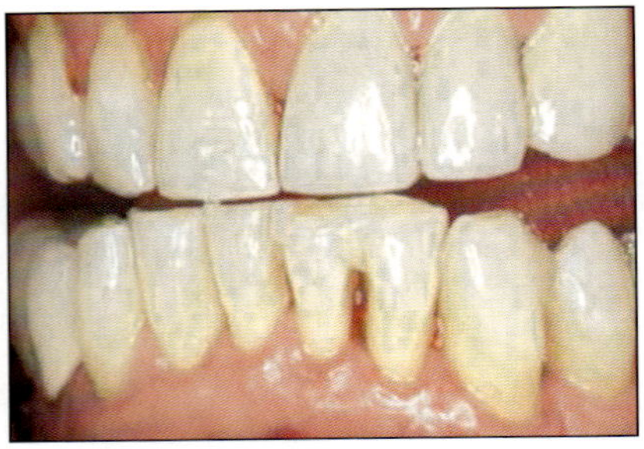

Fig 10-2c One month following the gingivectomy, the healed mandibular gingiva has excellent marginal contours. (Case courtesy of Dr Stuart Coleton, White Plains, NY.)

Purpose of the procedure	Removal of drug-induced hyperplastic gingiva
The gingival contour is refined following removal of the excess tissue.	

Wavelength and settings

CO_2 laser set to 7 W, continuous wave, with an 800 μm ceramic tip.

Alternate wavelengths that may be used

Since this tissue is not as hyperplastic as the tissue in case 1, this procedure could be performed using a diode or Nd:YAG laser with less concern about deep thermal damage to the surrounding tissues. Due to the poor oral hygiene and edematous tissue quality, use of an Er laser is not recommended because of the difficulty in maintaining adequate hemostasis.

Aphthous Ulcer: Case 1

Treatment of an aphthous ulcer on the lower lip of a female patient

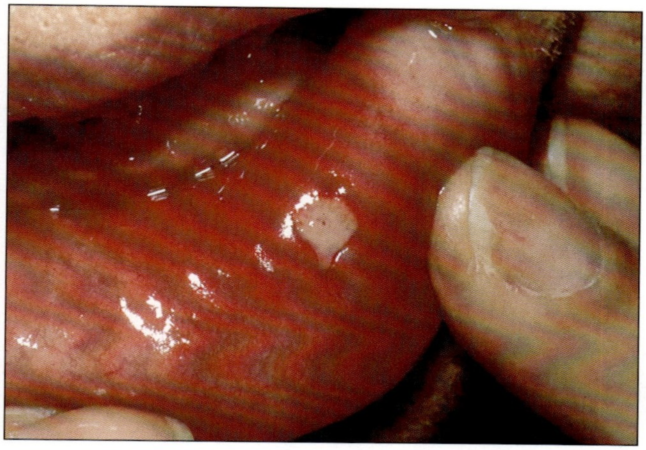

Fig 10-3a Large recurrent aphthous ulcer on the mucosa inside the lower lip.

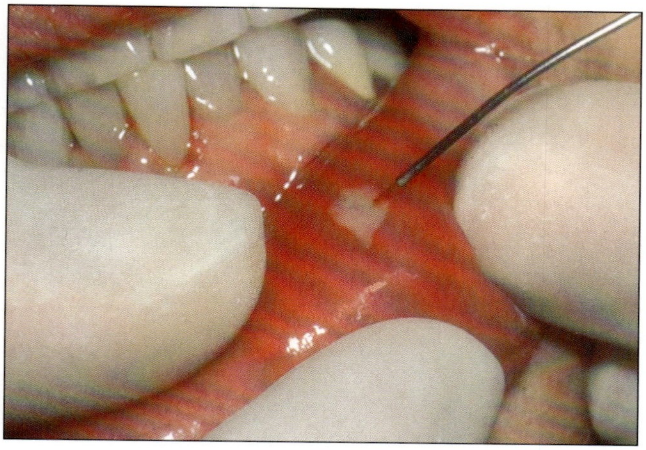

Fig 10-3b A Nd:YAG laser is used to treat the ulcer.

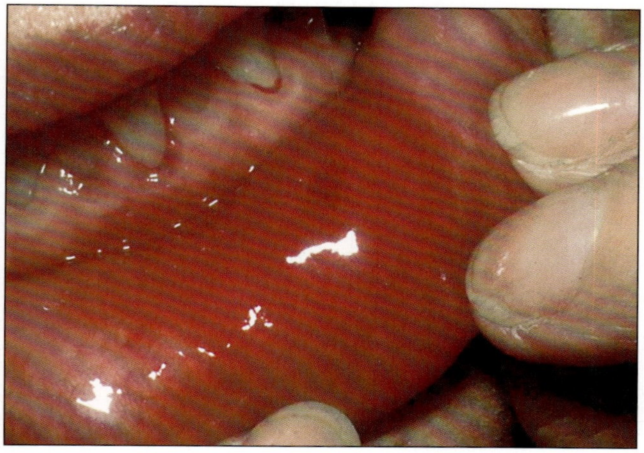

Fig 10-3c Postoperative view immediately following laser treatment.

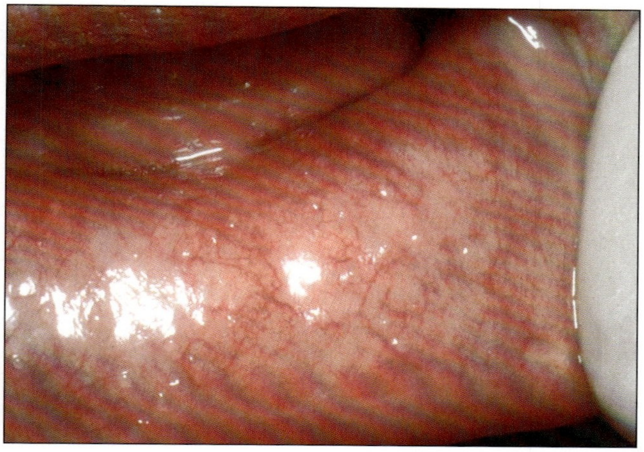

Fig 10-3d There is no sign of the ulcer 1 week after treatment.

Purpose of the procedure	Palliation of a recurrent aphthous ulcer
Laser treatment successfully removed the aphthous ulcer.	

Wavelength and settings

Nd:YAG laser set to 30 mJ, 60 Hz, defocused, with a 320 μm fiber.

Alternate wavelengths that may be used

Any laser can be used to perform this procedure.

Clinical tip

Laser treatment of recurrent aphthous ulcers can be performed with or without analgesia. Without analgesia, a defocused laser set to low power is placed between 6 and 8 cm from the ulcer and slowly circled in toward the lesion. If the patient begins to feel discomfort, the clinician slowly circles the laser 0.5 cm away from the lesion before slowly recircling in toward the lesion. This process is repeated until the clinician can touch the laser to the lesion without patient discomfort. The lesion is "painted" with the laser fiber, making certain that the entire area of ulcerated mucosa is exposed to the laser energy. The lesion may bleed slightly, then coagulate. Once the lesion has been completely covered by a film of coagulum, the treatment is completed.

When using infiltration or topical analgesia, the clinician can immediately place the laser 1 mm from the lesion and "paint" the numb ulcerated area until the entire lesion has been covered.

Though most cases of this type may be treated without analgesia, the use of analgesia should be discussed with the patient before treatment is initiated.

Aphthous Ulcer: Case 2

Treatment of an aphthous ulcer on the floor of the mouth.

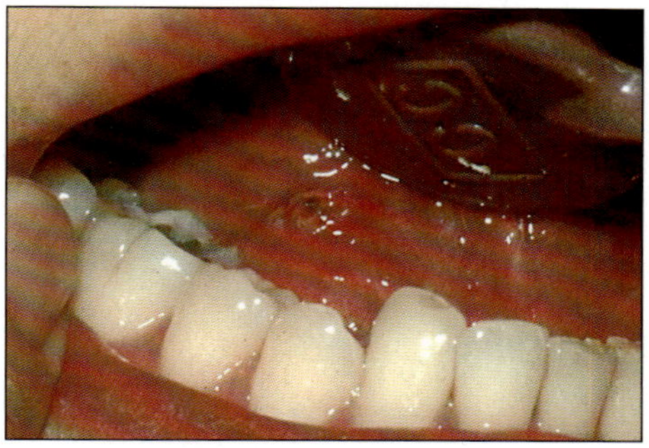

Fig 10-4a Large recurrent aphthous ulcer on the floor of the mouth.

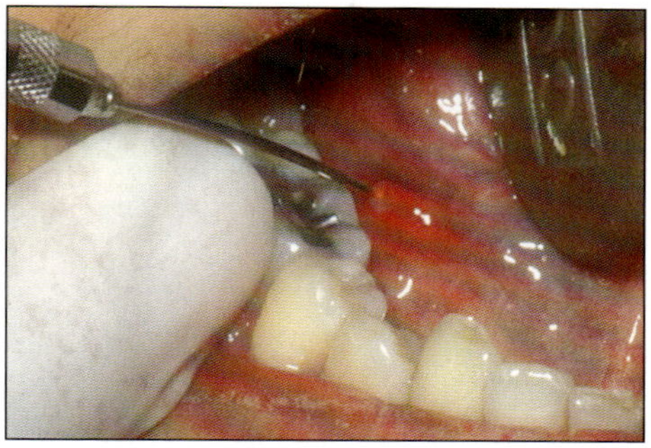

Fig 10-4b A laser is used to treat the sublingual ulcer.

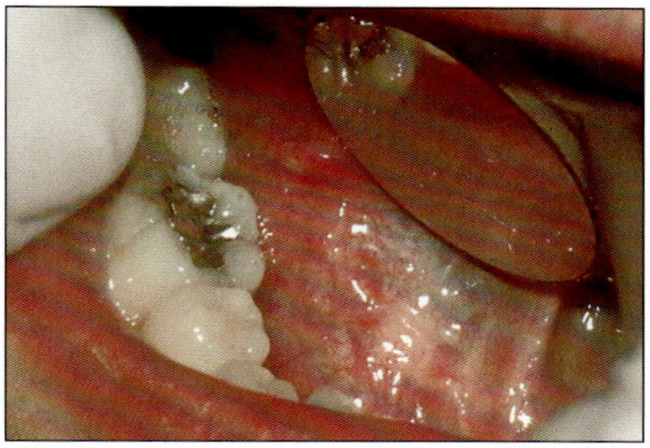

Fig 10-4c Aphthous lesion immediately following laser treatment.

Purpose of the procedure	Treatment of recurrent aphthous ulcer
Laser treatment successfully removes the aphthous ulcer.	

Wavelength and settings

Nd:YAG laser set to 30 mJ, 60 Hz, defocused, with 320 μm fiber.

Alternate wavelengths that may be used

Any laser can be used to perform this procedure.

Aphthous Ulcer: Case 3

Treatment of an aphthous-like lesion on the lower lip in an HIV-positive patient.

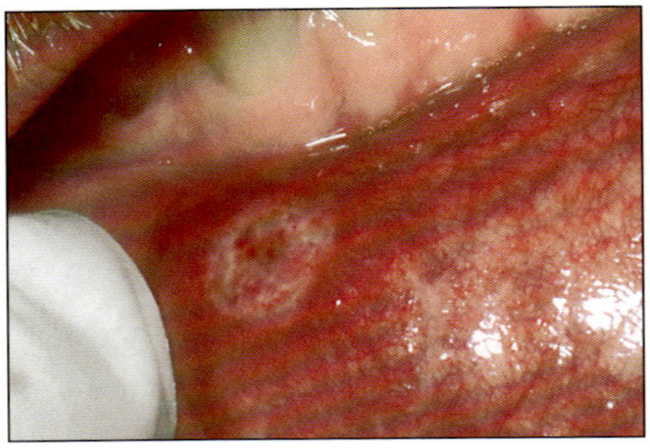

Fig 10-5a Large aphthous-like lesion on the mucosa inside the lower lip.

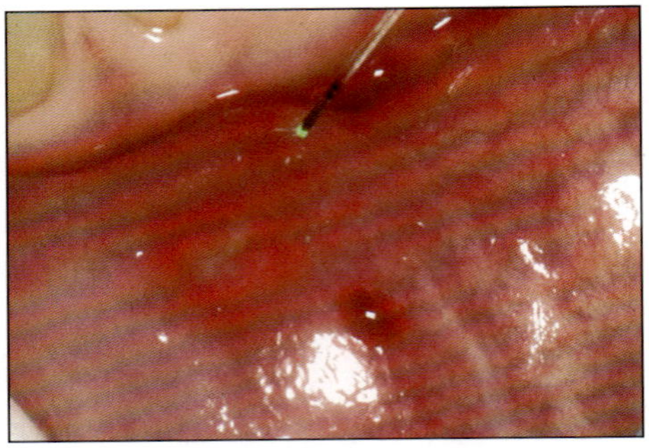

Fig 10-5b The laser begins the lesion treatment.

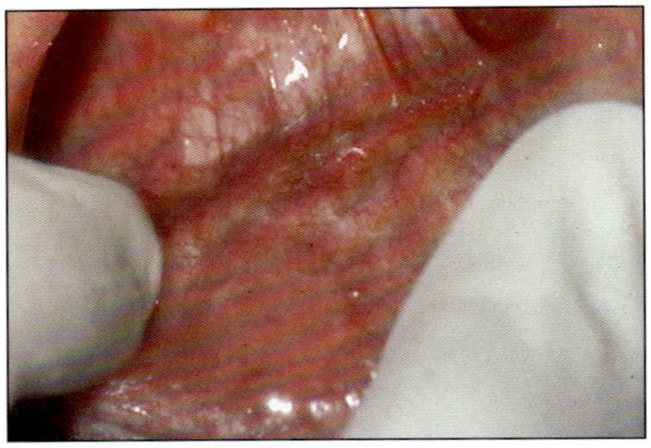

Fig 10-5c Two days following the treatment, the lesion on the lower lip has completely healed.

Purpose of the procedure

Palliation of an aphthous-like lesion

Laser treatment successfully removed the lesion.

Wavelength and settings

Nd:YAG laser set to 100 mJ, 50 Hz, defocused, with a 320 μm fiber.

Alternate wavelengths that may be used

Any laser can be used to perform this procedure.

Clinical discussion

This patient was extremely anxious about dental treatment and requested to be anesthetized for the treatment; note the blood from the pinprick of the needle (see Fig 10-5b). The laser settings used on this patient are much higher than in case 2 because the patient had been anesthetized.

Herpetic Lesion: Case 1

Treatment of a herpetic lesion in a female patient.

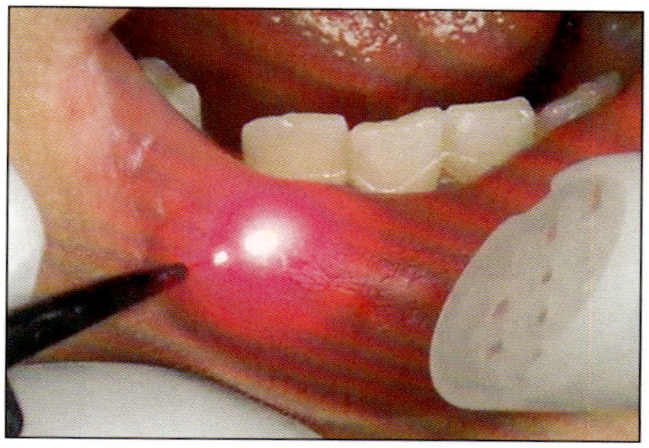

Fig 10-6a A diode laser ablates a herpetic lesion forming on the lower lip.

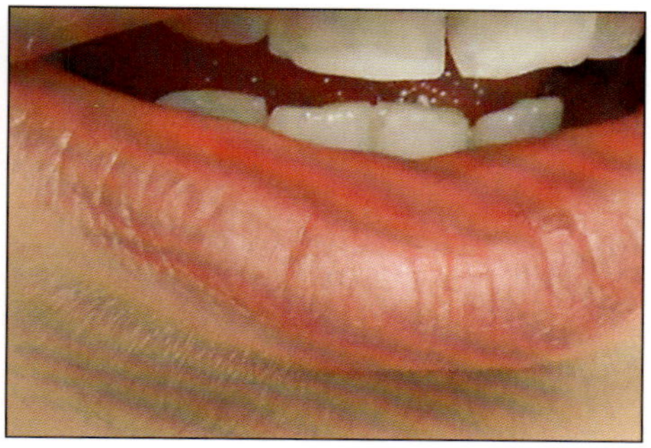

Fig 10-6b Immediate postoperative view of lip.

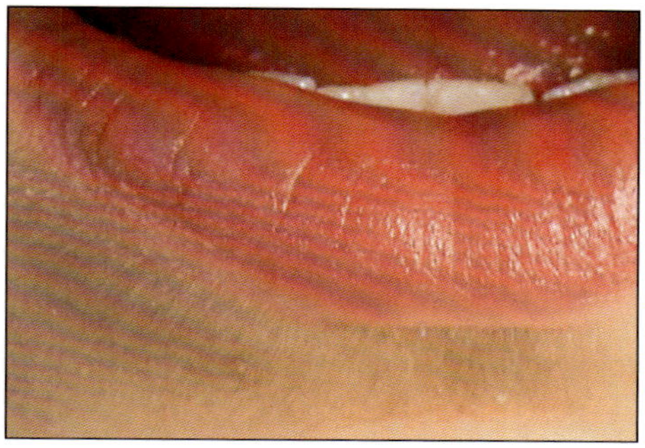

Fig 10-6c There is no evidence of the herpetic lesion 1 day after laser treatment. (Case courtesy of Dr Philip Hudson, Spokane, WA.)

Purpose of the procedure	Treatment of a herpetic lesion
Laser ablation disinfects the lesion, allowing for complete healing.	

Wavelength and settings

Diode laser set to 0.4 W, continuous wave defocused and incrementally increased to 0.7 W.

Alternate wavelengths that may be used

Any laser can be used to perform this procedure.

Pericoronitis: Case 1

Treatment of pericoronitis around a mandibular third molar.

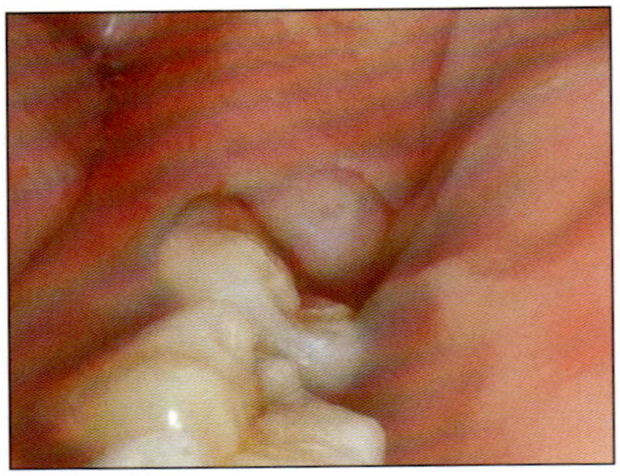

Fig 10-7a Inflamed pericoronal tissue around a partially erupted mandibular left third molar.

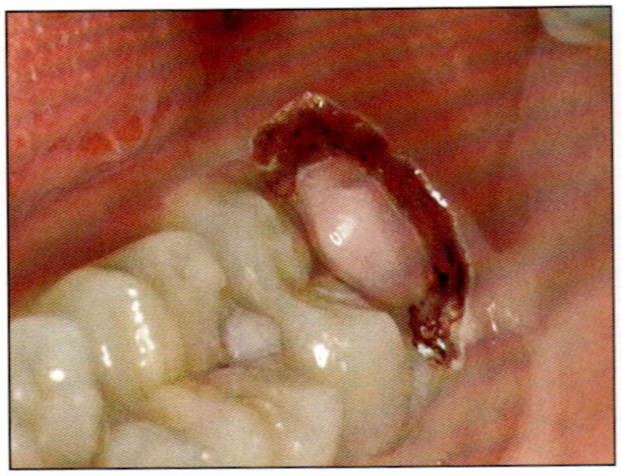

Fig 10-7b The laser has been used to make a semilunar incision over the partially erupted tooth.

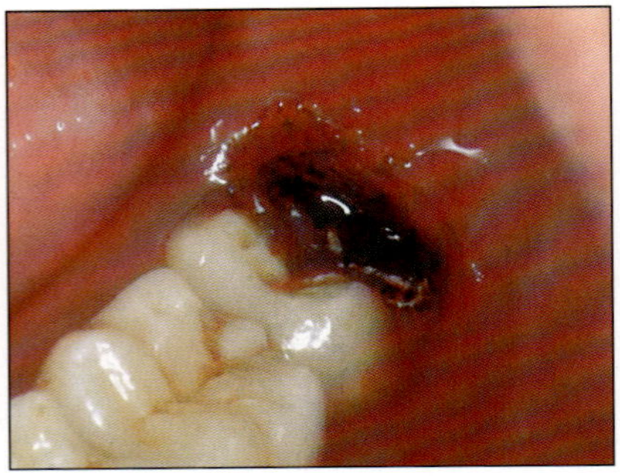

Fig 10-7c Immediate postoperative view showing a completely exposed third molar.

Purpose of the procedure	Treatment of pericoronitis
Ablation of inflamed pericoronal tissue exposes the mandibular left third molar.	

Wavelength and settings

CO_2 laser set to 4 W, continuous wave, with an 800 μm ceramic tip.

Alternate wavelengths that may be used

Any laser can be used to perform this procedure.

Clinical tip

This procedure treated the pericoronitis. Since pericoronitis is primarily a bacterial infection, use of the laser is preferred over a scalpel due to the laser's bactericidal capability. Once the inflamed tissue is removed, the clinician can decide if the mandibular left third molar should be extracted. In some cases, excision of the tissue will allow the tooth to completely erupt into the mouth, with no further treatment needed.

Gingival Abscess: Case 1

Drainage of an abscess around the mandibular right canine.

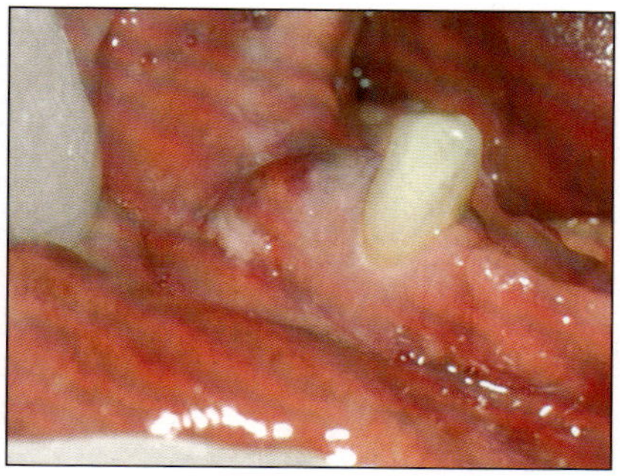

Fig 10-8a Fluctuant swelling around the mandibular right canine due to a combined periodontic and endodontic abscess.

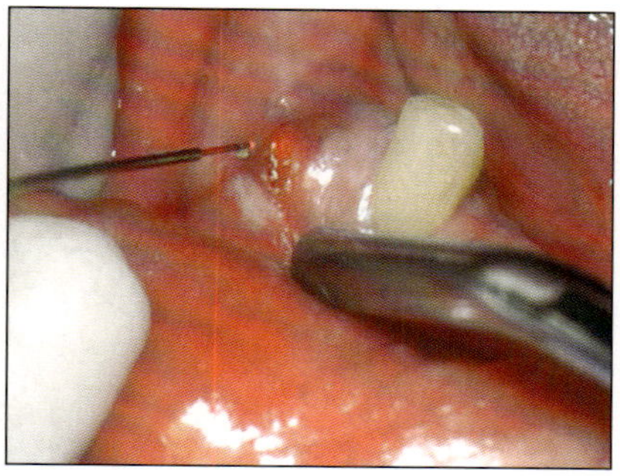

Fig 10-8b To make the incision, the laser fiber approaches the height of the fluctuant area.

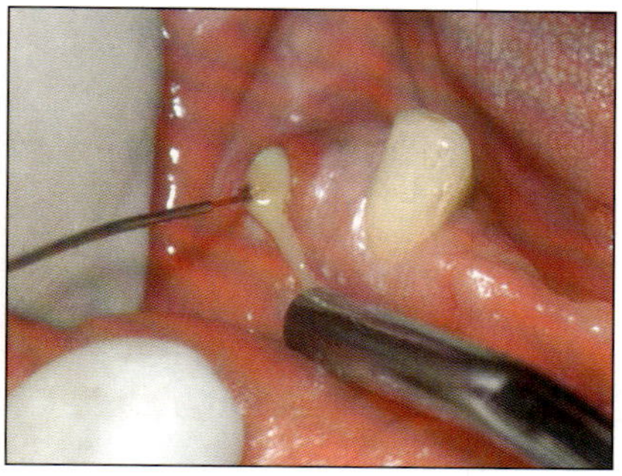

Fig 10-8c Once the incision has been made, the abscess begins to drain, and exudate flows freely from the incision.

Purpose of the procedure	Drainage of an abscess
Swelling is relieved once an incision is made and the abscess is drained.	

Wavelength and settings

Nd:YAG set to 100 mJ, 50 Hz, with a 320 μm fiber.

Alternate wavelengths that may be used

Any laser can be used to perform this procedure.

Clinical tip

As with aphthous ulcers, this procedure may be performed either with or without analgesia. Whether a laser or a scalpel is used, the procedure follows the same technique. The instrument is placed at the height of the fluctuant mass and an incision is quickly made down to the bone. The abscess should begin to drain immediately. The clinician must decide about placement of a drain as well as prescription of an antibiotic for the patient. An appointment for definitive treatment should be scheduled as soon as possible.

Kaposi Sarcoma Lesion: Case 1

Treatment of a Kaposi sarcoma lesion in the maxilla of an HIV-positive patient.

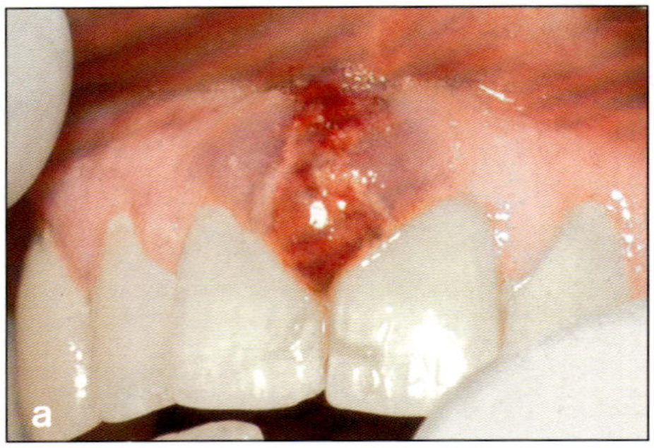

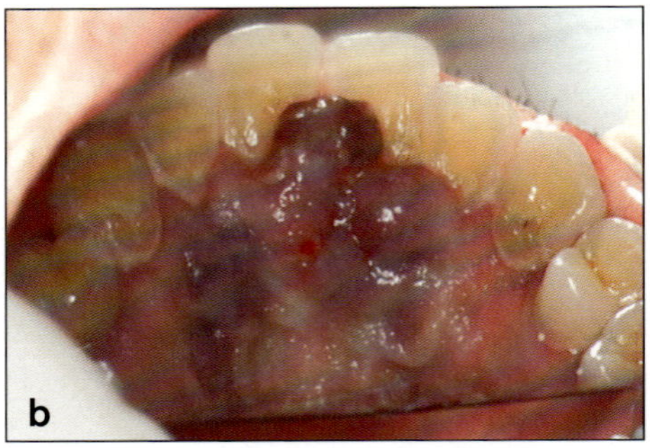

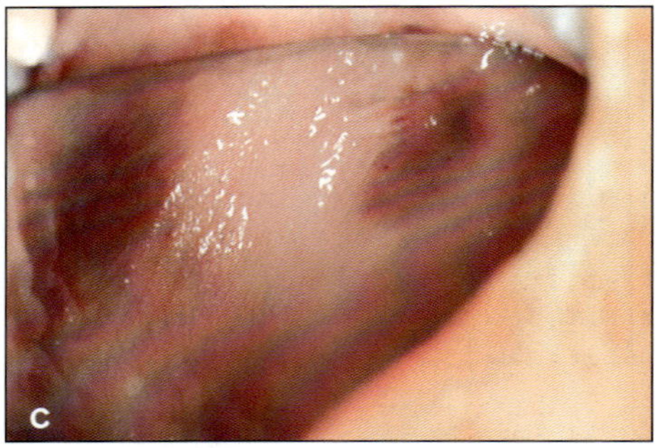

Figs 10-9a to 10-9c Preoperative facial *(a)*, anterior palatal *(b)*, and posterior palatal *(c)* views of an HIV-positive patient with a Kaposi sarcoma lesion extending through the embrasure from the facial aspect to the palate.

Purpose of the procedure	Treatment of Kaposi sarcoma

Laser treatment successfully ablates the Kaposi sarcoma lesion.

Wavelength and settings

CO_2 laser set to 5 W, continuous wave, with an 800 μm ceramic tip.

Alternate wavelengths that may be used

Although any laser may be used to perform this procedure, the CO_2 laser is most effective given its superior hemostatic ability and the highly vascular nature of these lesions. The Er family of lasers is least effective.

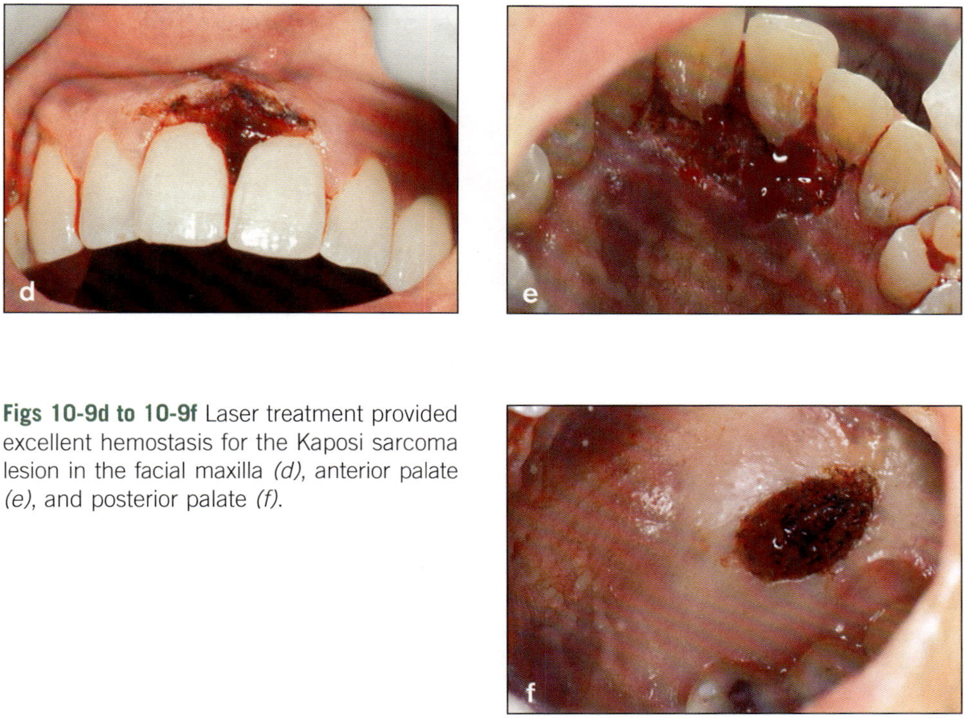

Figs 10-9d to 10-9f Laser treatment provided excellent hemostasis for the Kaposi sarcoma lesion in the facial maxilla *(d)*, anterior palate *(e)*, and posterior palate *(f)*.

Clinical tip

As with any laser procedure, it is imperative that the clinician and staff practice universal safety precautions, including appropriate methods of controlling laser plume. Along with high-speed suction, a smoke evacuator further minimizes exposure to the plume. A well-fitting laser plume mask (0.1 μm filtration) is mandatory for all clinical laser procedures.

Lichen Planus: Case 1

Treatment of lichen planus on the left cheek.

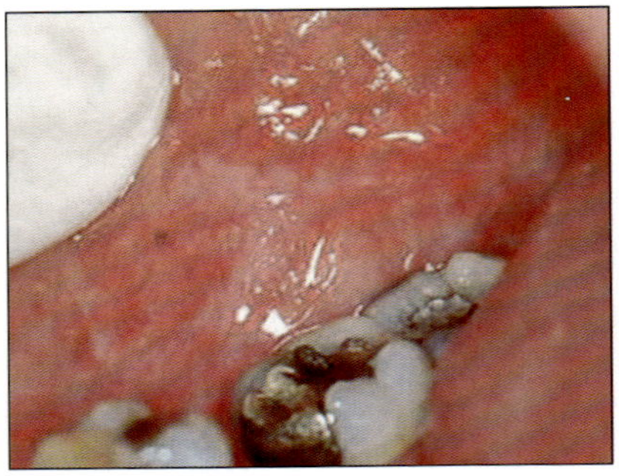

Fig 10-10a An area of lichen planus is visible on the mucosa inside the right cheek.

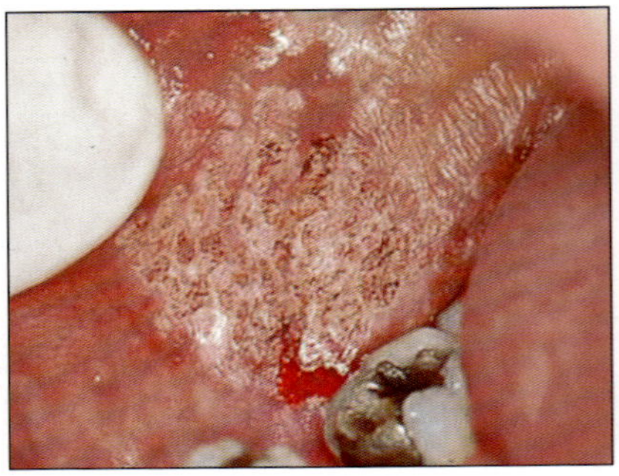

Fig 10-10b Immediate postoperative view of the right cheek.

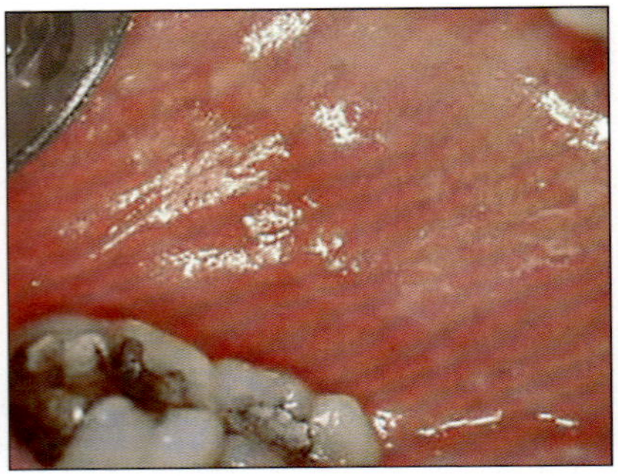

Fig 10-10c Two weeks following treatment, the lichen planus is gone.

Purpose of the procedure

Treatment of lichen planus

Laser ablation of the lichen planus removes the lesion.

Wavelength and settings

CO_2 set to 2 W continuous wave, with a 600 µm tip.

Alternate wavelengths that may be used

Any laser can be used to perform this procedure.

Clinical tip

It is imperative that a clinical diagnosis be made before soft tissue is ablated. If a diagnosis has not been established, a biopsy should be performed to determine a diagnosis before laser treatment is begun.

Premalignant Lesion: Case 1

Treatment of a premalignant lesion in the buccal vestibule.

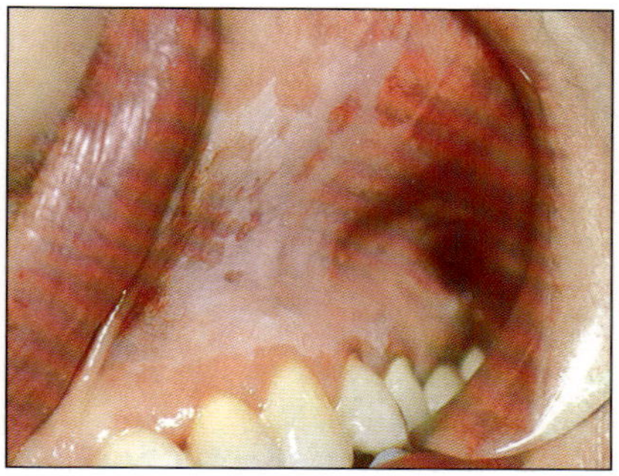

Fig 10-11a Preoperative view of a premalignant lesion extending along the buccal vestibule, from the right pterygomandibular raphe to the left pterygomandibular raphe.

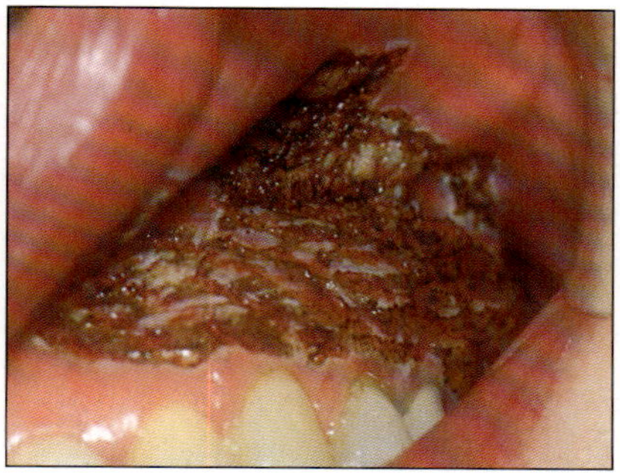

Fig 10-11b The immediate postoperative view demonstrates the hemostasis achieved during laser ablation of the lesion.

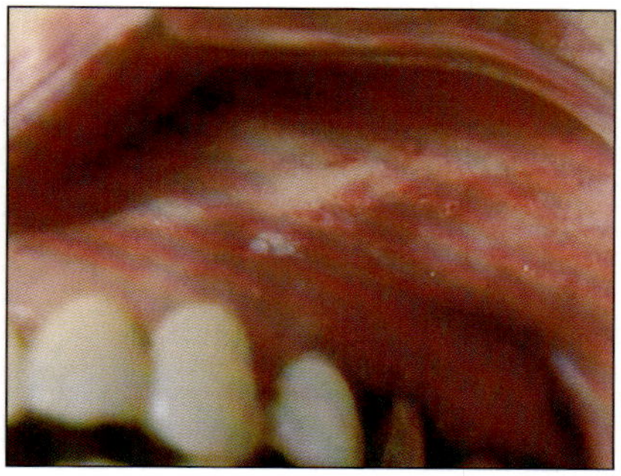

Fig 10-11c Healing of the buccal vestibule is evident 1 week following treatment.

Purpose of the procedure

Treatment of a premalignant lesion

Laser ablation successfully removes a premalignant lesion.

Wavelength and settings

CO_2 laser set to 5 W, continuous wave, with an 800 μm ceramic tip.

Alternate wavelengths that may be used

Any laser can be used to perform this procedure.

Clinical tip

Multiple incisional biopsies were previously performed on this lesion. Once the definitive diagnosis was made via biopsy, the oral pathologist determined that the lesion should be removed in toto. Treatment options of either conventional stripping of the mucosa with a scalpel or laser ablation were discussed with the patient. Due to the extent of the lesion, conventional stripping would have been a difficult task requiring sedation and risking blood loss and postoperative discomfort. Laser treatment did not require sedation, blood loss was insignificant, and postoperative discomfort was negligible.

Biopsy: Case 1

Biopsy of a tongue lesion in a patient taking an oral anticoagulant.

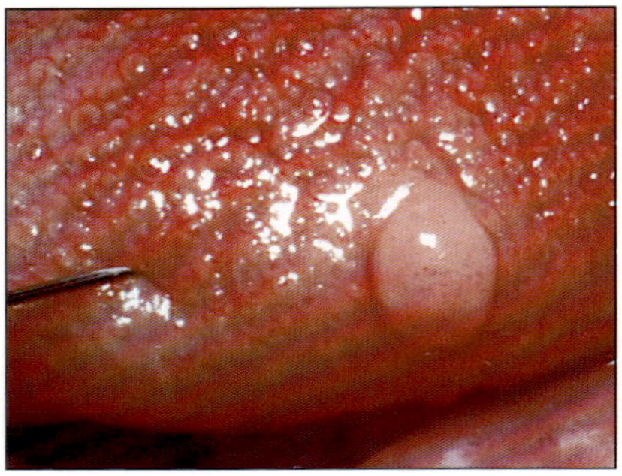

Fig 10-12a Anesthesia is deposited near a tongue lesion in preparation for a biopsy.

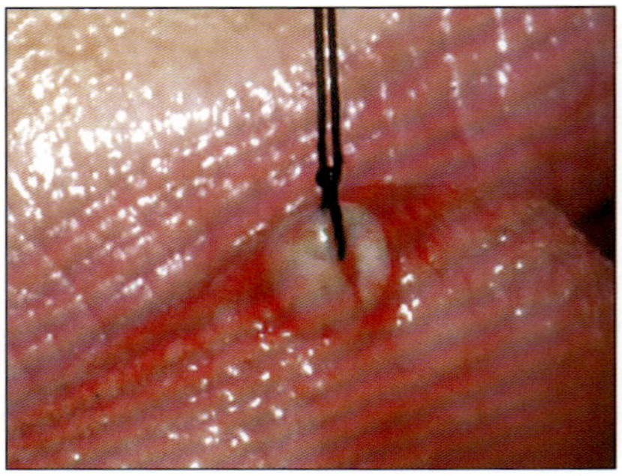

Fig 10-12b A purse string suture is placed through the lesion.

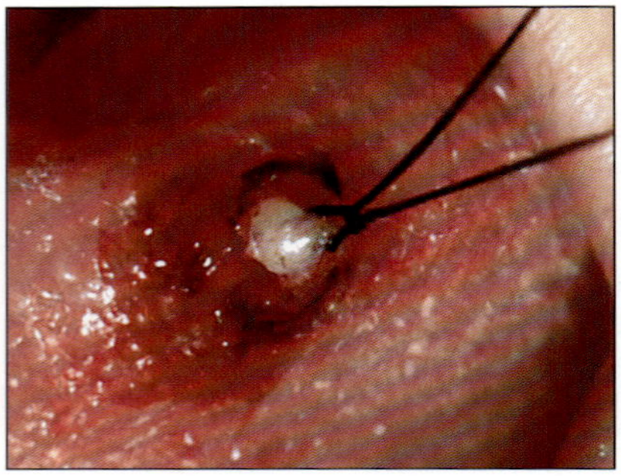

Fig 10-12c The purse string suture retracts the lesion while it is undermined through laser ablation.

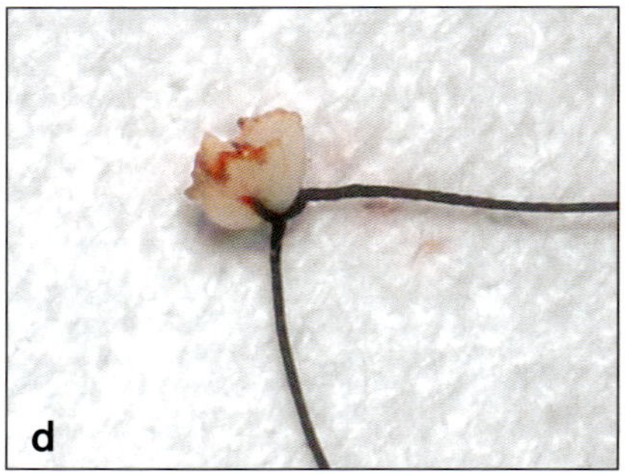

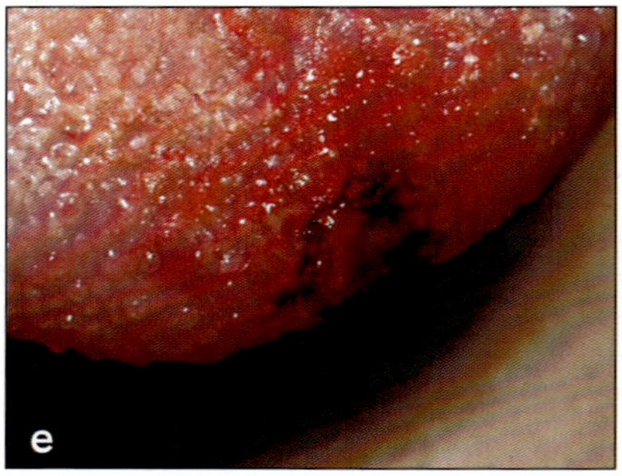

Figs 10-12d and 10-12e Immediate postoperative views showing the separated lesion *(d)* and the surgical site *(e)*. Even though the patient is taking an oral anticoagulant (ie, 5 mg of Coumadin), the laser provided excellent hemostasis.

Purpose of the procedure

Biopsy of a tongue lesion

Wavelength and settings

CO_2 laser; settings for the initial excision: 4 W with an 800 µm ceramic tip; settings for undermining the lesion: 3 W with a 250 µm tip.

Alternate wavelengths that may be used

Any laser can be used to perform this procedure.

Clinical tip

Deposition of anesthetic solution is an important consideration when performing laser biopsies. If anesthetic is irregularly deposited around the lesion, tissue absorbtion of the laser energy could be irregular, resulting in inconsistent laser penetration depth around the lesion. For efficient ablation, the anesthetic solution should be deposited at least 1 cm from the borders of the incision.

Purse string sutures make it easy to hold the lesion and maintain countertraction during biopsy. A single suture is placed through the lesion and then held as the lesion is undermined.

Biopsy: Case 2

Biopsy of a mucocele on the lower lip in a female patient.

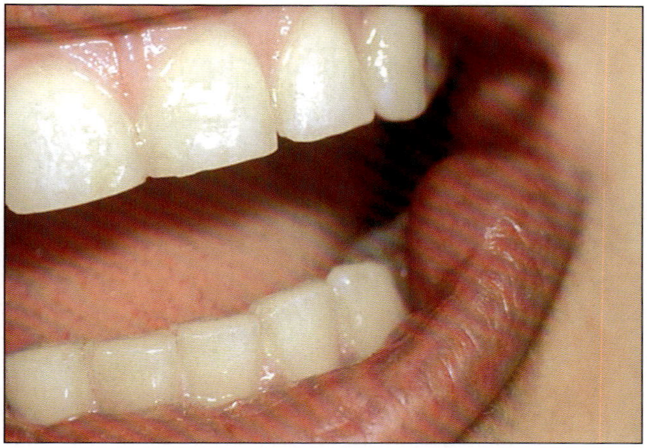

Fig 10-13a A large mucocele is located inside the patient's lower lip on the left side.

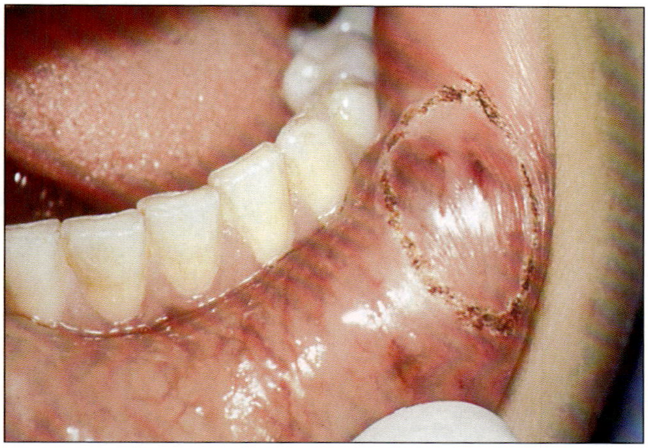

Fig 10-13b The wide borders of the biopsy are outlined using a laser at low power.

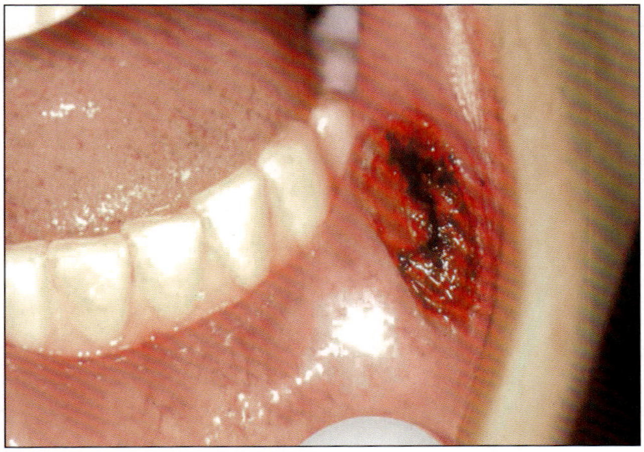

Fig 10-13c The lesion is removed with the laser instrument.

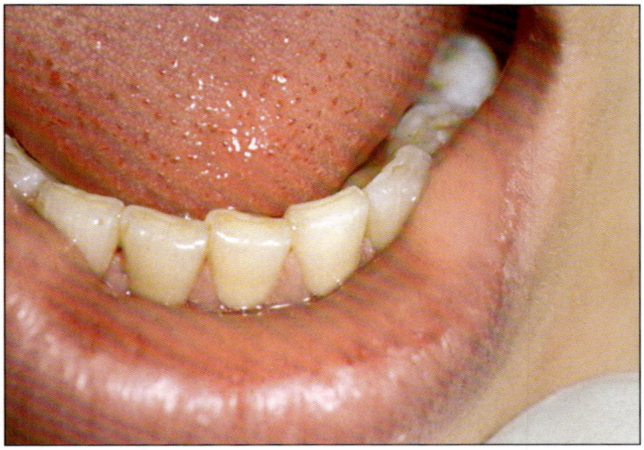

Fig 10-13d Secondary intention healing is complete 2 weeks after the laser biopsy.

Purpose of the procedure	Biopsy of a mucocele on the lower lip

Wavelength and settings

CO_2 laser; settings to outline the lesion: 3 W, pulsed, with an 800 µm ceramic tip; settings to remove the lesion: 3 W, continuous wave, with an 800 µm ceramic tip.

Clinical tip

When an excisional biopsy is performed, no matter what technique is being used—scalpel, electrosurgical instrument, or laser—it is imperative to plan wide borders that incorporate the entire lesion as well as some normal tissue surrounding the lesion. The pathologist must be able to read all of the margins of the biopsy without interference from thermal damage to the specimen. When a laser is used for any incision or excision, it is important to evaluate the effect of the laser parameters on the tissue to prevent inadvertent damage to the tissue.

The biopsy technique shown in this case illustrates the techniques of taking a wide border and of evaluating the tissue response to the laser. By first outlining the borders, the clinician can determine if the margins are too wide or narrow and change the outline before continuing. Likewise, if the laser parameters result in an insufficient or excessive incision depth or charring of the specimen, the parameters can be modified without affecting the clinical result. Once the clinician is satisfied with the borders, the laser setting is changed from a pulsed to a continuous wave mode to begin excision. Biopsy sites are generally left to heal by secondary intent, with no sutures. These surgical sites heal with no postoperative discomfort.

Biopsy: Case 3

Biopsy of a gingival lesion on the patient's maxilla.

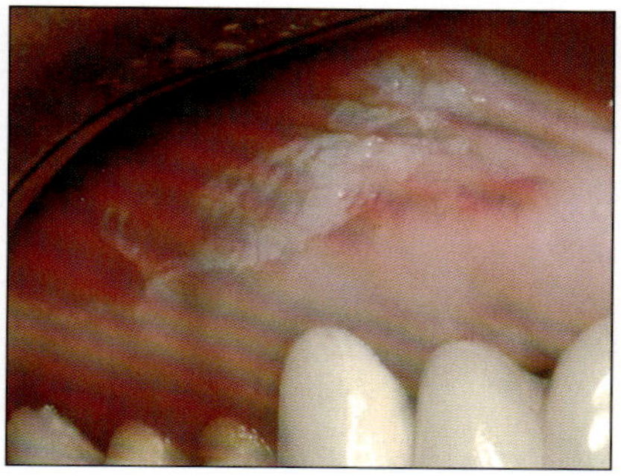

Fig 10-14a Preoperative view of a white lesion on the right side of the patient's maxilla.

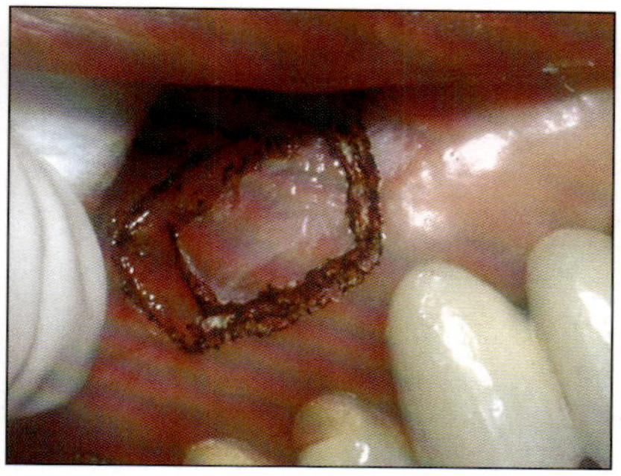

Fig 10-14b The laser was used to outline the biopsy margins.

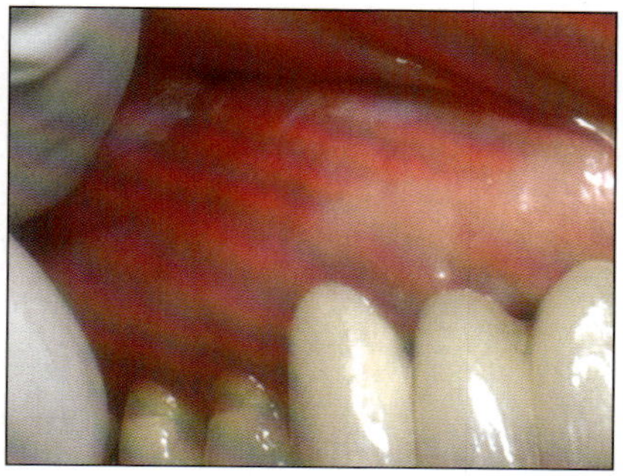

Fig 10-14c Two-week postoperative view showing complete healing.

Purpose of the procedure	Biopsy of a white lesion

Wavelength and settings

CO_2 laser set to 5 W, continuous wave, with an 800 µm ceramic tip.

Alternate wavelengths that may be used

Any laser can be used to perform this procedure.

Clinical tip

Unlike case 2, the technique for this procedure did not follow recommended protocol. The outline of the lesion was performed with a laser at high power in a continuous wave mode, rather than with a laser at low power, which resulted in charred and irregular borders. Despite these errors, Fig 10-14c shows excellent clinical results. Even using less than ideal technique, no damage was done to the tissue, and the clinical result was excellent. CO_2 lasers have a shallow penetration depth of only a few hundred microns. The evident charring in Fig 10-14b remains on the superficial layers of mucosa, and, because there is no thermal damage to the underlying tissue, the clinical result is unaffected.

Biopsy: Case 4

Biopsy of an irritation fibroma on the inside of the cheek.

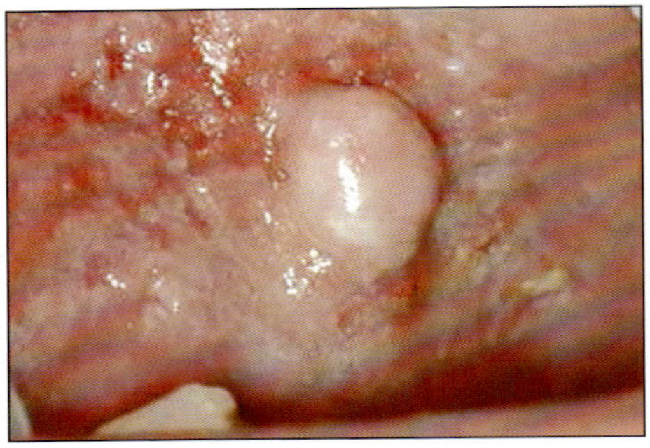

Fig 10-15a An irritation fibroma has formed on the inside of the cheek.

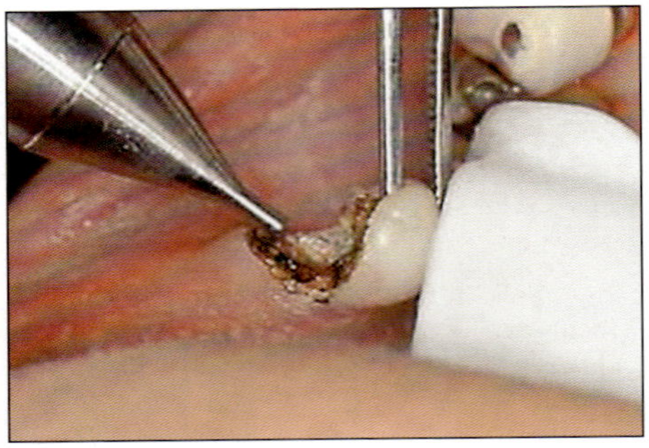

Fig 10-15b A laser is used to remove the fibroma while it is held by a metal instrument.

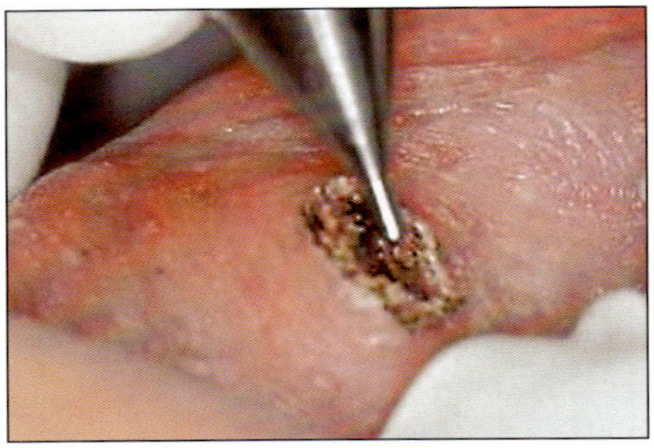

Fig 10-15c Immediate postoperative view of the surgical site.

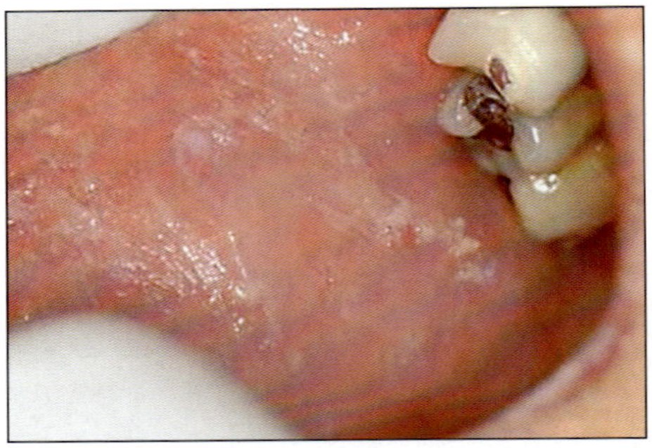

Fig 10-15d Two weeks following treatment, the surgical site is completely healed. (Case courtesy of Dr Steven Parker, Harrogate, North Yorkshire, England.)

Purpose of the procedure

Biopsy of an irritation fibroma

Wavelength and settings

CO_2 laser set to 2.5 W, continuous wave, with a 600 μm metal tip.

Alternate wavelengths that may be used

Any laser can be used to perform this procedure.

Clinical tip

Rather than a purse string suture, a metal instrument is used to hold the irritation fibroma during the biopsy. There are many instruments that may be used, including college pliers, a hemostat, and Adson-type forceps.

Biopsy: Case 5

Biopsy of an irritation fibroma on the tongue.

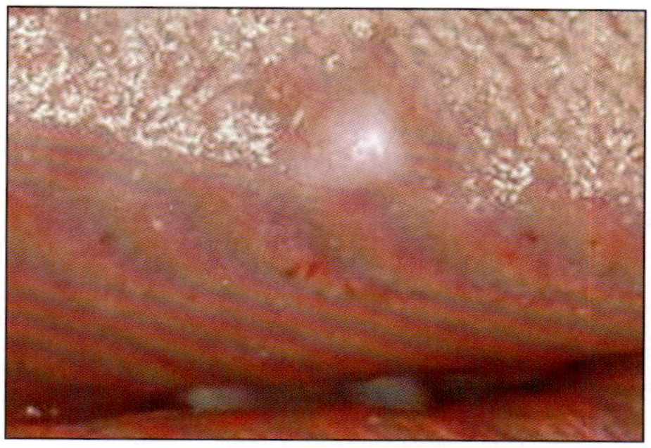

Fig 10-16a An irritation fibroma on the lateral border of the tongue.

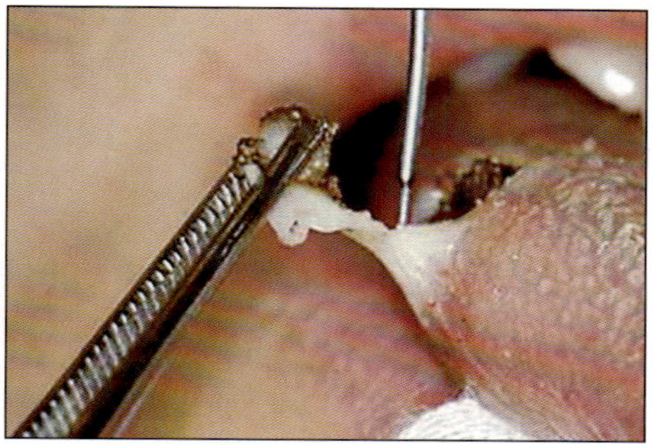

Fig 10-16b The laser undermines the fibroma while the lesion is held by a metal instrument.

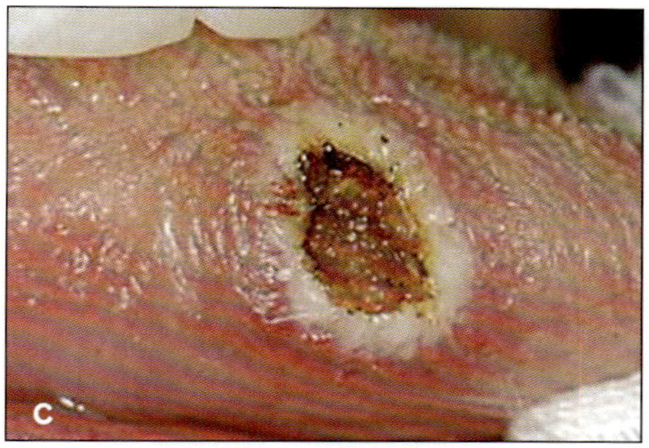

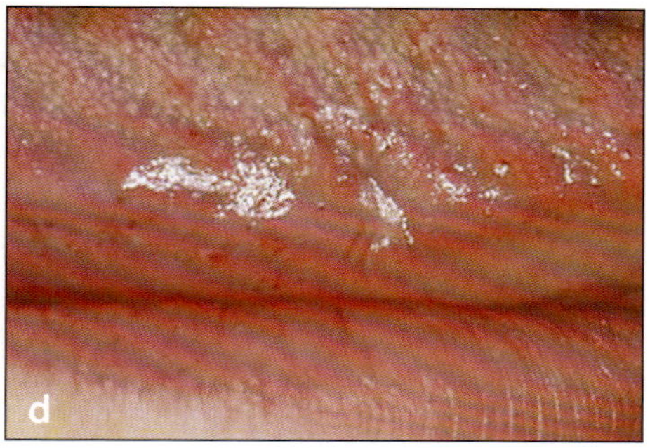

Figs 10-16c and 10-16d The surgical site immediately *(c)* and 3 weeks *(d)* after the biopsy.

Purpose of the procedure

Biopsy of an irritation fibroma on the tongue

Wavelength and settings

Nd:YAG laser set to 100 mJ, 20 to 30 Hz, with a 320 µm fiber.

Alternate wavelengths that may be used

Any laser can be used to perform this procedure.

Clinical tip

This case illustrates the efficiency of using an instrument such as a hemostat to grasp the lesion during laser surgery.

Biopsy: Case 6

Biopsy of a gingival giant cell granuloma.

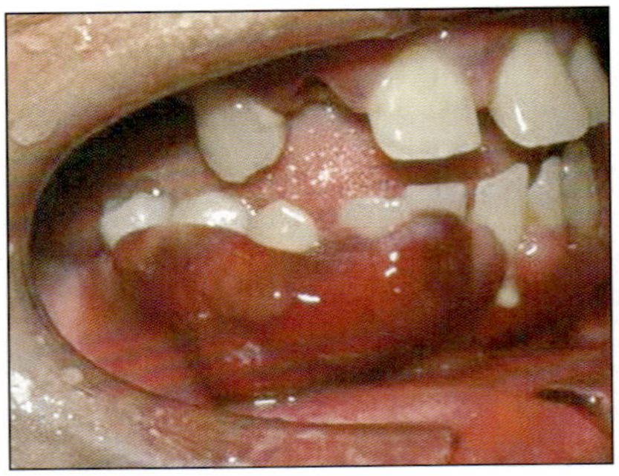

Fig 10-17a A peripheral giant cell granuloma on the mandibular gingiva.

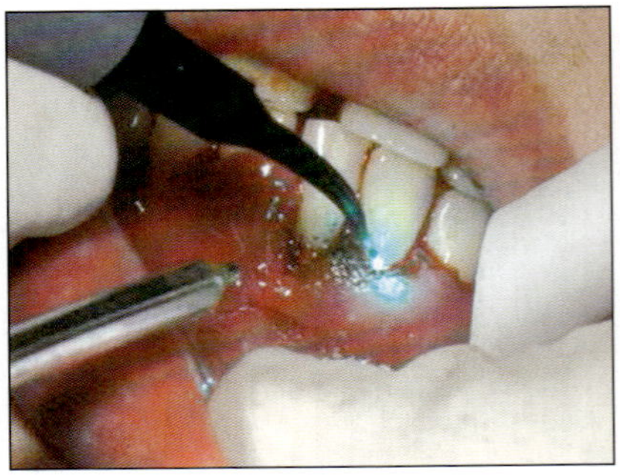

Fig 10-17b A laser begins to remove the gingival growth from the anterior region of the mandible.

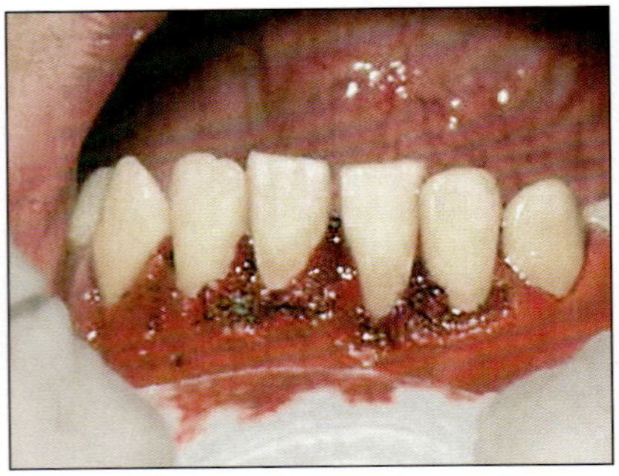

Fig 10-17c Immediately following surgery, the laser has accomplished adequate hemostasis.

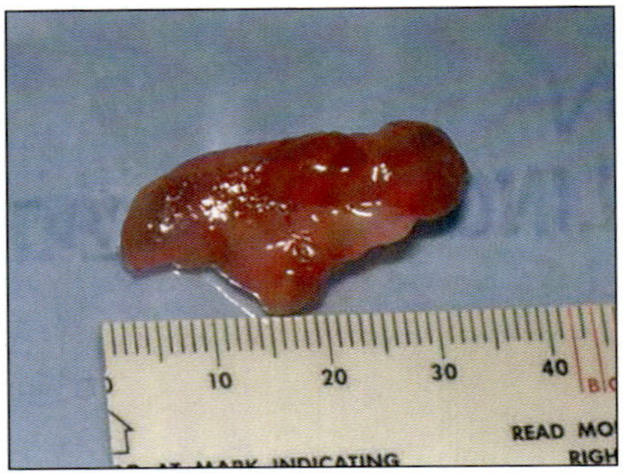

Fig 10-17d Biopsy specimen of the giant cell granuloma.

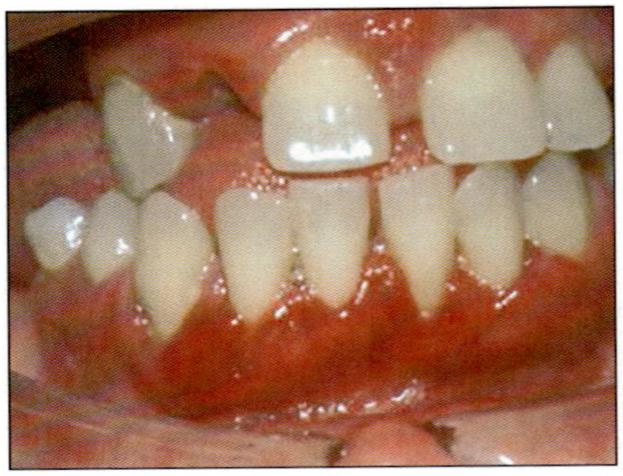

Fig 10-17e Two weeks after surgery, the mandibular gingiva is healed. (Case courtesy of Dr David Roshkind, West Palm Beach, FL.)

Purpose of the procedure	Biopsy of a giant cell granuloma

Wavelength and settings

Ar laser, 514 nm, set to 1.5 W, continuous wave.

Alternate wavelengths that may be used

Any laser can be used to perform this procedure.

Biopsy: Case 7

Biopsy of a palatal pyogenic granuloma in a female patient.

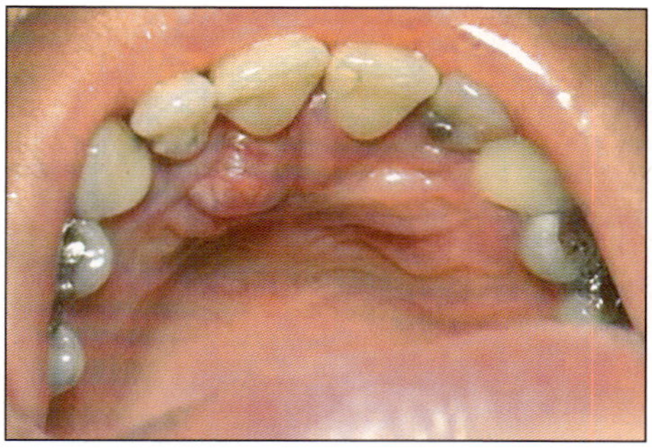

Fig 10-18a Pyogenic granuloma on the patient's maxillary palate apical to the maxillary right central incisor.

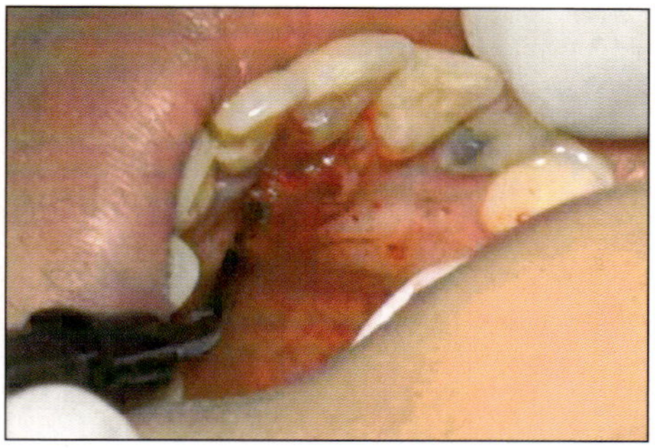

Fig 10-18b A Nd:YAG laser is used to remove the palatal lesion.

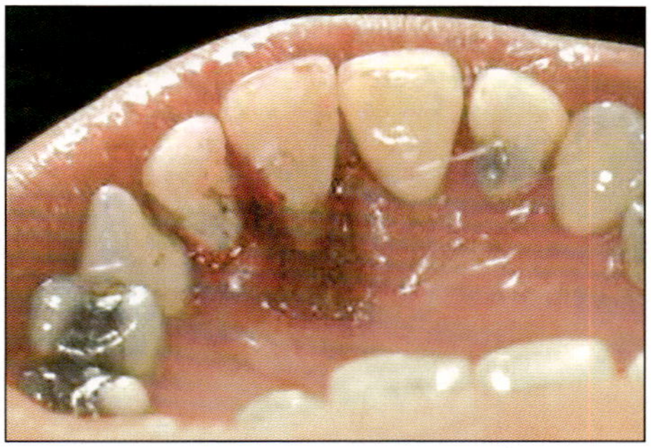

Fig 10-18c The immediate postoperative view of the surgical site shows hemostasis.

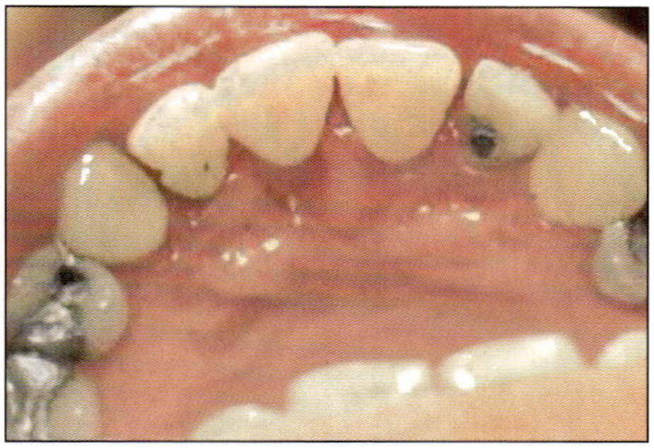

Fig 10-18d The surgical site has completely healed 2 weeks after the laser biopsy. (Case courtesy of Dr David Roshkind, West Palm Beach, FL.)

Purpose of the procedure	Biopsy of a pyogenic granuloma

Wavelength and settings
Nd:YAG laser set to 100 mJ, 20 Hz, with a 320 μm fiber.
Alternate wavelengths that may be used
Any laser can be used to perform this procedure.

Biopsy: Case 8

Biopsy of an irritation fibroma on the inside of the cheek.

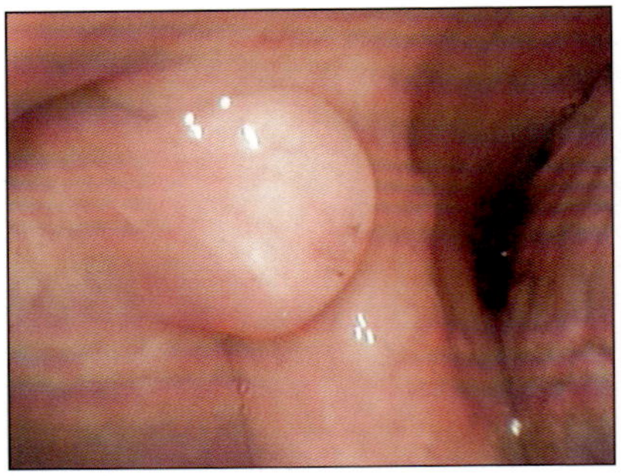

Fig 10-19a A large irritation fibroma on the inside of the posterior cheek.

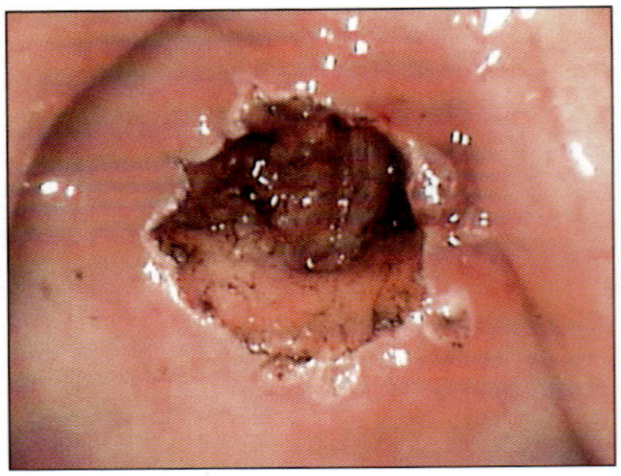

Fig 10-19b A CO_2 laser was used to remove the fibroma.

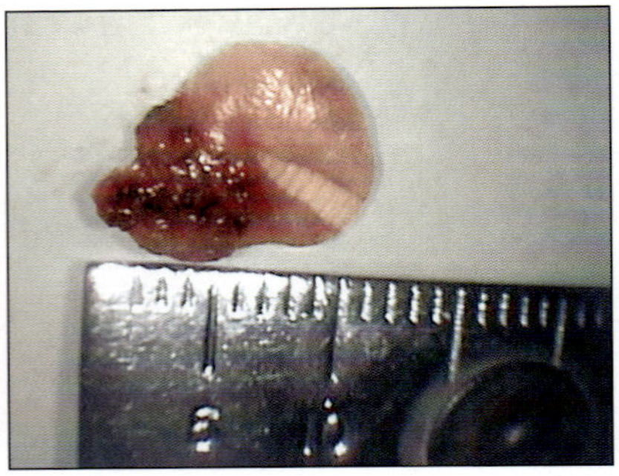

Fig 10-19c Biopsy specimen immediately following removal.

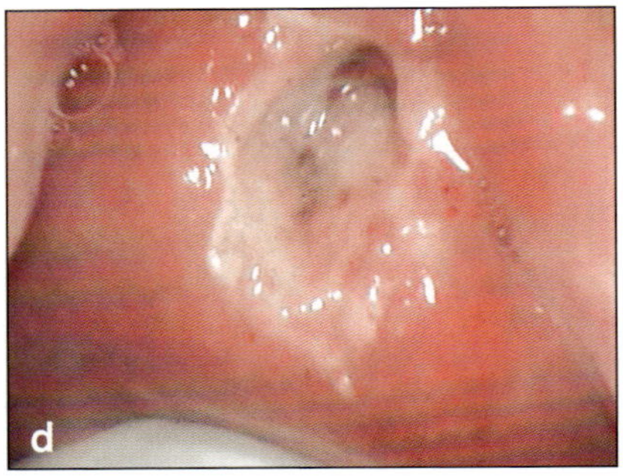

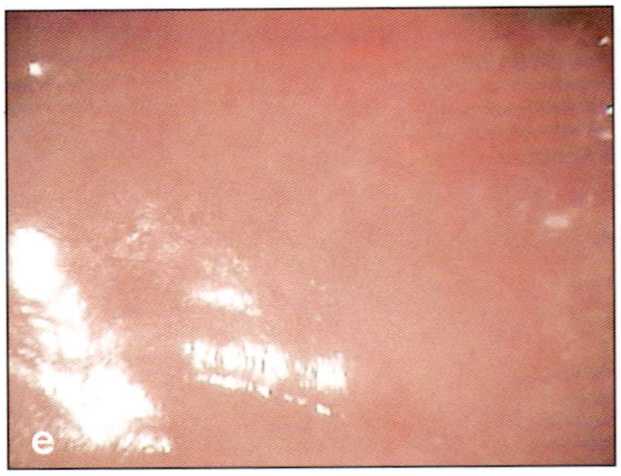

Figs 10-19d and 10-19e Postoperative views 1 day *(d)* and 1 week *(e)* following laser biopsy. (Case courtesy of Dr Dennis Pietrini, Franklin Park, IL.)

Purpose of the procedure	Biopsy of an irritation fibroma

Wavelength and settings
CO_2 laser set to 4 W, continuous wave.
Alternate wavelengths that may be used
Any laser can be used to perform this procedure.

Biopsy: Case 9

Biopsy of a hemangioma fibrous lesion on the inside of the lower lip.

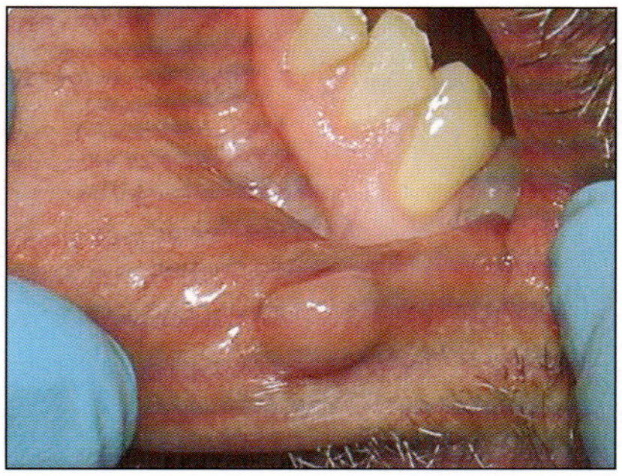

Fig 10-20a A vascularized lesion has formed on the inside of the patient's lower lip.

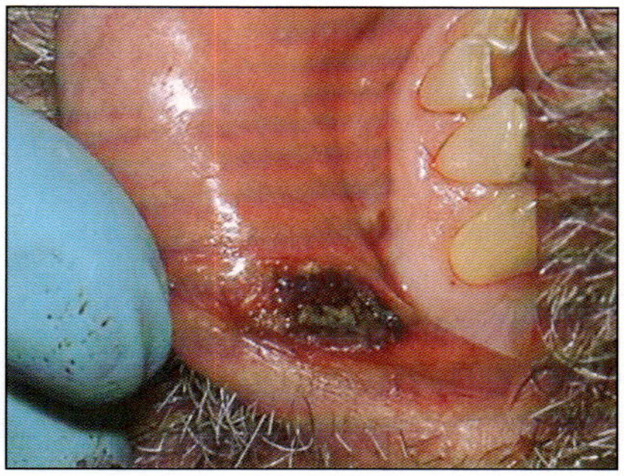

Fig 10-20b An Er laser was used to remove the lesion.

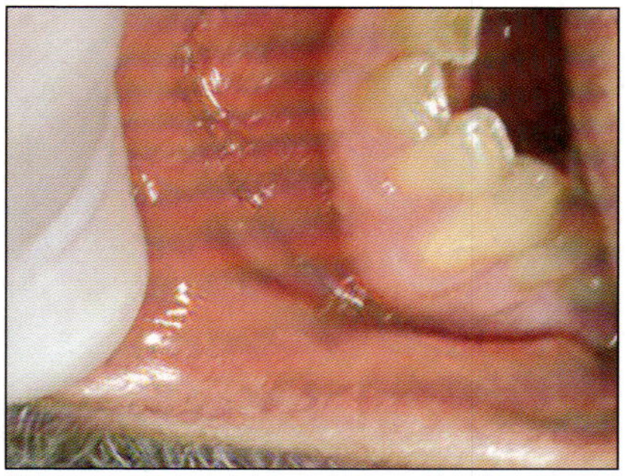

Fig 10-20c Two months following biopsy, there is no scar or evidence of surgery.

Purpose of the procedure	Biopsy of a hemangioma

Wavelength and settings

Er laser set to 30 Hz, 80 mJ, with a 600 μm tip and no water spray.

Alternate wavelengths that may be used

Any laser can be used to perform this procedure.

Clinical tip

The Er family of lasers can achieve hemostasis, although the shallow penetration depth limits bleeding control. When Er lasers are used, the water spray should be turned off. In addition, the laser beam should be defocused, which provides a larger spot size for distributing the laser energy to a wider area and aids in hemostasis.

References

1. Wigdor HA, Walsh JT Jr, Featherstone JD, Visuri SR, Fried D, Waldvogel JL. Lasers in dentistry. Lasers Surg Med 1995;16:103–133.
2. Wlodawsky R, Strauss RA. Intraoral use of lasers in oral maxillofacial surgery. Oral Maxillofac Surg Clin North Am 2004;16:149–163.
3. Strauss RA. Lasers in oral and maxillofacial surgery. Dent Clin North Am 2000;44:851–874.
4. Fisher SE, Frame JW. The effects of the carbon dioxide surgical laser on oral tissues. Br J Oral Maxillofac Surg 1984;22:414–425.
5. Niamtu J 3rd. The treatment of vascular and pigmented lesions in oral and maxillofacial surgery. Oral Maxillofac Surg Clin North Am 2004;16:239–254.
6. Abu-Serriah M, Critchlow H, Witters CJ, Ayoub A. Removal of partially erupted third molars using an erbium (Er):YAG laser: A randomised controlled clinical trial. Br J Oral Maxillofac Surg 2004;42:203–208.
7. Minton JP. The laser in surgery. A 23 year perspective. Am J Surg 1986;151:725–729.
8. Zimmermann I, Stern J, Frank F, Keiditsch E, Hofstetter A. Interception of lymphatic drainage by Nd:YAG laser irradiation in rat urinary bladder. Lasers Surg Med 1984;4:167–172.
9. Lanzafame RJ, McCormack CJ, Rogers DW, Naim JO, Herrera HR, Hinshaw JR. Mechanisms of reduction of tumor recurrence with carbon dioxide laser in experimental mammary tumors. Surg Gynecol Obstet 1988;167:493–496.
10. Lanzafame RJ, Rogers DW, Naim JO, Herrera HR, DeFranco C, Hinshaw JR. The effect of CO_2 laser excision on local tumor recurrence. Laser Surg Med 1986;6:103–105.
11. Lanzafame RJ, Rogers DW, Naim JO, DeFranco CA, Ochej H, Hinshaw JR. Reduction of local tumor recurrence by excision with the CO_2 laser. Laser Surg Med 1986;6:439–441.

11

LASER APPLICATIONS IN PEDIATRIC DENTISTRY

Dental lasers are an extremely valuable tool in many pediatric dental procedures.[1–3]

A variety of laser wavelengths may be used to perform soft tissue surgeries, such as exposure of unerupted teeth; revision and repositioning of the frenum[4,5]; removal of inflamed, hyperplastic, or granulomatous gingival tissue during orthodontic treatment; treatment of soft tissue proliferation due to drug therapy (eg, immunosuppressant drugs); or incision and drainage of soft tissue abscesses.[6] The use of lasers in these procedures offers clinical benefits that include bacterial reduction at the wound area, good coagulation of blood vessels, and precise control in the amount of tissue removed.[7–12]

Erbium (Er) lasers are highly effective in removing tooth structure and can be used for tooth preparation.[13–15] The laser is an excellent tool for treating young children and children who present with physical or cognitive challenges that may limit communication and prevent their understanding of necessary dental procedures. When a patient moves unexpectedly, the risk of injury from a dental laser is far lower than from a dental handpiece. Additionally, using the Er family of lasers does not usually require local anesthesia for treatment of carious tooth structure, eliminating the potential for injury from cheek or lip biting. The need for sedation may also be reduced, since many of these patients can accept dental care when they understand that alternative instrumentation can be used.

Exposure of Unerupted Teeth: Case 1

Exposure of unerupted teeth in an 11-year-old male.

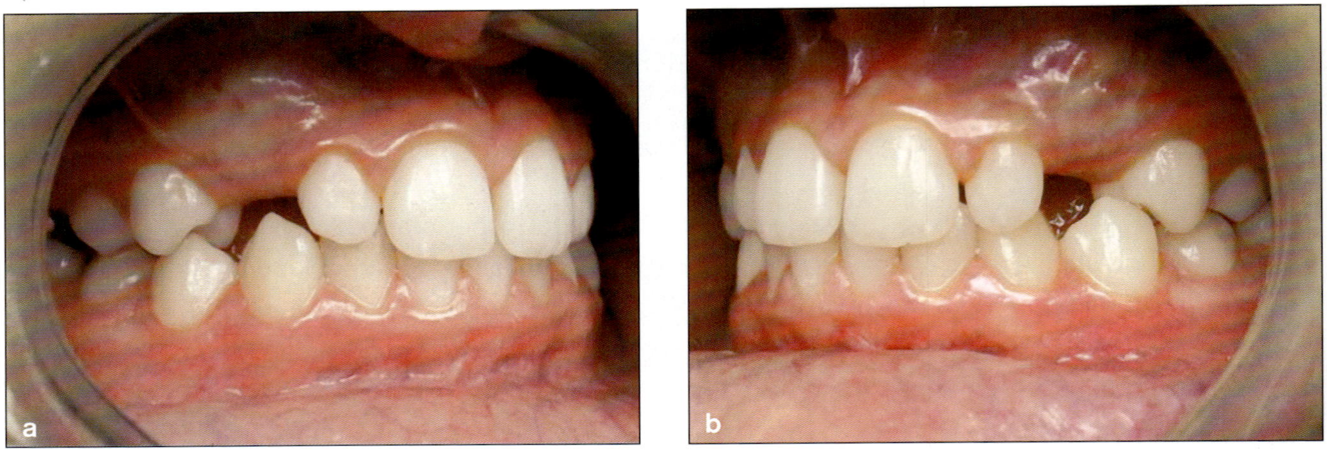

Figs 11-1a and 11-1b Preoperative bilateral views of unerupted maxillary canines.

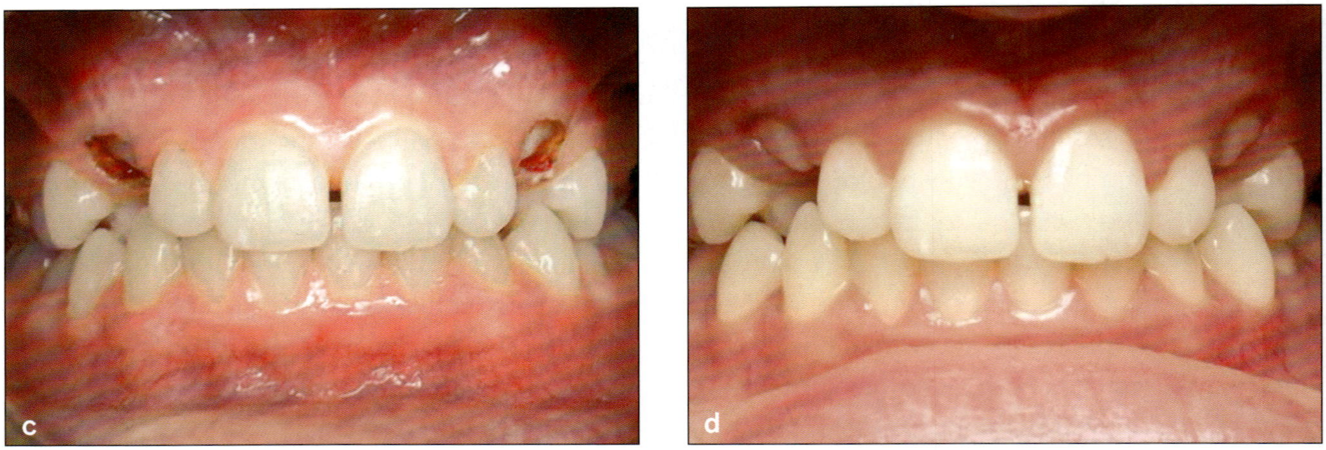

Figs 11-1c and 11-1d Postoperative views of canines immediately following removal of gingival tissue *(c)* and 2 weeks later *(d)*. Exposure of canines allows for natural eruption to proceed.

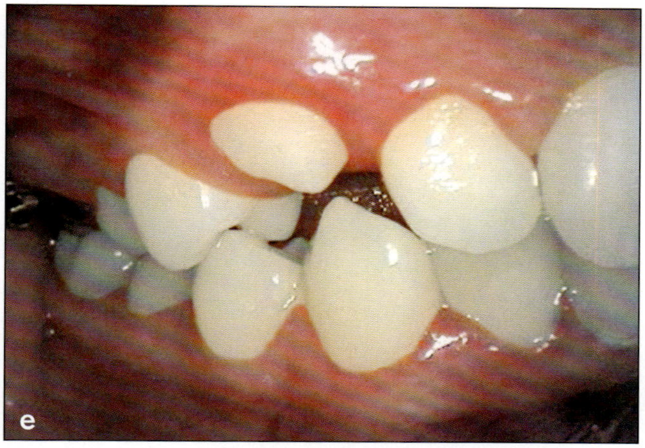

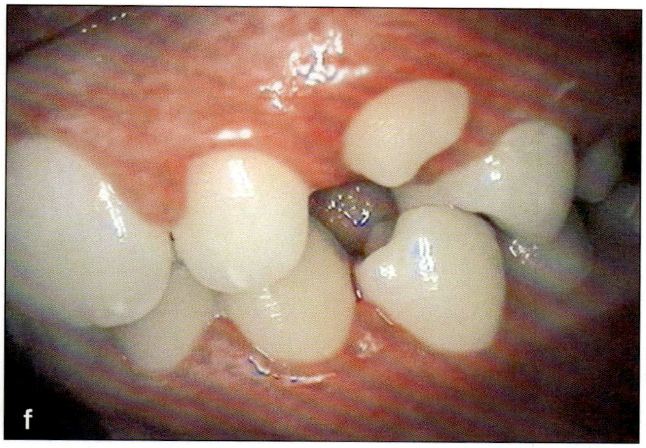

Figs 11-1e and 11-1f Six-week postoperative views of the progression of the canines. (Case courtesy of Dr Philip Hudson, Spokane, WA.)

Purpose of the procedure	Exposure of unerupted teeth
Once exposed, the path of eruption can be guided orthodontically. Alternatively, natural movement may be monitored over time.	

Wavelength and settings

Diode laser, 810 nm, set to 1 W, continuous wave, with a 400 μm fiber.

Alternate wavelengths that may be used

While any soft tissue laser can accomplish the same procedure, care must be taken when using CO_2 and Er lasers because their wavelengths can ablate the enamel tissue if too much power is used during the procedure. These instruments can be safely used if the beam is kept parallel to the long axis of the tooth and directed toward the soft tissue.

Clinical tip

Currettes can be used to explore the area and determine the precise location of unerupted teeth as well as to remove tissue tags during exposure.

Exposure of Unerupted Teeth: Case 2

Exposure of unerupted teeth in a 12-year-old male.

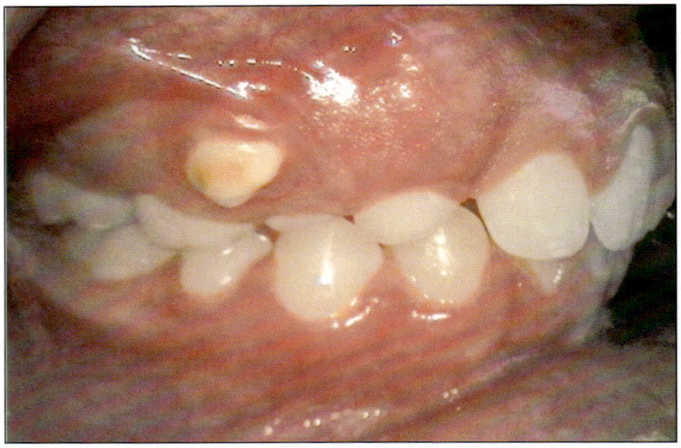

Fig 11-2a Partially erupted maxillary right first premolar and several overretained primary teeth.

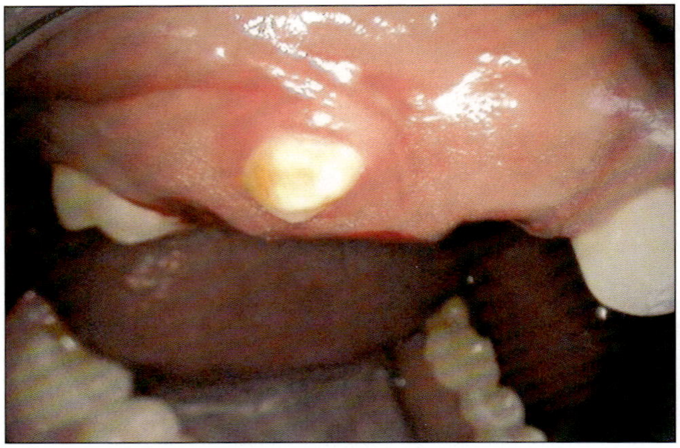

Fig 11-2b Postoperative view following conventional extraction of the primary teeth.

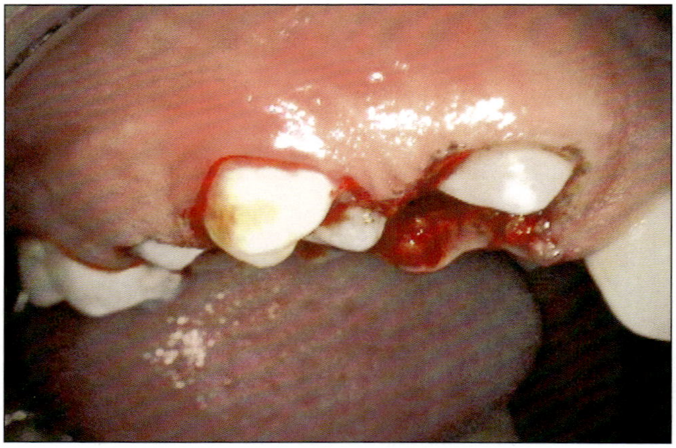

Fig 11-2c Removal of gingival tissue to expose the permanent teeth and aid eruption.

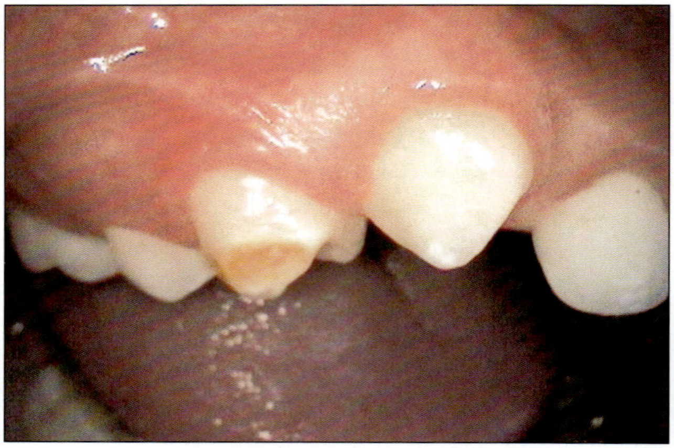

Fig 11-2d Developing occlusion 3 months postoperative. (Case courtesy of Dr Philip Hudson, Spokane, WA.)

Purpose of the procedure	Exposure of unerupted teeth

Following extraction of overretained primary teeth and surgical exposure of the permanent teeth, the maxillary right canine and premolars emerge naturally into the dental arch.

Wavelength and settings

Diode laser, 810 nm, set to 1 W, continuous wave, with a 400 μm fiber.

Alternate wavelengths that may be used

While any soft tissue laser can accomplish the same procedure, care must be taken when using CO_2 and Er lasers because their wavelengths may ablate the enamel tissue if too much power is used during the procedure. These instruments can be safely used if the beam is kept parallel to the long axis of the tooth and directed toward the soft tissue.

Exposure of Unerupted Teeth: Case 3

Exposure of an unerupted tooth and repositioning of the labial frenum in a 13-year-old female.

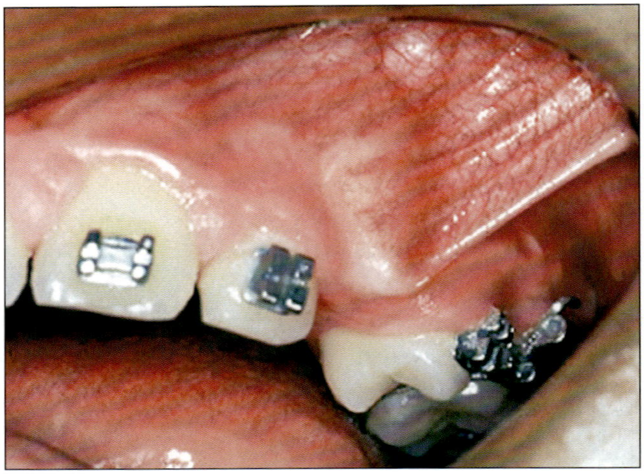

Fig 11-3a Unerupted maxillary left canine covered by thin gingiva attached to a labial frenum.

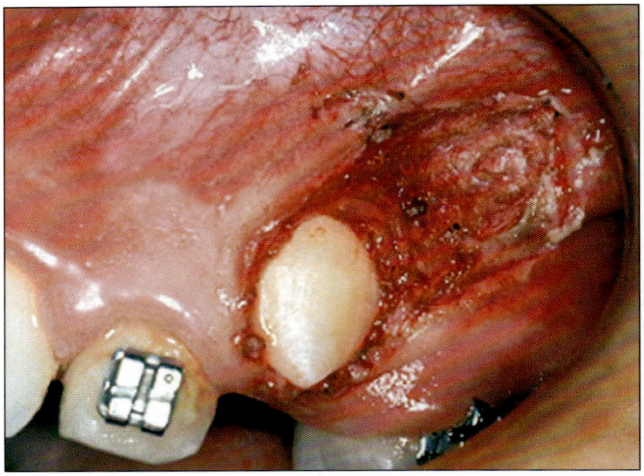

Fig 11-3b Postoperative view immediately following exposure of the canine and repositioning of the frenum.

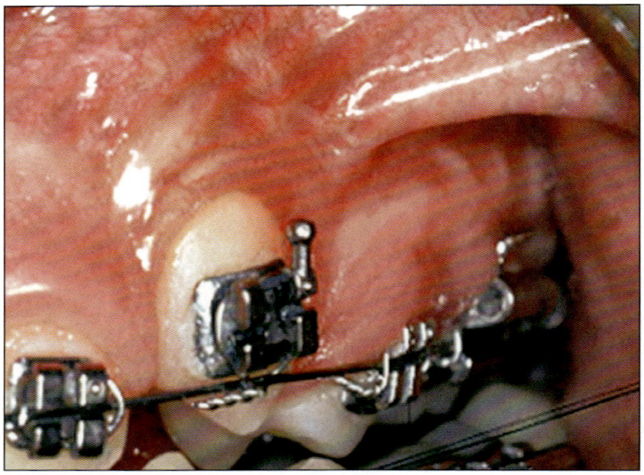

Fig 11-3c Ten days postsurgery, the canine is emerging into position in the dental arch with orthodontic guidance.

Purpose of the procedure

Exposure of an unerupted tooth

Removing the thin gingival covering and repositioning the labial frenum allows the canine's eruption to be guided via orthodontic movement.

Wavelength and settings

Nd:YAG laser set to 100 mJ, 20 Hz, 2 W, with a 320 μm fiber.

Alternate wavelengths that may be used

While any soft tissue laser can accomplish the same procedure, care must be taken when using CO_2 and Er lasers because they may ablate enamel tissue if too much power is used during the procedure. These instruments can be safely used if the beam is kept parallel to the long axis of the tooth and directed toward the soft tissue.

Exposure of Unerupted Teeth: Case 4

Exposure of an unerupted tooth in an 11-year-old male.

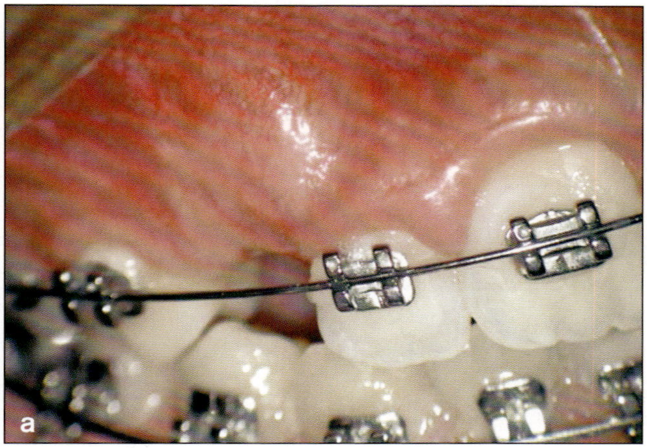

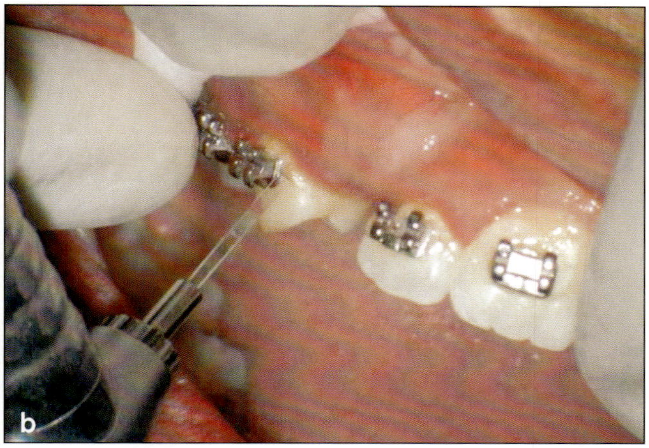

Figs 11-4a and 11-4b Preoperative *(a)* and intraoperative *(b)* views of the maxillary right canine area.

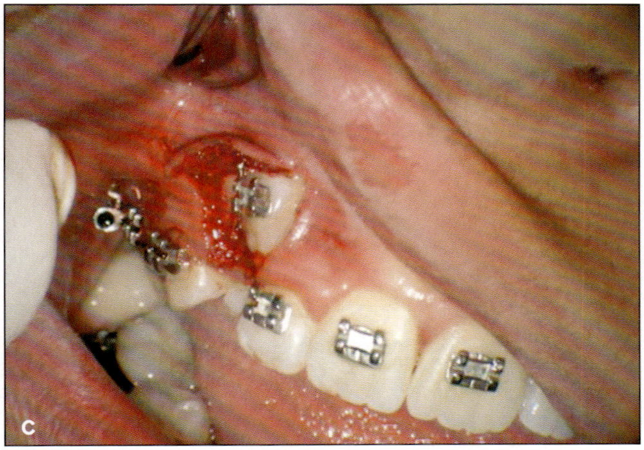

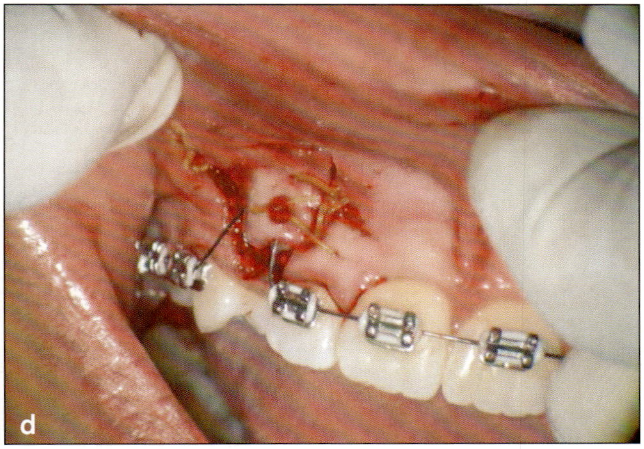

Figs 11-4c and 11-4d Following the lateral retraction of a gingival flap, an orthodontic bracket was bonded to the exposed canine *(c)*. The gingival flap was resutured over the tooth *(d)* to allow for an orthodontically guided eruption.

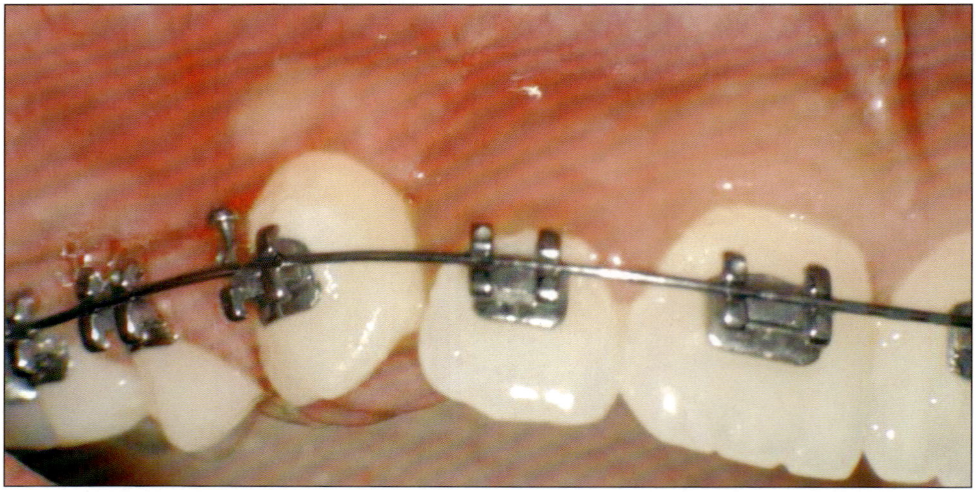

Fig 11-4e Three-month postoperative view showing the erupted canine in its appropriate position in the dental arch. (Case courtesy of Dr Glenn van As, North Vancouver, BC, Canada.)

Purpose of the procedure

Exposure of an unerupted tooth.

Orthodontic movement was used to create room in the dental arch for the unerupted tooth. A gingival flap was created so that an orthodontic bracket could be attached to the unerupted tooth to guide its path of eruption following exposure.

Wavelength and settings

Er:YAG laser set to 30 mJ, 30 Hz, with a 600 μm sapphire tip and no water spray.

Alternate wavelengths that may be used

While any soft tissue laser can accomplish the same procedure, care must be taken when using CO_2 and Er lasers because their wavelengths may ablate the enamel tissue if too much power is used during the procedure. These instruments can be safely used if the beam is kept parallel to the long axis of the tooth and directed toward the soft tissue.

Clinical tip

Exposure of an unerupted tooth in cases 3 and 4 required removal of gingiva to place orthodontic brackets on the exposed tooth. To prevent periodontal problems, the clinician must preserve an adequate amount of attached gingiva.

Frenectomy

The position and extension of frena influence both periodontal health and the alignment of the permanent dentition. In pediatric patients, irregular frenal attachment is most common for maxillary labial and mandibular lingual frena. A diastema may develop between the maxillary or mandibular incisors when the frenum extends too far coronally. In addition, an abnormal position of the lingual frenum may cause ankyloglossia, which can lead to difficulties in eating, swallowing, and maintaining oral hygiene. In newborns, ankyloglossia can prevent latching onto the breast during breastfeeding.

Frenectomies can be performed with various laser wavelengths. Some clinicians place a suture at the new termination point prior to repositioning the frenum, while others find this step unnecessary when using a laser. Occasionally, interproximal bone must be removed when a labial frenum extends through the papilla onto the palate. When osseous surgery is required, only the Er family of lasers can be used to correct the bony architecture.

Frenectomy: Case 1

Repositioning of the labial frenum in a 15-year-old male.

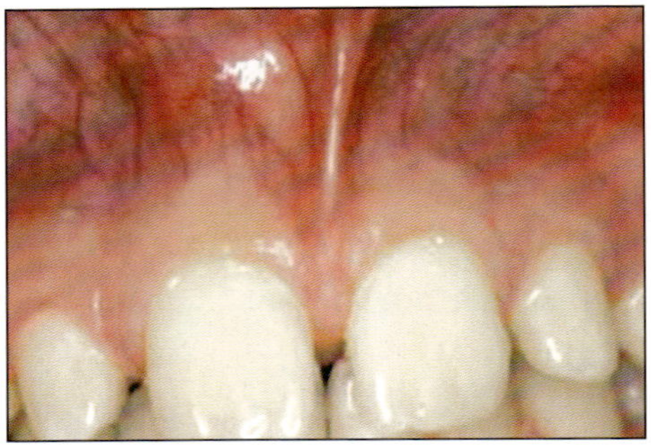

Fig 11-5a Maxillary labial frenum extending through the papilla between the central incisors to the palate.

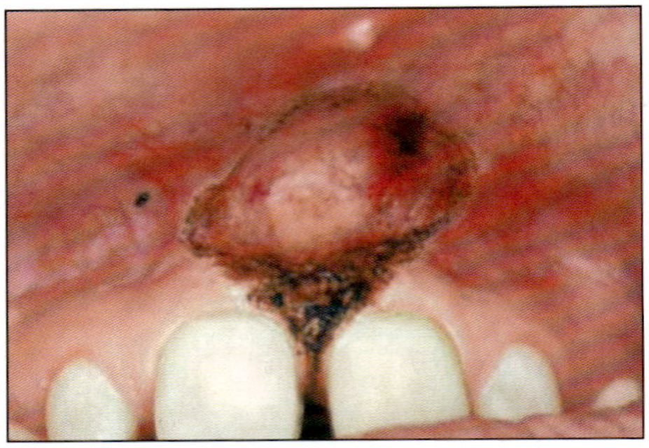

Fig 11-5b Postoperative labial view immediately following the frenectomy.

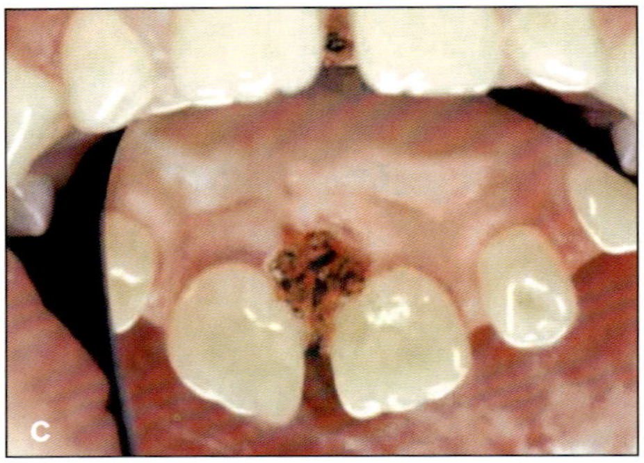

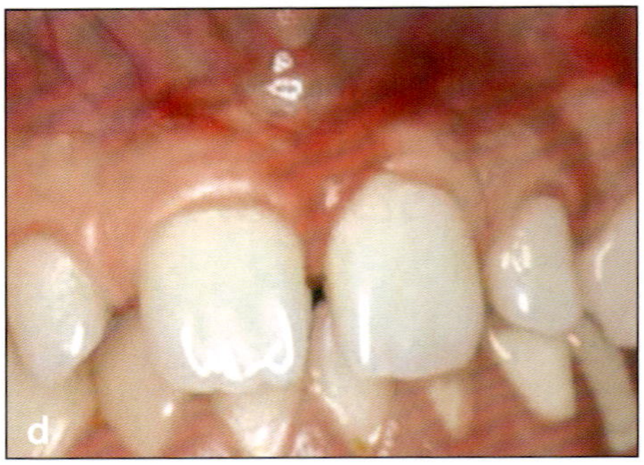

Figs 11-5c and 11-5d *(c)* Postoperative lingual view. *(d)* Three weeks after surgery, the area is completely healed. (Case courtesy of Dr Stuart Coleton, White Plains, NY.)

Purpose of the procedure	Repositioning of a labial frenum
The diastema between the central incisors can be closed once the maxillary labial frenum is repositioned.	

Wavelength and settings
CO_2 laser set to 5 W, continuous wave, with an 800 μm ceramic tip.
Alternate wavelengths that may be used
Any laser can be used to perform this procedure.

Frenectomy: Case 2

Repositioning of lingual frenum in a 13-year-old female.

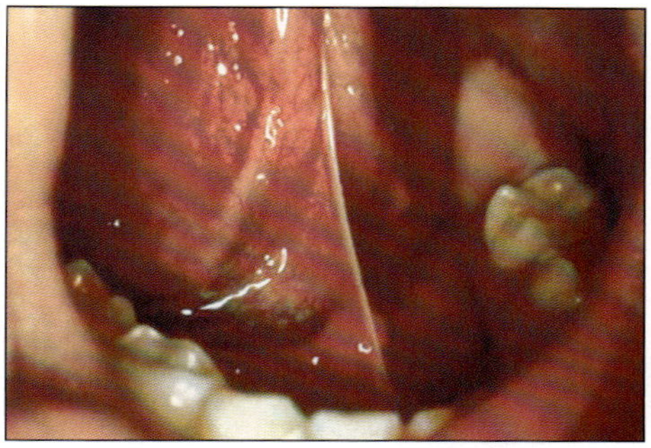

Fig 11-6a Preoperative view of a lingual frenum.

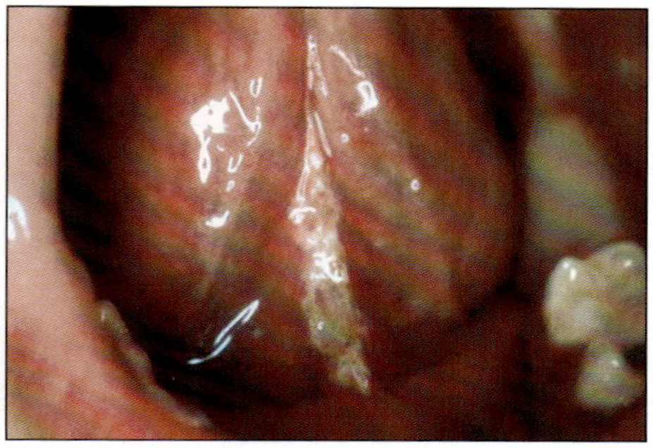

Fig 11-6b Postoperative view immediately following the frenectomy.

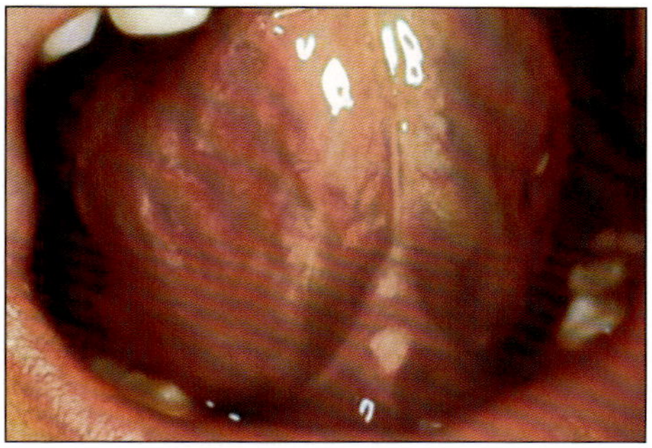

Fig 11-6c Complete healing is evident 2 weeks following the surgery. (Case courtesy of Dr Hector Martinez Arizpe, Monterrey, Mexico.)

Purpose of the procedure

Repositioning of the lingual frenum

Tongue mobility is increased by repositioning of the lingual frenum.

Wavelength and settings

Nd:YAG laser set to 100 mJ, 20 Hz, with a 320 μm fiber.

Alternate wavelengths that may be used

Any laser can be used to perform this procedure.

Clinical tips

Although any laser can be used to successfully perform a frenectomy, achieving acceptable hemostasis is difficult when using Er lasers because of their free-running pulse and shallow tissue penetration. If Er lasers are used, the clinician can facilitate coagulation by using maximum hertz with no water spray.

Stabilization of the frenum during incision and ablation can be accomplished using an instrument such as a hemostat. In addition, the clinician can maintain tension on the frenal tissue by retracting the lip or tongue.

It is especially important to remove the full extent of the frenal attachment nearest the teeth, as shown in case 1.

Frenectomy: Case 3

Repositioning of the lingual frenum in a 3-month-old infant.

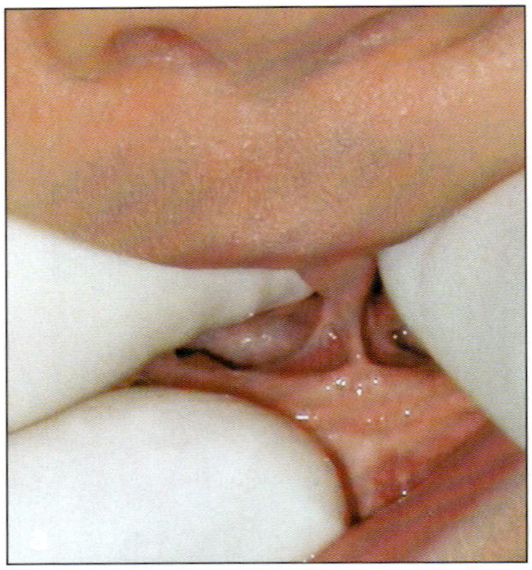

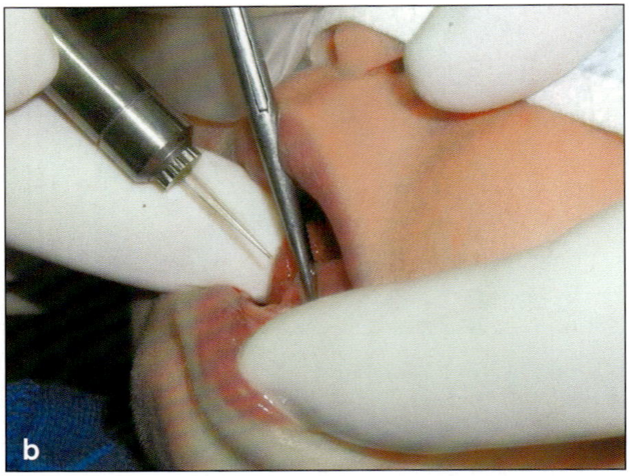

Figs 11-7a and 11-7b Preoperative *(a)* and intraoperative *(b)* views of an infant with ankyloglossia. The infant had difficulty nursing due to the abnormal lingual frenum.

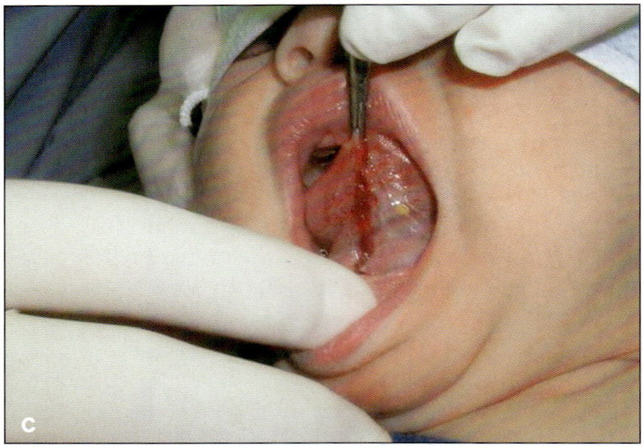

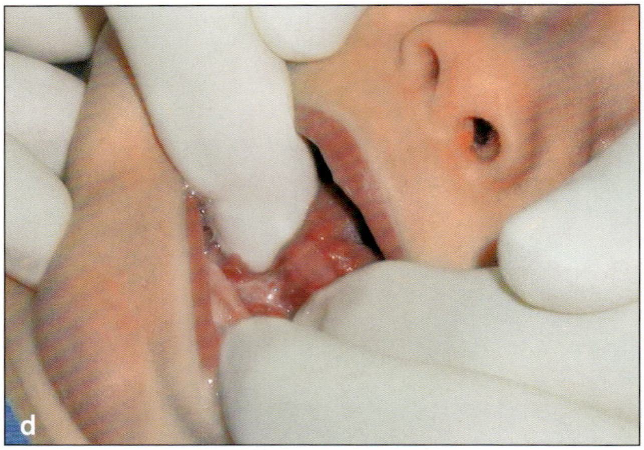

Figs 11-7c and 11-7d Immediate *(c)* and 10-day *(d)* postoperative views. (Case courtesy of Dr Lawrence Kotlow, Albany, NY.)

Purpose of the procedure	Repositioning of the lingual frenum

The increased tongue mobility provided by the frenectomy successfully treated the ankyloglossia in this infant, allowing her to latch onto the breast during feeding.

Wavelength and settings

Er laser set to 60 mJ, 10 Hz, with a soft tissue sapphire tip and no water spray.

Alternate wavelengths that may be used

While other wavelengths can be used, deeper-penetrating wavelengths (eg, diode, Nd:YAG) might cause thermal damage to the delicate soft tissues of the infant's mouth.

Clinical tip

Studies report that ankyloglossia is relatively common in newborns and infants and can be manifested by problems with nursing and nutrition. Repositioning the lingual frenum increases the freedom of tongue movement and can alleviate nursing difficulty associated with ankyglossia. When the frenectomy is performed, the infant is laid on the lap of the clinician or assistant. The infant's tongue is held by the clinician's fingers or retracted by a hemostat or grooved tongue positioner to stabilize the frenum (Fig 11-8). Local anesthesia is usually unnecessary. The procedure takes less than a minute and provides approximately 8 to 10 mm of increased tongue movement. As with all laser procedures, protective eyewear must be worn by the patient (Fig 11-9).

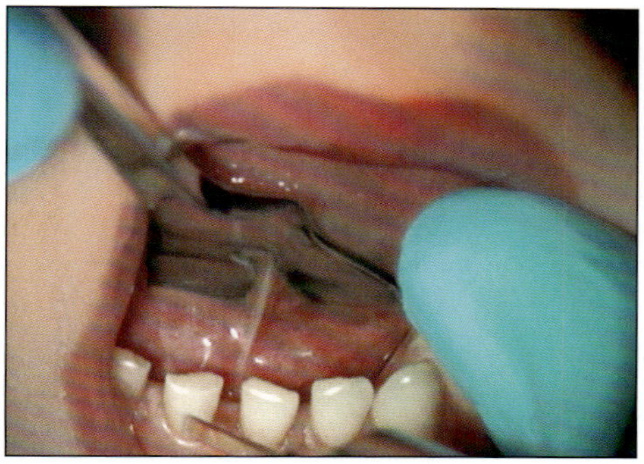

Fig 11-8 Grooved tongue positioner retracting the tongue and stabilizing the frenum. (Courtesy of Dr Lawrence Kotlow, Albany, NY.)

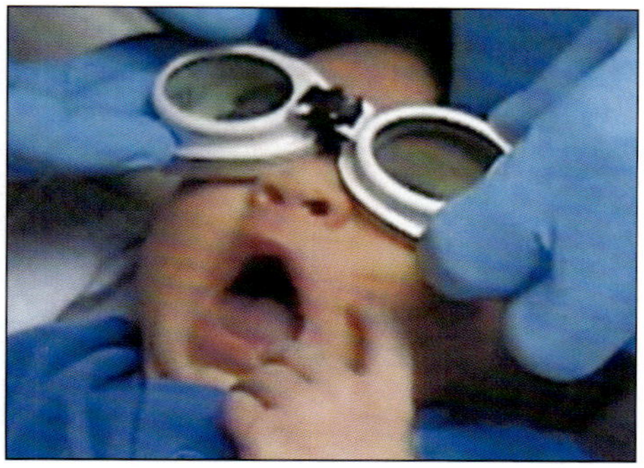

Fig 11-9 Protective goggles used during laser surgery. (Courtesy of Dr Lawrence Kotlow, Albany, NY.)

Gingivectomy

When fibrous tissue develops around teeth and prevents proper tooth emergence into the dental arch, lasers may be used to remove the excess fibrous tissue.

During orthodontic treatment, some pediatric patients experience hypertrophy of gingival tissue. This condition usually results from poor oral hygiene or mouth breathing. Lasers can easily remove excess tissue and restore the proper gingival contour, and patients must be instructed in oral hygiene and maintenance.

Laser treatment may also be required for patients who are prescribed certain drugs that cause gingival hyperplasia as a common side effect. Phenytoin (ie, Dilantin) is used to treat many seizure disorders in pediatric patients. Calcium-channel blockers (eg, nifedipine, verapamil, diltiazem), though not commonly prescribed for pediatric patients, also may cause gingival enlargement. Cyclosporine and other immunosuppressive drugs, commonly used after solid-organ transplant surgery to prevent rejection of the transplanted organ, are used in pediatric organ recipients.

Gingivectomy: Case 1

Removal of excess fibrous tissue in a 16-year-old male.

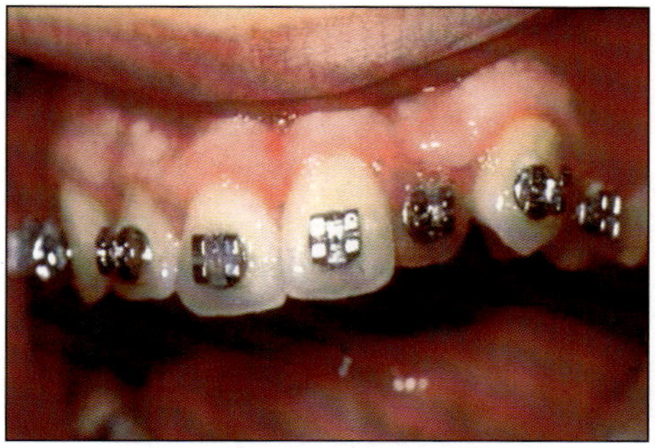

Fig 11-10a Preoperative view showing an abnormal lingual position of the left lateral incisor due to excess fibrous tissue.

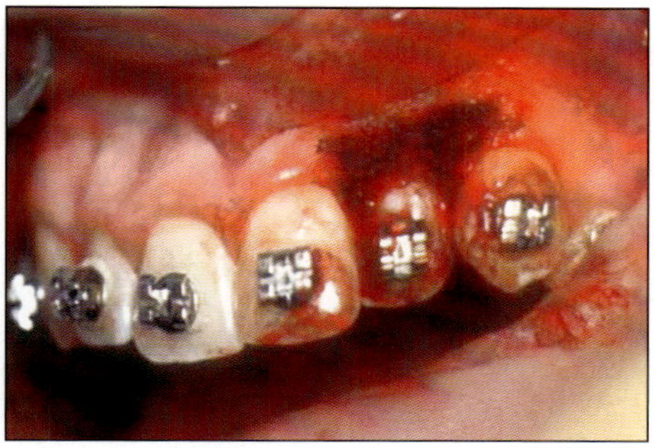

Fig 11-10b Postoperative view immediately following tissue removal.

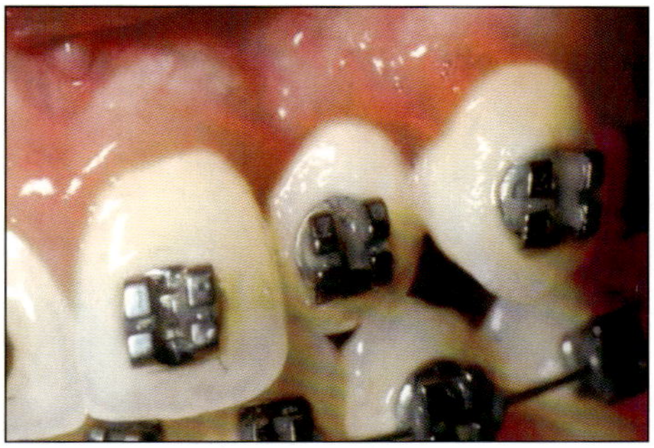

Fig 11-10c Two-week postoperative view showing complete gingival healing.

Purpose of the procedure	Removal of excess fibrous tissue

Once excess fibrous tissue is removed and the gingival margin is recontoured, the left lateral incisor can be orthodontically guided into a better position in the arch.

Wavelength and settings

CO_2 laser; settings to remove excess tissue: 3 W, continuous wave, with an 800 µm ceramic tip; settings to contour the gingival margin: 2 W, continuous wave, with a 250 µm metal tip.

Alternate wavelengths that may be used

Any laser can be used to perform this procedure.

Gingivectomy: Case 2

Removal of hyperplastic gingival tissue in a 14-year-old male.

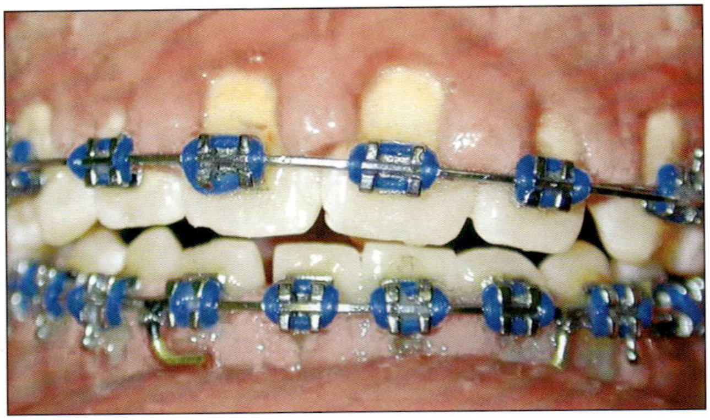

Fig 11-11a Hyperplastic gingiva in both arches.

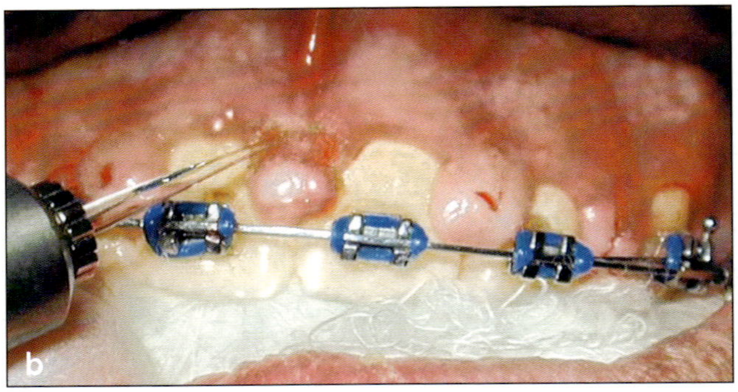

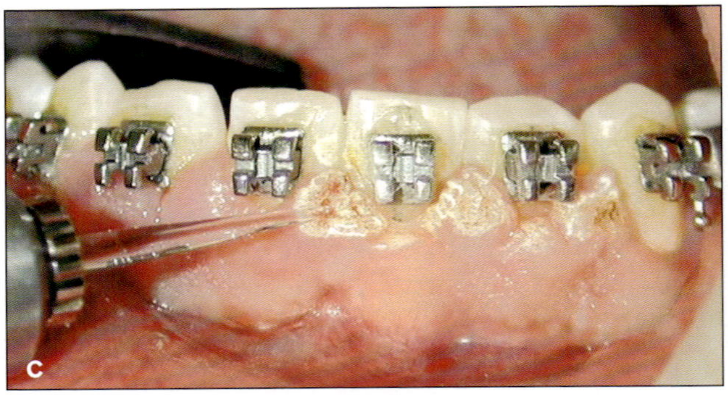

Figs 11-11b and 11-11c Intraoperative views of soft tissue ablation in the maxilla *(b)* and mandible *(c)*.

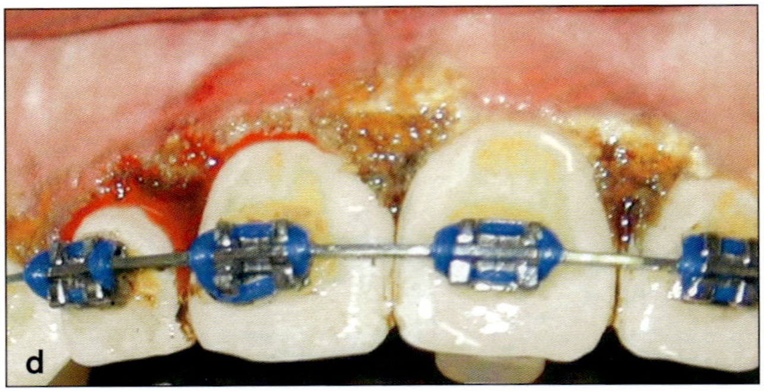

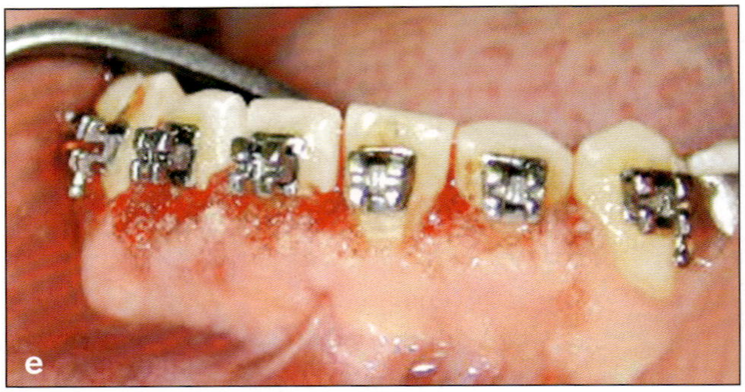

Figs 11-11d and 11-11e Postoperative views immediately following the tissue removal in the maxilla *(d)* and mandible *(e)*.

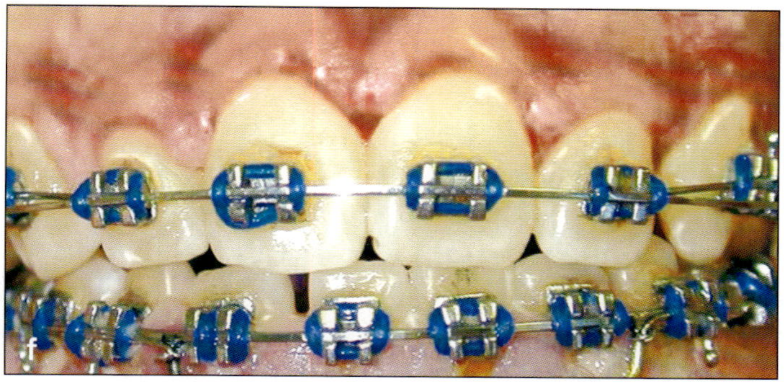

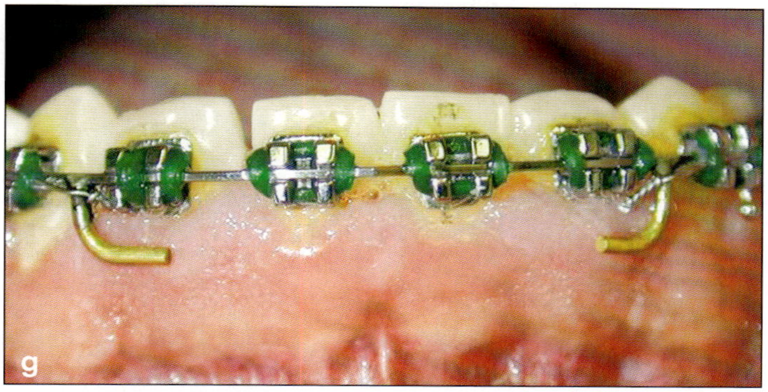

Figs 11-11f and 11-11g Gingival healing is evident in the maxilla *(f)* and mandible *(g)* only 1 week following surgery. (Case courtesy of Dr Lawrence Kotlow, Albany, NY.)

Purpose of the procedure	Removal of hyperplastic tissue during orthodontic therapy.
The natural gingival contour is restored by removing the hyperplastic tissue.	

Wavelength and settings

Er:YAG laser set to 55 mJ, 30 Hz, with a tapered sapphire tip and no water spray.

Alternate wavelengths that may be used

Any laser can be used to perform this procedure.

Gingivectomy: Case 3

Removal of hyperplastic gingiva in a 15-year-old kidney transplant patient.

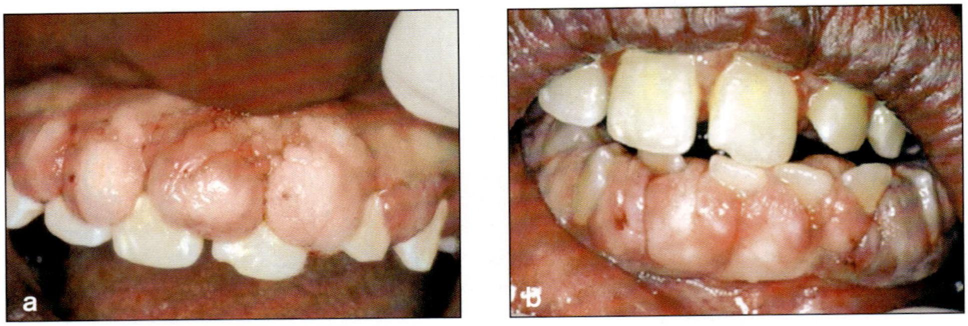

Figs 11-12a and 11-12b Preoperative views of severe drug-induced gingival hyperplasia in the maxilla *(a)* and mandible *(b)* due to cyclosporine use.

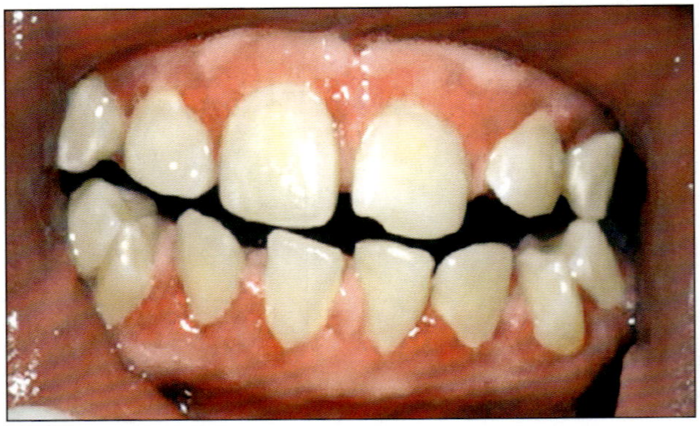

Fig 11-12c Healing of gingiva following laser surgery: 2 weeks postoperative in the maxilla and 1 week postoperative in the mandible.

Purpose of the procedure	Removal of hyperplastic gingiva secondary to cyclosporine use

Once the excess gingiva is removed, the contour can be refined at the gingival margin.

Wavelength and settings

CO_2 laser; settings for tissue removal: 4 W, continuous wave, with an 800 μm ceramic tip; settings for contouring gingival margins: 3 W, continuous wave, with a 250 μm metal tip.

Alternate wavelengths that may be used

Although any laser can be used, removing large amounts of hyperplastic gingiva requires laser wavelengths that remove soft tissue efficiently and provide adequate hemostasis. The Er family of lasers may not provide adequate hemostasis during the procedure. When either diode or Nd:YAG lasers are used for soft tissue excision, the depth of laser penetration requires care to avoid overheating the tissue with the laser energy.

Alternate technique

The ideal protocol for removing hyperplastic gingiva would be a combined technique of gross soft tissue debulking with a scalpel followed by soft tissue recontouring using a laser with a small fiber-optic, ceramic, or metal tip. Hemostasis would then be obtained with the laser.

Drainage of a Gingival Abscess: Case 1

Drainage of an abscess superior to a maxillary central incisor in a 3.5-year-old patient.

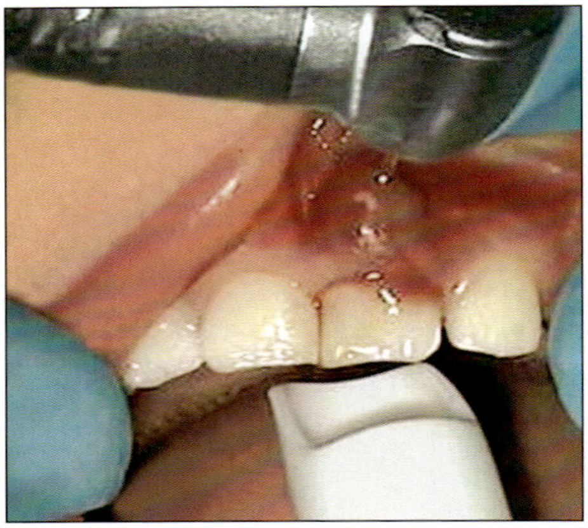

Figs 11-13a Intraoperative view showing the laser in position over a gingival abscess.

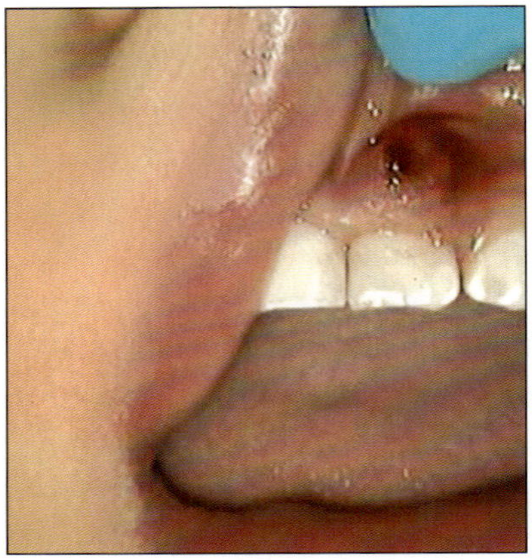

Figs 11-13b Once an incision is made, the gingival abscess is drained. (Case courtesy of Dr Barry L. Jacobson, Fort Lee, NJ.)

Purpose of the procedure	Drainage of a gingival abscess
Swelling is relieved once an incision is made and the gingival abscess is drained.	

Wavelength and settings

Er,Cr:YSGG laser set to 2 W with a soft tissue tip.

Alternate wavelengths that may be used

Any laser can be used to perform this procedure.

Restorative Dentistry

The Er family of lasers is particularly effective in removing caries and preparing primary teeth for pediatric restorations. Studies have demonstrated significant reduction in the amount of bacteria on the walls of the cavity preparation, the absence of a smear layer on the dentinal surface, and pulpal benefits compared to the use of a dental handpiece.[16–22] These advantages translate into improved patient comfort and minimal postoperative sensitivity.

Strip Crown Restoration: Case 1

Preparation of primary anterior teeth for strip crowns in a 4-year-old patient.

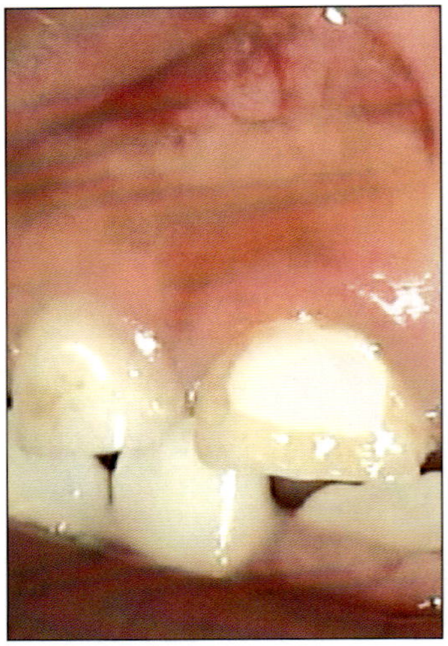

Fig 11-14a Preoperative view of severe caries lesions on primary maxillary left central and lateral incisors.

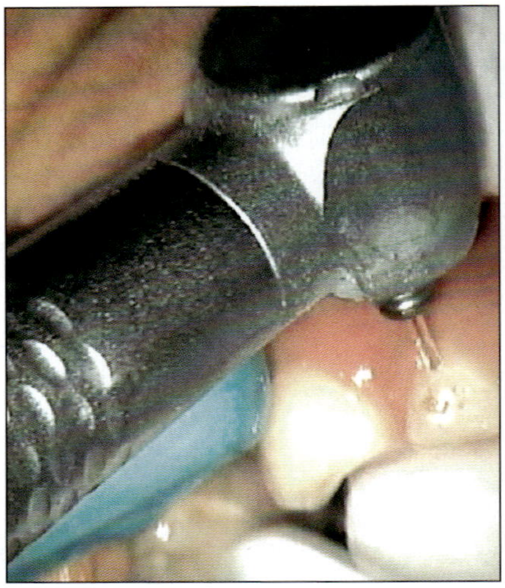

Fig 11-14b Intraoperative view of tooth preparation on the maxillary left central incisor.

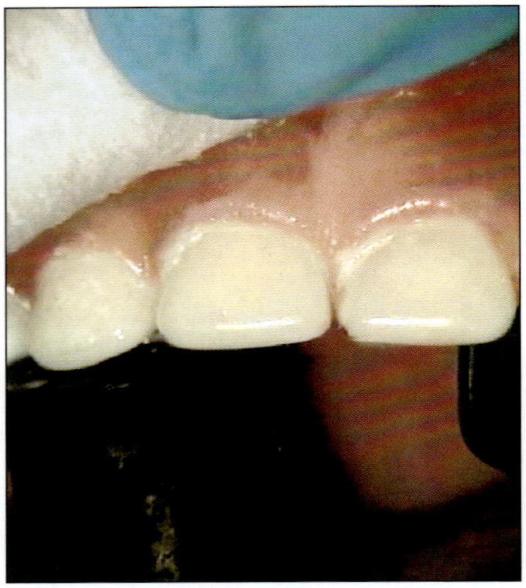

Fig 11-14c Postoperative view showing the primary maxillary incisors restored with resin composite strip crowns. (Case courtesy of Dr Barry L. Jacobson, Fort Lee, NJ.)

Purpose of the procedure	Preparation of primary anterior teeth for strip crowns

Once the tooth preparations are completed, the strip crown forms are filled with resin composite and placed over the preparations. The restorations can be finished and polished once the strip crown forms are removed.

Wavelength and settings

Er,Cr:YSGG laser set to 5.5 W, with 75% water and 75% air.

Alternate wavelengths that may be used

Only the Er family of lasers can be used for tooth preparation.

Restoration of Leaking Sealants: Case 1

Restoration of a second molar in young male patient.

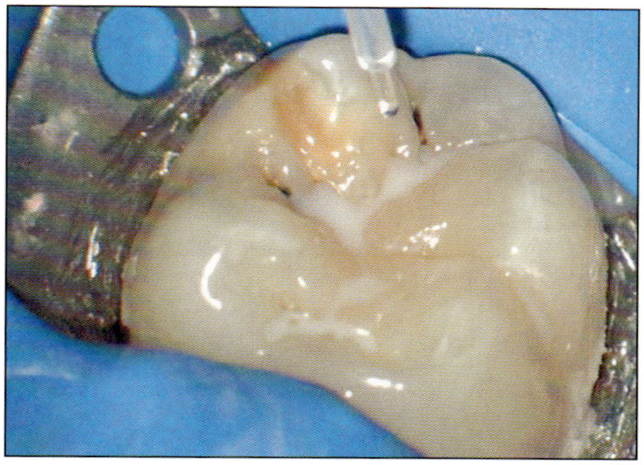

Fig 11-15a Permanent second molar showing a leaking occlusal sealant and recurrent decay. The Er laser tip is in place to begin ablation.

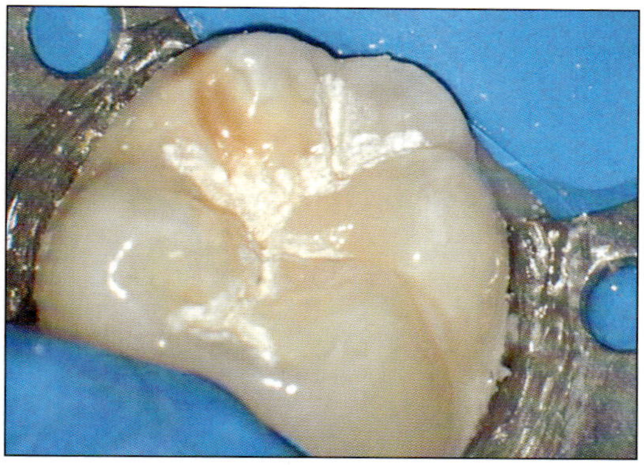

Fig 11-15b Postoperative view immediately following removal of occlusal sealant and excavation of carious tooth structure.

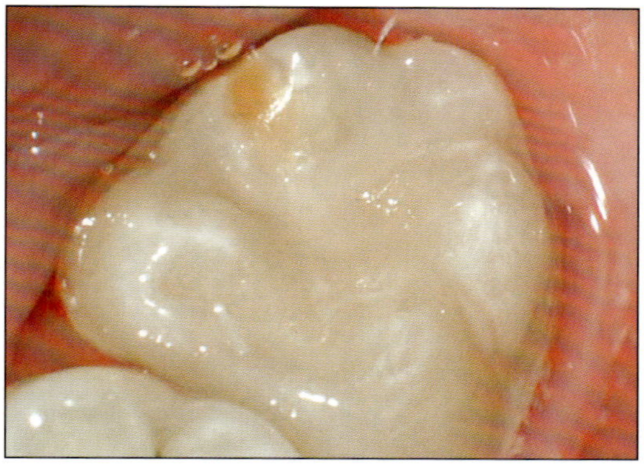

Fig 11-15c Definitive restoration. (Case courtesy of Dr Glenn van As, North Vancouver, BC, Canada.)

Purpose of the procedure

Class I restoration

The second molar is restored once the caries and defective sealant are removed.

Wavelength

Er laser.

Alternate wavelength that may be used

Only the Er family of lasers can be used for tooth preparation.

Clinical tip

The Er wavelengths easily ablate resin composite and similar restorative materials. Using the proper laser settings is critical to the success of the procedure. The laser was used on high power to remove the sealant and then on reduced power for caries removal. As with any good clinical technique, the finished tooth preparation should be as conservative as possible.

Pulpotomy

Pulpotomies can be performed successfully using various laser wavelengths. Studies have shown that lasers are as effective in root canal disinfection for pediatric pulpotomies as conventional medicaments (eg, formocresol).[23] In addition, if the tooth is vital, use of an Er family laser will ensure that some vital tissue remains intact in the apical portion of the root canal system. The use of other wavelengths to perform pulpotomies (ie, diode and carbon dioxide [CO_2]), readily achieve hemostasis but may remove too much pulpal tissue because of deeper penetration.

Pulpotomy: Case 1

Pulpotomy in a primary molar.

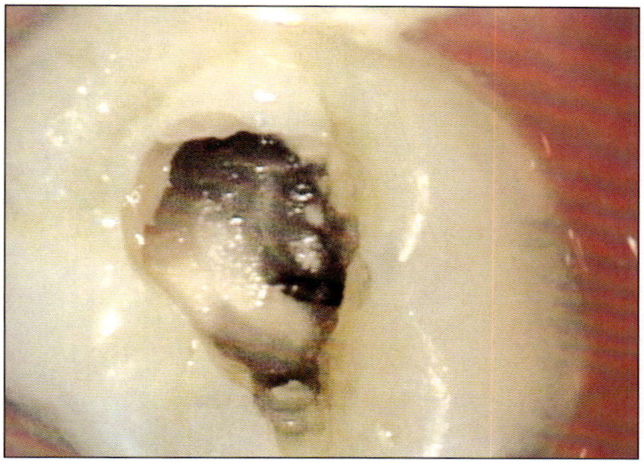

Fig 11-16a Postoperative view of hemostasis immediately following coronal pulp removal.

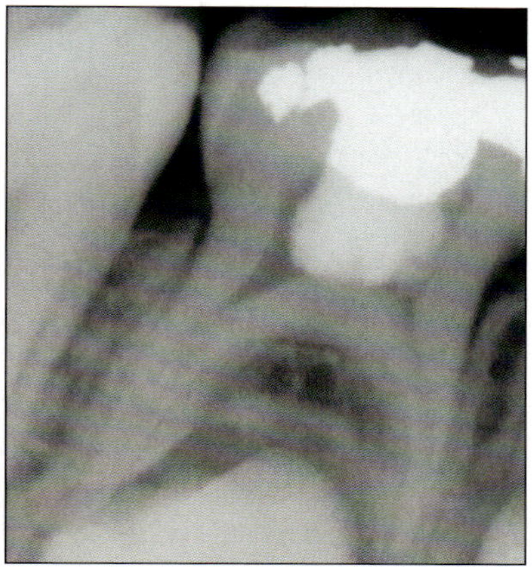

Fig 11-16b Eighteen months following endodontic surgery, a radiograph shows a stable molar with normal periodontium and periapical tissues. (Case courtesy of Dr Lawrence Kotlow, Albany, NY.)

Purpose of the procedure

Vital pulpotomy

An Er laser was used to remove caries and disinfect the root canal in preparation for obturation.

Wavelength and settings

Er laser; settings for caries removal: 50 mJ, 30 Hz, with a 600 μm tip with water spray; settings for pulpal tissue ablation: 30 mJ, 50 Hz, with a 600 μm tip and no water spray.

Alternate wavelengths that may be used

While other lasers can be used for pulpotomies, deeper-penetrating wavelengths (ie, diode and CO_2) might ablate too much pulpal tissue.

References

1. Kotlow L. The use of the erbium hard and soft tissue laser in the pediatric dental practice. J Southeast Soc Pediatr Dent 2001; 17:12–14.
2. Martens L. Laser-assisted pediatric dentistry: Review and outlook. J Oral Laser Applications 2003;3:203–209.
3. Parkins F. Lasers in pediatric and adolescent dentistry. Dent Clin North Am 2000;44: 821–830.
4. Kotlow LA. Ankyloglossia (tongue tie): A diagnostic and treatment quandary. Quintessence Int 1999;30:259–262.
5. Fernando C. Tongue Tie—From Confusion to Clarity: A Guide to the Diagnosis and Treatment of Ankyloglossia. Sidney, Australia: Tandem Publications, 1998.
6. Guelmann M, Britto LR, Katz J. Cyclosporin-induced gingival overgrowth in a child treated with CO_2 laser surgery: A case report. J Clin Pediatr Dent 2003;27:123–126.
7. Goharkhay K, Moritz A, Wilder-Smith P, et al. Effects on oral soft tissue produced by a diode laser in vitro. Lasers Surg Med 1999; 25:401–406.
8. Rowson JE. The contact diode laser—A useful instrument for excising oral lesions [abstract]. Br J Oral Maxillofac Surg 1995;33:123.
9. White JM, Goodis HE, Rose CL. Use of the pulsed Nd:YAG laser for intraoral soft tissue surgery. Lasers Surg Med 1991;11:455–461.
10. Baraldi CE, Puricelli E, Kulkes S, Martins GL. Er:YAG laser in oral soft tissue surgery [abstract 59]. J Oral Laser Appl 2001;1:24.
11. Watanabe H, Ishikawa I, Suzuki M, Hasegawa K. Clinical assessments of the erbium:YAG laser for soft tissue surgery and scaling. J Clin Laser Med Surg 1996; 14:67–75.
12. Wilder-Smith P, Arrastia AM, Liaw LH, Berns M. Incision properties and thermal effects of three CO_2 lasers in soft tissue. Oral Surg Oral Med Oral Pathol Oral Radiol Endod 1995;79:685–691.
13. DenBesten PK, White JM, Pelino JP, Furnish G, Silveira A, Parkins FM. The safety and effectiveness of an Er:YAG laser for caries removal and cavity preparation in children. Med Laser Appl 2001;16:215–222.
14. Kato J, Moriya K, Jayawardena JA, Wijeyeweera RL. Clinical application of Er:YAG laser for cavity preparation in children. J Clin Laser Med Surg 2003;21:151–155.
15. Matsumoto K, Hossain M, Hossain MM, Kawano H, Kimura Y. Clinical assessment of Er,Cr:YSGG laser application cavity preparation in children. J Clin Laser Med Surg 2002; 20:17–21.
16. Hibst R, Stock K, Gall R, Keller U. Controlled tooth surface heating and sterilization by Er:YAG laser radiation. In: Altshuler GB, Chiesa F, Geschwind HJ, et al (eds). Laser Applications in Medicine and Dentistry. San Jose, CA: International Society of Optical Engineering, 1996:119–126.
17. Sharon-Buller A, Block C, Savion I, Sela M. Reduced bacteria levels in cavities prepared by Er:YAG laser. J Oral Laser Applic 2003; 3:153–155.
18. Lee BS, Lin CP, Hung YL, Lan WH. Structural changes of Er:YAG laser-irradiated human dentin. Photomed Laser Surg 2004;22: 330–334.
19. Glockner K, Rumpler J, Ebeleseder K, Stadtler P. Intrapulpal temperature during preparation with the Er:YAG laser compared to the conventional burr: An in vitro study. J Clin Laser Med Surg 1998;16:153–157.
20. Oelgiesser D, Blasbalg J, Ben-Amar A. Cavity preparation by Er-YAG laser on pulpal temperature rise. Am J Dent 2003;16:96–98.
21. Cavalcanti BN, Lage-Marques JL, Rode SM. Pulpal temperature increases with Er:YAG laser and high-speed handpieces. J Prosthet Dent 2003;90:447–451.
22. Eversole LR, Rizoiu I, Kimmel AI. Pulpal response to cavity preparation by an erbium, chromium:YSGG laser-powered hydrokinetic system. J Am Dent Assoc 1997;128:1099–1106.
23. Liu JF, Chen LR, Chao SY. Laser pulpotomy of primary teeth. Pediatr Dent 1999;21: 128–129.

DENTAL COLLECTION